# CISM COURSES AND LECTURES

*Series Editors:*

*The Rectors of CISM*
Sandor Kaliszky - Budapest
Mahir Sayir - Zurich
Wilhelm Schneider - Wien

*The Secretary General of CISM*
Giovanni Bianchi - Milan

*Executive Editor*
Carlo Tasso - Udine

The series presents lecture notes, monographs, edited works and
proceedings in the field of Mechanics, Engineering, Computer Science
and Applied Mathematics.
Purpose of the series is to make known in the international scientific
and technical community results obtained in some of the activities
organized by CISM, the International Centre for Mechanical Sciences.

INTERNATIONAL CENTRE FOR MECHANICAL SCIENCES

COURSES AND LECTURES - No. 375

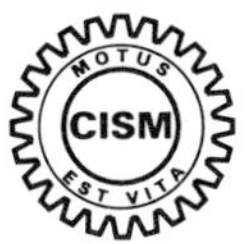

# HUMAN AND MACHINE LOCOMOTION

EDITED BY

A. MORECKI
WARSAW UNIVERSITY OF TECHNOLOGY

K.J. WALDRON
OHIO STATE UNIVERSITY

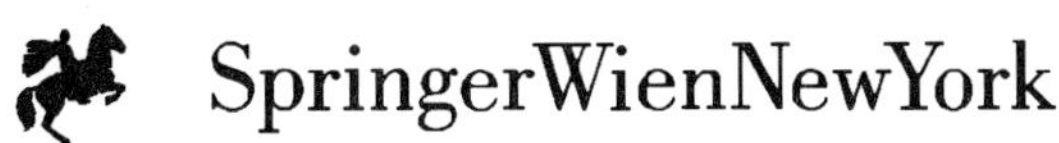

Springer Wien New York

Le spese di stampa di questo volume sono in parte coperte da
contributi del Consiglio Nazionale delle Ricerche.

This volume contains 166 illustrations



In order to make this volume available as economically and as
rapidly as possible the authors' typescripts have been
reproduced in their original forms. This method unfortunately
has its typographical limitations but it is hoped that they in no
way distract the reader.

ISBN 3-211-82905-9 Springer-Verlag Wien New York

# PREFACE

*A major trend in the study of legged locomotion systems is the creation of better mathematical models and their use in combination with more effective kinematic and dynamic analysis techniques to provide a more precise description. Those same models may also be used as the bases of numerical simulation techniques for use in the design and control of artificial legged locomotion systems. A new possibility is to reverse the process by the construction of artificial mechanical systems that serve as physical models of biological systems, allowing access to parameters that are not directly accessible in biological systems.*

*Traditionally, studies of locomotion biomechanics have been directed at providing basic information that can be used in clinical settings for diagnostic and therapeutic purposes. While this continues to be a major theme, recent technological advances have broadened the applicability of information from such studies.*

*In the past few years many successful walking and running machines have been constructed and tested. This work has led to many new insights into the fundamentals of legged locomotion. Although, to date, practical applications have been few in number, there is great potential, as demonstrated by biological systems. One recurring theme is the construction of a biped machine with human dimensions to provide mobility in constrained environments designed for human beings. Another is the design of orthotic assistance devices to replace functions lost by human patients due to injury. In these cases, a more complete understanding of the biological system is an essential foundation.*

*Legged locomotion systems have considerable potential for providing in severe terrain conditions, and where damage to the environment from the locomotion system must be minimised. Here animal models may be more appropriate since systems with four, six or eight legs are presently favoured.*

*We observe in the last years some progress in the design of the more efficient algorithms as well as control methods (behavioural type). Walking mili, micro and nano machines are at present one of the most fascinating field. Different kinds of actuators, legs, sensors are used during the design process of such a machines.*

*In this book we attempt to cover the state of the art in both biological and artificial legged locomotion systems. The seven chapters focus on a range of topics ranging from very detailed modelling of the musculo-skeletal system, through mathematical modelling and simulation to theories applicable to locomotion mechanics and control. The final two chapters deal with the mechanics, control and design of artificial legged locomotion systems.*

*The contents of this book are based on materials presented during the Advanced School "Modelling and Simulation of Human and Walking Robots Locomotion" which took place at CISM, the International Centre for Mechanical Sciences, Udine, Italy, July 8-12, 1996. The lecturers were the authors of the chapters of this book.*

*A. Morecki*
*K. Waldron*

# CONTENTS

# MODELLING AND SIMULATION OF HUMAN
# AND WALKING ROBOT LOCOMOTION


## A. Morecki

### Warsaw University of Technology, Warsaw, Poland


# ABSTRACT


Legged locomotion of vertebrates as well as biological classification of locomotion type are presented. Biomechanical modelling of human locomotion, plane model with 11 D.O.F., reduced order dynamic models of computer analysis of human gait, muscle drives and control system are given.

Next biomechanical bipeds, design of own electromechanical biped, computer model of a human musculoskeletal model, anthropomorphic biped robot, method of reference trajectory generations are discussed.

In the second part multi-legged walking robots, old walking machines, old Chinese machine, contemporary four-legged machines, design and testing of MK-4 walking machine, new design of four-legged machine are given.

Six legged walking machines, insect locomotion, description of selected machines are discussed.

Six legged walking robot - HERMES and some experimental results dealing with identification of its properties are given.

In the third part micromechanisms and microwalking robots, basic terms and definitions, present state of research of mobile micromachines like fourlegged microwalking machine driven by electromagnetic force, micromobile robot driven by gas turbine and finally possible applications and perspectives are discussed.

# 1. INTRODUCTION

The word locomotion originates from two Latin words: locus-place and motio-motion. Locomotion is a cyclic movement of animals involving change of place at which they currently find themselves. Such movements as, let us say, scratching, burying or curling-up are not locomotive movements. Animal locomotion proceeds in water, in mud, on land, underground, on trees and in the air [1].

Locomotion takes place by means of pseudopodia, whole body, tail, or limbs. Legs upper in the phylogenetic development of animals first in arthropodia. Parallel to arthropodia there appear the transversely striated muscles which are very powerful, owing to which arthropodia can move about equally well in water, on land and in the air.

Will shortly describe the legged locomotion of vertebrates, as well as biological classification of locomotion types.

## 1.1 Legged locomotion  of vertebrates

## 1.1.1 Biological classification of locomotion types

The evolution of locomotion in vertebrates is presented by examples in Fig. 1 and diagrammatically in Fig. 2. and Fig.3. Fish, the lowest vertebrate class, live mainly in water but a few of their representatives (the lungfish species) can also move on land and even in trees. there are moreover certain fish species which can jump out of water and fly some distance. Amphibians and reptiles are amphibious animals. Some of the species climb trees (frogs and chameleons). The first vertebrates to fly were reptiles (pterodactyls). They originated the bird class (Fig. 2a). Also mammals derive from reptiles, though from those which lived only on land. Both classes (birds and mammals) live in all environments, their constant blood temperature, giving a high strength per unit body weight, significantly contributing here.

Along with phylogenetic development (from fish to mammal) the  vertebrates have perfected their movement organs. Fish move practically only by means of the tail (an exception is lungfish). Amphibians and reptiles use the trunk and the extremities for locomotion. Only those which have secondarily lost their extremities (legless amphibians and snakes) move using the entire vertebral column.. The two highest organized classes, birds and mammals, move almost exclusive by means of their extremities (Fig. 2b). Only mammals living in water, owing to which their extremities have become vestigial (whale, seal and dolphin), are exceptions.

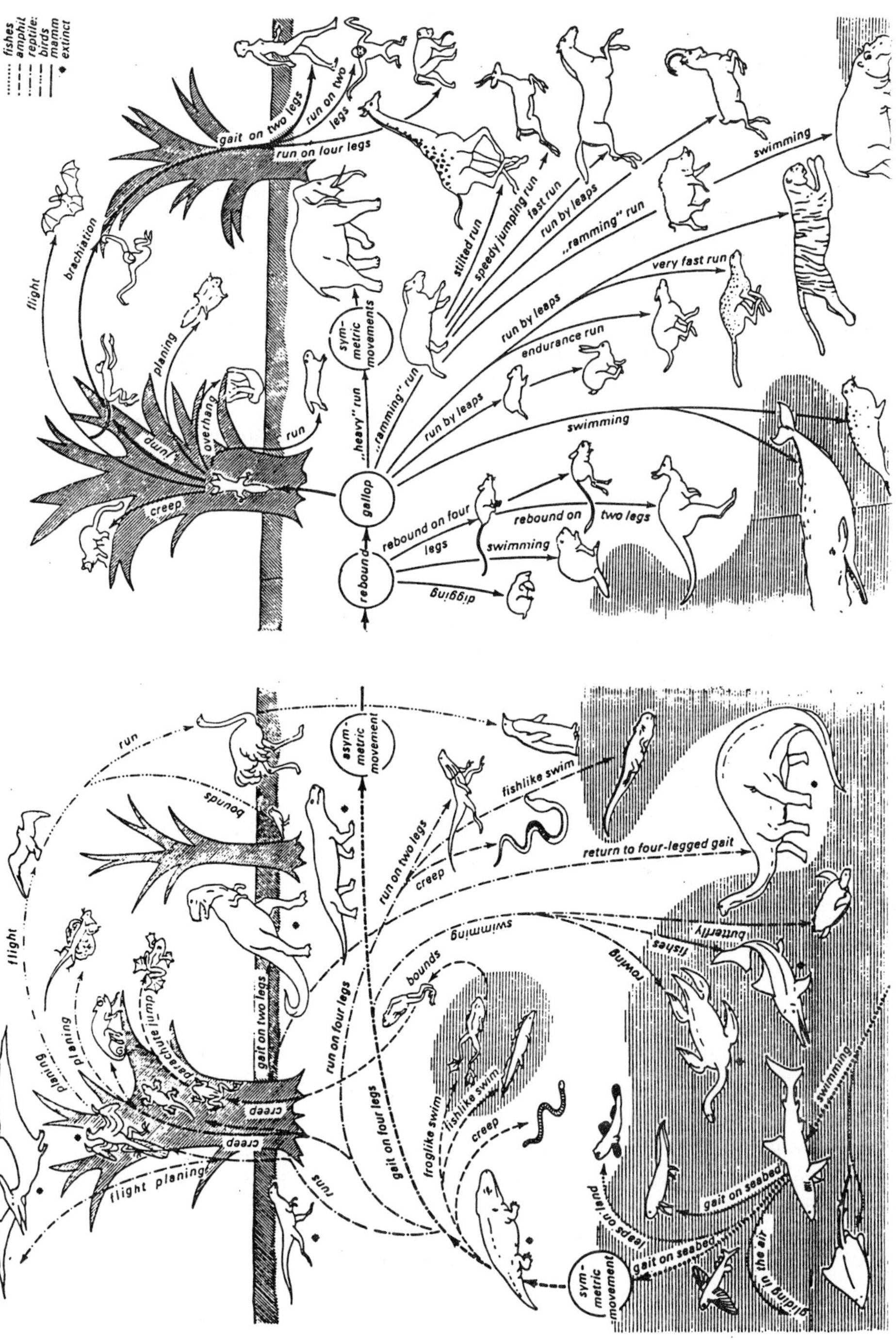


Fig. 1. Diagram of evolution in vertebrate.

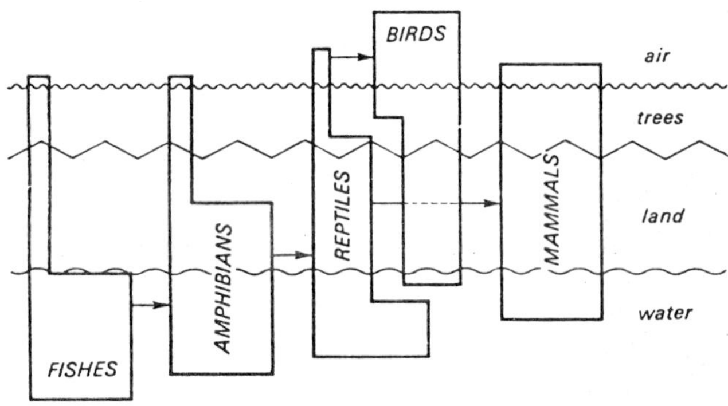



Fig.2. Diagram of development of vertebrates and environments in which they move.

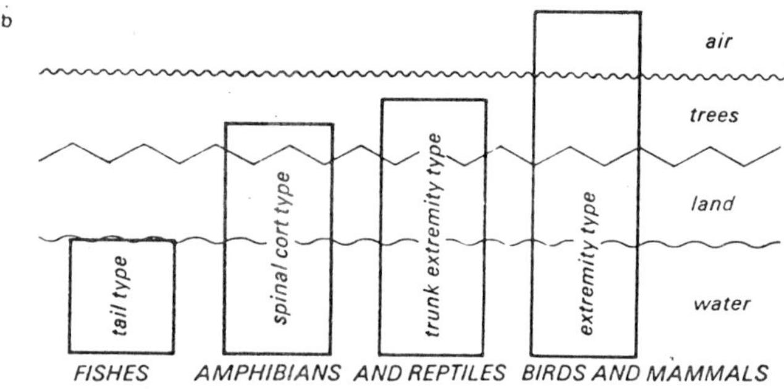



Fig.3. Diagram of types of travel of vertebrates in various environments

Coming back to the Fig.1 we like to comment the problem of the beginning of the evolution of life on earth. Many scientists are in favour with the hypothesis that life started in the water. In the last time new facts arrived, which support it. According to the last announcements about 420 million years ago, the creatures in the freshwater pools near the east of what is today Western Australia must have decided there might be more food in the next pool.

The footprints and feeding burrows the bizarre creatures left behind preserved in the rich red sandstones of the kalbarri National Park, about 600 km north of Perth, mark the first known occasion when life emerged from the water to walk on the land - at least 30 millions years earlier than scientists previously thought.(Fig.4.).

A dream find for scientists (University of Western Australia geologist Roger Buick, one of the team that found the ancient landscape) the creatures that lurked in Western Australia's primeral waters were the stuff of night moves when they were alive: amphibious scorpions up to 2 m long and giant centipedes that could grow even longer. [2]

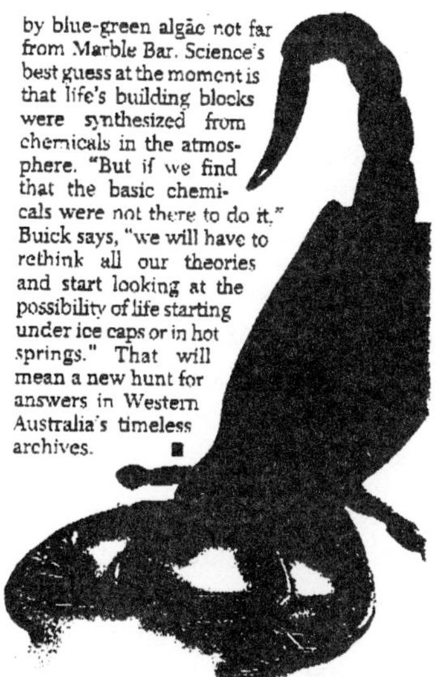


Fig. 4. Giant see scorpions made their mark in pioneering forays onto dry land about 420 millions years ago.

The legged type of locomotion is most efficient on land, in trees and in the air. Let us consider more closely some of the terrestrial types of locomotion in vertebrates. [1]

There are two basic types of locomotion on land, namely the walk and the run. The walk is characterised by sidewise alternating movement of legs which develop the vertical component of the ground reaction force less than $2Q$ ($Q=$ body weight), owing to which the flying phase is non-existent. Moreover, the time of movement of all the legs is identical. An example of slow walk is that of the turtle (Fig. 5a) in which there legs are all the time in contact with the ground, thus providing good body stability in motion.

Increasing the frequency of movement of the legs, not only the gait velocity but also the number of legs in the swing phase is increased. An example of quick walk is that of the elephant (Fig. 5b).

In man, the most economical gait for walking is 90-110 steps per minute. The vertical component of the ground reaction force then keeps in the range $(0.8$-$1.2)Q$. At frequency of 195-200 steps per min, the vertical component of the ground reaction force of the base grows above the value $2Q$ and the walk turns into a run.

The run is characterised by asymmetrical movement of legs and only half of their number can simultaneously touch the ground (two legs in quadrupeds and one leg in bipeds), whereas in flight all the legs together with the body keep in the air. During a run the time of the flight phase is about twice as long as of the support phase. While running, a very strong rebound of the hind limbs may take place (the ground reaction force of the base is several times as great as $Q$) and then the time of the flight phase is lengthened while the stance phase is shortened. This form of movement is characteristic of the leap.

The fastest form of run is the gallop (Fig. 5e). In the gallop, the animal attains the flight phase after a stance of both the hind - and forelegs. This is result of their asymmetric and asynchronous work, with only one (hind and fore) extremity slowing down the forward movement of the body for as brief period following which it immediately (after setting the other leg on the ground) thrusts the body upward and forwards bringing about the flight phase.

The intermediate forms of locomotion between walk and run are the trot, the amble and the ricochet.

The trot is characterized by sidewise alternating movement of the extremities whereas the amble, by one-sided movement of the extremities (for example, two left ones) (Fig. 5d). At slow movements the flight phase is non-existent (walk) and at fast movements, it does occur but is much shorter than the stance phase (run).

The ricochet characterized by asymmetric and asynchronous work of the legs, due to which in one phase all of them are on the ground and in the other the body rises into the air (the flight phase). Since in the ricochet the forelimbs slow down the flight of the body only after landing, they have become vestigial in some species (jerboa, kangaroo) (Fig. 5e).

Amphibians and reptiles move exclusively by the walk and the trot (excepting the frog which leaps) where by virtue of the sidewise alternating movement of the extremities they additionally make use of the lateral movements of the spine. Moreover, their spinal column prevents movements in the saggital plane. Birds and mammals use in locomotion (leaps and run) very powerful extensor and flexor muscles of the spine.

In some animals, intermediate forms between leap and run occur, for example, in the hare, antelope or chamois, which greatly helps them negotiate various land obstacles (bushes, ditches, rocks) while maintaining a high locomotive velocity of the animal. A run by leaps is perfectly suited to changes in length and height of steps, coupled with change of the rhythm of movements. These changes are made possible by the fact that during a walk the ground reaction force is never maximum as against leaping when the animal can change at will the value of the impulse force up the maximum.


## 1.2. Biomechanical modelling of human locomotion

### 1.2.1. Biomechanical modelling

Biomechanical modelling of human locomotion bas been attempted many times (Pandy and Berme 1989, Leo Cappozzo and Pedotti 1975, Morecki and others 1975, Seireg and Arvicar 1975). However, it is beset by several serious difficulties. Firstly, it is not possible to accurately measure or estimate many of the critical variables, like force exerted by any given muscle as a function of time. In the some manner, key control variables cannot accurately estimated. The human system employs a very large number of sensors feeding back to the CNS by many nerve pathways. Various investigators have attempted to simulate human locomotion on the computer over a period of many years, satisfactory results have proved elusive. This is not solely a result of the difficulties cited above. In order to simulate a multiply actuated system like the human body it is necessary to postulate algorithms for co-ordination and control. However, the co-ordination of the human system is not well understood.

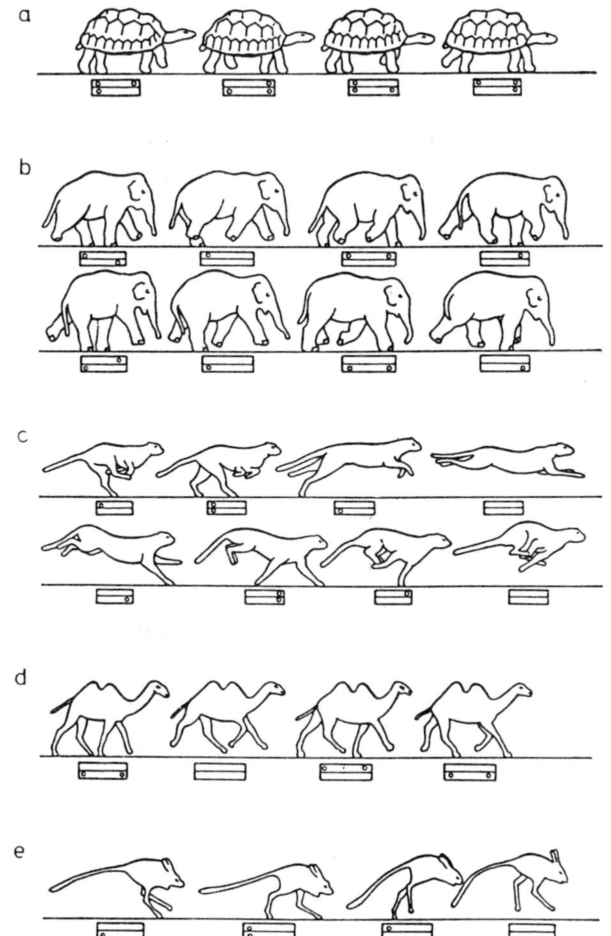

Fig.5.
Basic forms of land
locomotion of
vertebrates,
a - slow gait;
c - gallop;
d - amble;
e - ricochet.

Various dynamic models, less or more advanced, are used lately for the study of locomotive movements, specifically walking and running.

As it was mentioned above the live organisms are very complicated systems adapted to performing many different functions. Thus, starting modelling, a purpose to be served by the model should be defined. The first step after the purpose was settled is to choose a structural scheme and define the number of degrees of freedom. The next step is to determine the number of drives, their layout and principle of operation. The mathematical description of model's motion may be conducted by means of energetic methods which however, for more number of degrees of freedom, are hardly effective when using numerical solutions (A. Morecki and others 1975). In the previously published works (A. Morecki et al.1969) the construction of structural scheme of a whole man with his limbs was described. For this purpose, bones are replaced by rigid links and joints by kinematic pairs belonging to the 3rd, 4th and 5th class with rotary motions exclusively. Such a system has w = 240 to 250 degrees of freedom (Fig.6a). Mobility of the limbs amounts to 120 and mobility of the hands and feet amounts to 92. The first rough simplification usually assumed when building the model of the whole man, is to replace the whole trunk and head with one or two degrees of freedom. Moreover, if 22 degrees of freedom of each hand and foot is given up, the model with w = 29 - 30 degrees of freedom is obtained (Fig.6b). When resigning in turn one degree of freedom in hip and knee joints the model of 25 DOF is obtained. Such a model was suggested by I. Kato (1973). In the last years a new version of robot musician with 50 DOF was proposed (Kato 1985).

Many different models were proposed in last years. Among them a 3-D models consists of 17 body segments and 44 DOF looks very interesting (Hatze 1980). More simple models were offered with 3, 4 and 5 links (Pedotti 78, Hemami and Jaswa 1978, Vukobratović and Jurcić 1969, McGee 1978). Fig. 7 illustrates some of existing models.

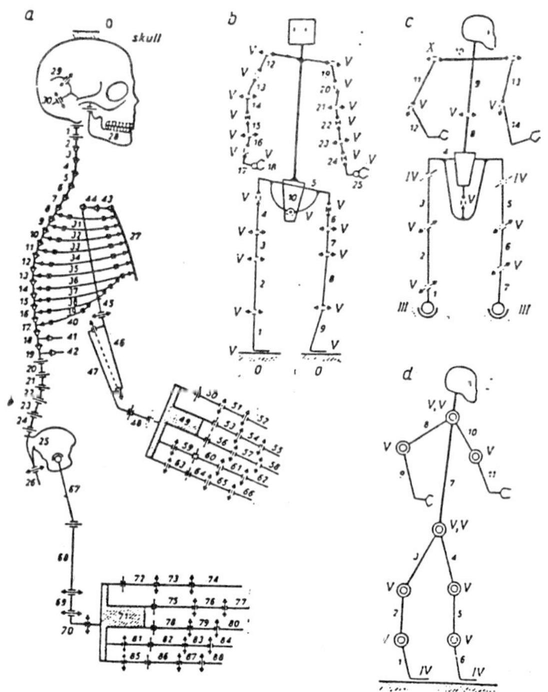

Fig. 6. Successive stages of simplifying man's structural model,

    a- complete model;

    b- model with w=25;

    c- model with w=20 or 23;

    d- model with w=11 (according to [3]).

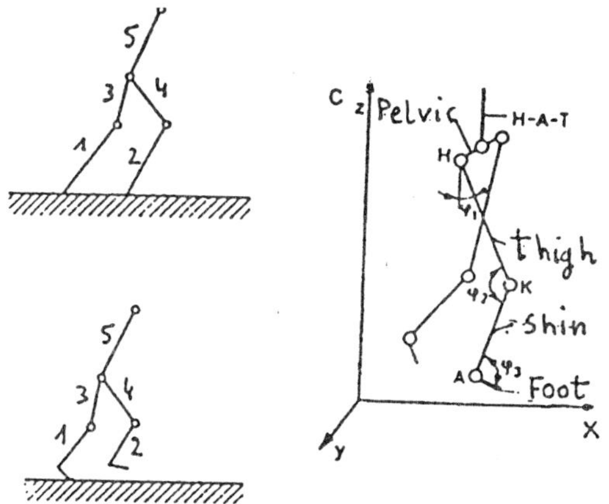


Fig 7.
Simples model
a) Five links model
b) Five links model with feets
c) 3-D model including pelvis

## 1.2.2. Plane model with 11D.O.F.

The walk and run belongs to two essential forms of displacement of the whole body by means of lower limbs. During the man's walk there appears two support form and lower limbs must secure the motion forward and backwards as well as left and right i.e. they must posses the mobility in both saggital and horizontal planes in relation to the body. Moreover, the whole body, in a spatial model, must have the possibility to incline to sides (the motion in the frontal plane) in order to balancing the moments of centrifugal forces arising when changing of the motion direction. The anthropomorphic model of motion - of the walk and run should under this assumptions enable following motions for the lower limbs: two motions in each hip joint, one motion in the knee and ankle joints, three motions when meeting the foot with the ground in the two-support phase, two motion of the trunk (rotation around the vertical axis and lateral bend), three motions for one limb in the model of run, one motion in the shoulder joint and one motion in the elbow joint. The mobility of a such model is w = 20 and for the model of run w = 23

The particular case of this model is a planar model (in the saggital plane) with w = 11 DOF. Further reducing the number of DOF seems to the inadmissible in consideration of the physical of modelling of the examined process (Fig.8).

Furthermore, the whole body treated as a three-dimensional model should allow reversal of the direction of movement (movement in frontal plane) to equilibrate the moments of the centrifugal forces produces by these changes.

These are the assumptions on which the model shown in Fig. 6c was proposed. The model has a mobility w = 20 for walking and w = 23 for running. A special case of this model is a plane model (the saggital plane) with a mobility w = 11 for the running phase (Fig. 8a). A further reduction of the number of degrees of freedom does not appear to be possible, if a similarity with the investigated process is to be maintained.

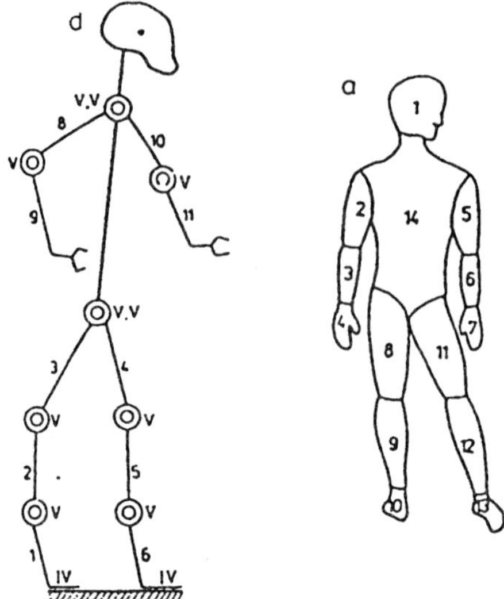


Fig. 8.
Minimal models
a) Plane model wit 11 or 12 DOF
b) Model with 14 segments

We now consider in detail the results obtained in the examination of the plane model (Fig. 8a) which is presented in working form in Fig. 9. In formulating the mathematical description of the model, further assumptions were accepted, namely:

⇒   the extremities and the trunk are treated as rigid elements:

⇒   all joints $0_i$, are treated as rotational kinematic pairs of class **V**,

⇒   the geometry of the system, i.e. the length of all links $l_i$, their position and the position of the centres of masses $s_i$, have been regarded as being given:

⇒   the angular velocities $\dot{\varphi}_i$ of all links are given,

⇒   the masses $m_i$, of all links and their moments of inertia $I_{0i}$ are given,

⇒   the centres of masses $s_i$, of i-th link are lying on the section $0_i$, $0_{i+1}$ and all the centres of masses are lying in one plane,

⇒   the moments of forces $M_i$, applied to each link are position, velocity and time function which means that:

$$M_i = M_i(\varphi_{i-2}, \varphi_{i-1}, \varphi_i, \varphi_{i+1}, \dot{\varphi}_{i-1}, \dot{\varphi}_i, t); \qquad (1)$$

⇒   wind resistance forces $W_i$ are neglected,

⇒   the base is assumed to be undistorable,

⇒   the joint $0_i$ transmits only the forces $F_x$ and $F_y$.

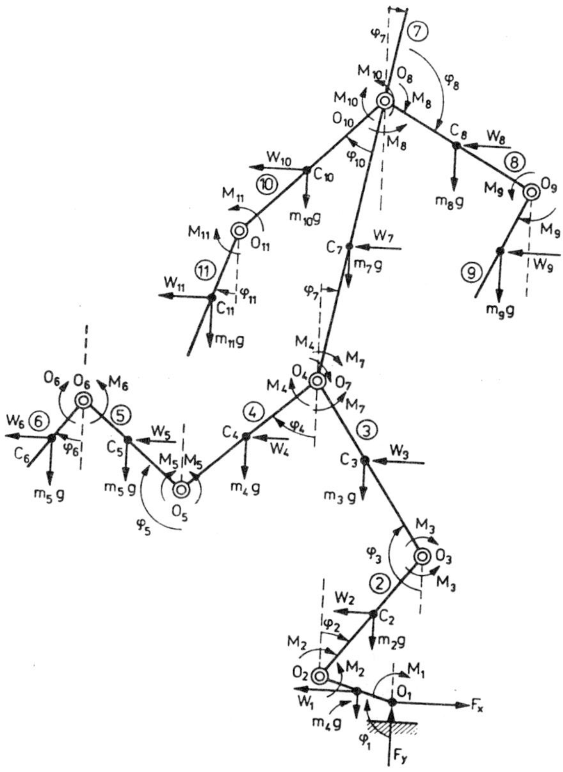


Fig.9. Plane model used for study of running (according to [1] ).

The classical procedure in laying the equations of movement using Lagrange's equations of the second kind proves rather ineffective in this case on account of the large number of degrees of freedom involved. For this reason, a new method, called the superposition of movements method, was developed in the case considered [1].

The equations of motion of the model are a set of eleven second-order non-linear differential equations of the form

$$\sum_{i=1}^{11} a_{ij}\ddot{\varphi}_j + \sum_{j=1}^{k} b_{ij}\dot{\varphi}2_j^2 - \sum_{j=k+1}^{11} b_{ij} - C_1 = 0 \qquad (2)$$

where:

$$a_{ij} = a_{ji}, \quad b_{ij} = b_{ji}, \quad k \le i,$$
$$i = 1,2, \quad \ldots, \quad 11;$$
$$S_j = m_j s_j + 1_j \sum_{k=j+1}^{11} m_k$$

$$a_{ij} = \begin{cases} l_j S_j \cos(\varphi_j - \varphi_i), & i \ne j \\ I_{oi} + l_i^2 \sum_{k=j+1}^{11} m_k, & i = j \end{cases} \qquad b_{ij} = \begin{cases} l_i S_j \sin(\varphi_j - \varphi)_{i,} & i \ne j \\ 0, & i = j \end{cases}$$

$C_i$ is a generalised force dependent on the force of gravity $m_i g$, resistance $W_1$ and moments $M_i$.

We obtain the solutions to the set equations (2), with the initial conditions, the elastic characteristic of the base and the moments of forces $M_i(t)$ being given, in the form of $\varphi_i(t)$ and $\dot{\varphi}_i(t)$. With the movement system given, i.e., $\varphi_i(t)$ and $\dot{\varphi}_i(t)$ the set of equations (2) is a set of eleven algebraic equations linear with respect to $M_i$, $F_x$ and $F_y$. We can then find the required values, for the moments of muscle forces in the joints and the components $F_x$ and $F_y$. The calculations can be made only numerically.

The second of the problems considered was solved, i.e., the values of $M_i(t)$ and of $F_x$ and $F_y$ were determined, in a study by J. Olszewski [1]. An experimental study was carried out to verify the numerical values obtained. Using chronocyclography and force-plate method the angular displacements in eleven principal joints were photographed during the running phase and the values of the component forces $F_x$ and $F_y$ were registered as the foot touched the force-plate. During the measurements a considerable influence of elasticity of the ground was observed as the foot of the man under test came in contact with it. Taking into account the displacements of this point, the number of degrees of freedom of the model should be increased to $w = 13$, i.e. two more degrees should be added.

The general view of the man under test is shown in Fig. 10 and an example of evaluating the results for the position just considered in Fig. 10b. In this graph, the dashed line gives the values of forces $F_{y1}$ in state $0_1$ calculated assuming non-deformability of the base, i.e., assuming the nulling of acceleration at the point $0_1$, whereas the curve $F_{y0}$ gives values with accelerations of the foot being considered. The curve $F_{yp}$ was platted from measurements. It follows from these curves that allowing for the deformability of the foot, a satisfactory conformity of results has been obtained.

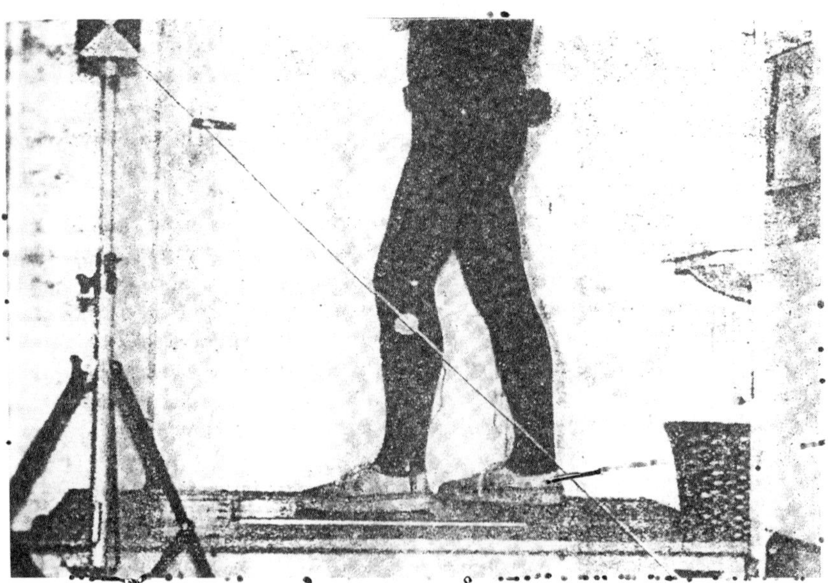

Fig. 10. Measuring in running.
a) Measuring stand for running

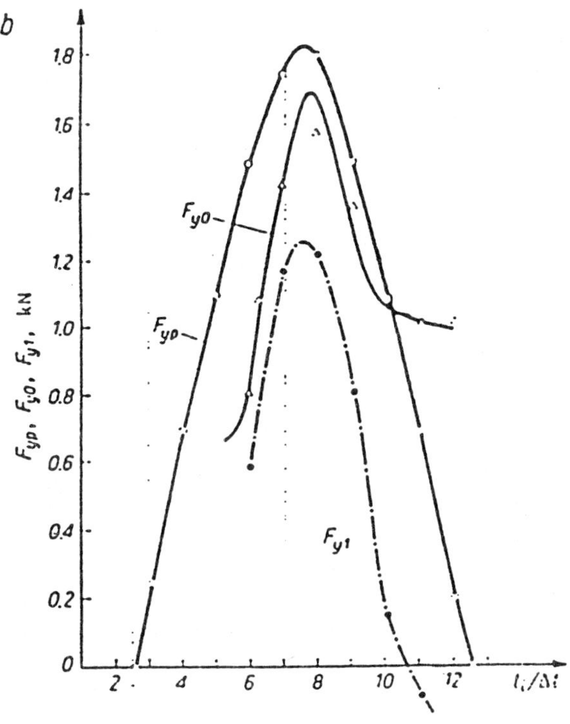


Fig. 10. Measuring in running.
b), c) Measurements results of vertical component of reaction force during stance phase.


## 1.3. Reduced order dynamic models for computer analysis of human gait

One general approach to the analysis of human gait is to make use of mathematical models in order to obtain estimates of variables not directly measurable by non-invasive means. In particular, estimated joint torques obtained from dynamic models derived from rigid body mechanics can be combined with EMG data to permit quantitative evaluation of neuro-muscular function during gait [4]. However, if such analysis is to be carried out on-line by a small computer, it is necessary to employ models which have been considerably simplified in comparison to the actual reality of musculoskeletal complexity. In view of this need, this item provides a brief description and a preliminary evaluation of two different types of simplified saggital plane models and their associated instrumentation.

It is important at the outset to distinguish between two distinctly different types of dynamic models for gait. The first type, which can be called a motion simulation model assumes that joint torques are determined by some specified feedback control law and employs principles of rigid body mechanics to determine the resulting limb segment accelerations. These are determined by some specified feedback control law and employs principles of rigid body mechanics to determine the resulting limb segment accelerations. These are then integrated numerically to obtain the system state, which is in turn needed to determine joint torques for the next computation cycle. In the other variety of mathematical model, called a motion analysis model or the „second problem of mechanics" limb segment motions are given and it is the joint torques or muscle forces which are to be determined. The gait analysis problem is thus in a certain sense the inverse of the gait simulation problem. While both types of models are useful, since the authors are primary interested in eventual clinical applications, this paper is entirely concerned with motion analysis.

## System using two force plates

At Warsaw Technical University, during the past several years, an intensive study of human locomotion has been undertaken. A mechanical model of the human body with 13 degrees  of freedom has been used for this purpose [1]. At the beginning of this investigations human motion during running was recorded by a  chronocyclographic method. The three components of ground reaction force were measured by a single force plate. The model was verified by these experiments and good results were obtained using off-line data analysis.

Mechanical model of the human body

The mechanical model of the human body described in  [1] has been  modified to include the double support phase of gait.

In the previously used model the system of co-ordinates was attached to the ankle joint, which caused the excessive numerical sensitivity during computations. For this reason the co-ordinates have been moved to the hip joint.

Investigation of walking, calls for an adequate model, mathematical description and methodology of experimental verification. The modified model used by the authors in investigations [4,5,6,7,8] is shown in Fig. 11.

The equations of motion for a planar model with 13 degrees of freedom are given in the matrix form (4) and (5).

The aim of the investigations presented in this work was to determine the static and dynamic torques acting in all joints, in function of time or relative angles.

Equations (4) and (5) are complemented with geometric data determining the positions of the centres of gravity and mass moments of inertia.

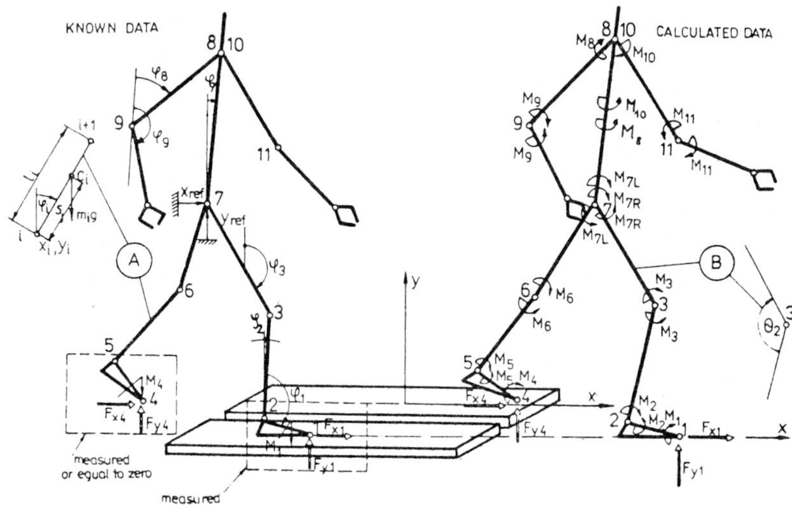


Fig. 11. Eleven-mass model for numerical and experimental analysis.

Moreover, is necessary to know the change of joint angles, $\phi_i$, their first and second derivatives, and two linear co-ordinates for the displacement of the hip joint axis. It is indispensable to know two components of the ground reaction ($F_{x4}$, $F_{y4}$) and the moment of $F_{y4}$ force about the axis of the metatarsus joint. The co-ordinates of the reference system attached to the hip joint are designated by ($x_{ref}$, $y_{ref}$) (Fig. 11).

$$
\begin{bmatrix}
a_{1,1} & a_{1,2} & a_{1,3} & \cdots & a_{1,13} \\
a_{2,1} & a_{2,2} & a_{2,3} & \cdots & a_{2,13} \\
\cdot & & & & \cdot \\
\cdot & & & & \cdot \\
a_{6,1} & a_{6,2} & a_{6,3} & \cdots & a_{6,13} \\
\cdot & & & & \cdot \\
\cdot & & & & \cdot \\
a_{12,1} & a_{12,2} & a_{12,3} & \cdots & a_{12,13} \\
a_{13,1} & a_{13,2} & a_{13,3} & \cdots & a_{13,13}
\end{bmatrix}
*
\begin{bmatrix}
\ddot{\phi}_1 \\
\ddot{\phi}_2 \\
\cdot \\
\cdot \\
\ddot{\phi}_6 \\
\cdot \\
\cdot \\
\ddot{\phi}_{12} \\
\ddot{\phi}_{13}
\end{bmatrix}
+
\begin{bmatrix}
b_{1,1} & b_{1,2} & b_{1,3} & \cdots & b_{1,13} \\
b_{2,1} & b_{2,2} & b_{2,3} & \cdots & b_{2,13} \\
\cdot & & & & \cdot \\
\cdot & & & & \cdot \\
b_{6,1} & b_{6,2} & b_{6,3} & \cdots & b_{6,13} \\
\cdot & & & & \cdot \\
\cdot & & & & \cdot \\
b_{12,1} & b_{12,2} & b_{12,3} & \cdots & b_{12,13} \\
b_{13,1} & b_{13,2} & b_{13,3} & \cdots & b_{13,13}
\end{bmatrix}
*
\begin{bmatrix}
\dot{\phi}_1^2 \\
\dot{\phi}_2^2 \\
\cdot \\
\cdot \\
\dot{\phi}_6^2 \\
\cdot \\
\cdot \\
\dot{\phi}_{12}^2 \\
\dot{\phi}_{13}^2
\end{bmatrix}
+
\begin{bmatrix}
c_{1,0} \\
c_{2,0} \\
\cdot \\
\cdot \\
c_{6,0} \\
\cdot \\
\cdot \\
c_{12,0} \\
c_{13,0}
\end{bmatrix}
=
\begin{bmatrix}
0 \\
0 \\
\cdot \\
\cdot \\
0 \\
\cdot \\
\cdot \\
0 \\
0
\end{bmatrix}
\quad (4)
$$

where:

$$a_{ij} = a_{ji}, \quad i, j \in \langle 1,13 \rangle, \quad b_{ij} = -b_{ji}, \quad i, j \in \langle 1,11 \rangle$$

$$a_{ij} = \begin{cases} 1_j s_j \cos(\varphi_j - \varphi_i), & \text{for } i \neq j \\ I_{oi} + l_i^2 \sum m_{k,} & \text{for } i=j \end{cases} \qquad b_{ij} = \begin{cases} l_i s_j \sin(\varphi_j - \varphi_i), & \text{for } i \neq j \\ 0, & \text{for } i=j \end{cases}$$

(5)

$$s_j = m_j s_j + l_j \sum m_k ,$$

$c$ - *a generalised force corresponding with the co-ordinate arising from forces of gravity $m_i g$ and moments $M_i$*

After substituting these data into eqs. (4) one obtains:

- reaction forces $F_{x1}$, $F_{y1}$ and torque $M_1$,

- moments of forces in function of time $M_i(t)$ and relative angles $M_i(\theta_k)$.

The purpose of experimental verification is to compare values of the measured quantities $F_{x1exp}$, $F_{y1exp}$ and $M_{1exp}$ with those calculated. In the experiment 2 force platforms were used. For small differences between the compare values it was assumed the model was adequate and the calculated values of the moments $M_i$ were close to real values.

The procedure followed in solving so formulated problem is given bellow:

(i)　After shooting a film of a given motion, one can obtain from the film Cartesian co-ordinates of chosen joints $(x_i, y_i)$ (where $i = 1,2,...,7$). Basing on these co-ordinates joint angles $\phi_i$ are calculated.

(ii)　Using the method of adjustment calculus velocities and accelerations are computed. In the same step $x_{ref}$ and $y_{ref}$ are calculated. In this case a symmetry of motion is assumed, which means that calculations are conducted for 6 angles $\phi_i$ ($\phi_1$, $\phi_2$, $\phi_3$, $\phi_7$, $\phi_8$, $\phi_9$) and the remaining are determined on the basis of these calculations.

(iii)　Using the two force platforms, vertical and horizontal components of the ground reaction are measured for the left and the right foot, and then moments $M_1$ and $M_4$ are determined in the numerical way.

Data $F_{X4}$, $F_{Y4}$ and $M_4$ are first substituted into eqs. (4) and then $F_{X1}$, $F_{Y1}$ and $M_1$ are calculated. Forces $F_{x1}$ and $F_{y1}$ are measured and moment $M_1$ is calculated with purpose to check the moments $M_i$ developed by muscles in individual joints.

The computations are conducted with use of a set of computer programmes named HLS (Human Locomotion System). The programmes are written in FORTRAN IV language and are intended for CYBER 70 computer system.

The instrumentation used in this system is as follows [7,8]:

(1)    PENTAZET-35 movie camera;

(2)    K-202 minicomputer with CPO-2 digital image processor;

(3)    CYBER-70/7216 model computer system;

(4)    HP-25 programmed calculator;

(5)    Two platforms;

(6)    Recorder for registering acceleration signals (from accelerometers) and ground reaction components (from the force platforms);

(7)    Stereocomparator.

The procedure runs the programs in the following sequence:

1.  Cartesian co-ordinates,

2.  Converter,

3.  Adjustment calculus,

4.  Force-point-moment,

5.  Moments in joints of a man,

6.  Comparator.

Program „Cartesian co-ordinates" computes the rectangular Cartesian co-ordinates for 7 chosen joints of a man. Program „Converter" converts information about co-ordinates of the joints axes. Angular co-ordinates, velocities and accelerations are determined by means of the „Adjustment calculus". The components of the floor reaction, and moments of those forces are calculated with use of the „Force-points-moment" program.

The values of components of the ground reaction for the assumed model are computed with use of the program „Moments in the joints of a man" and the results obtained from running the programs: „Cartesian co-ordinates", „Adjustment calculus" and „Force-point-moment".

The comparison of the results of computations made for the model with those obtained experimentally is performed with use of the program „Comparator".

Great attention is given to the problem of determining the moments of forces developed in the joints of a man in a function of relative angles.

HLS system enables to obtain the course of the time following quantities:

$F_{x1}, F_{y1}, M_1, M_i(t), M_i(\theta_k)$.

An example of relationship between the moment $M_3(\theta_2)$ of muscular forces acting in the knee joint and the relative angle between the shank and the thigh is given in Fig. 12. The graph closes on substitution of the 560th time interval.

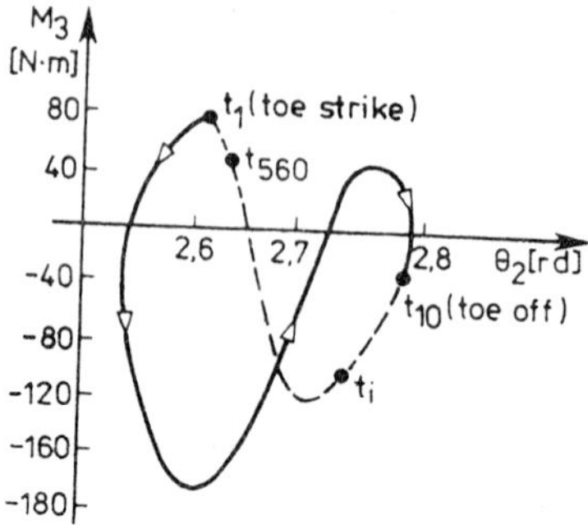



Fig.12.
Knee moment $M_3$ versus relative angle $\theta_2$ between thigh and shank.

## Force plates

Two special force plates capable of measuring all six components of ground reaction have been designed, constructed, and tested by the Biomechanics Team at Warsaw Technical University. Each plate is supported at three points in order to obtain a statically determined system. The specifications of each plate are:

1. Maximum horizontal force (X, Z): ±: 500 N,
2. Maximum vertical force Y : 5000N,
3. Linearity: <1% of full scale,
4. Error in centre of pressure co-ordinates:
   ± 2 mm lateral, ± 4 mm longitudinal,
5. Crosstalk $Y \rightarrow X$ ± 2%, $X \rightarrow Y$ < 1%%,
6. Least natural frequency: 75 Hz.

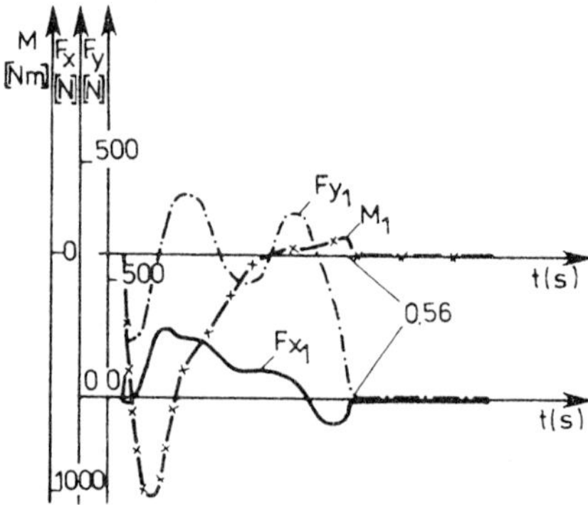



Fig. 13. Vertical $F_{x1}$, horizontal $F_{y1}$, ground reaction forces and moment $M_1$ associated with right leg during one gait cycle obtained from force.

Fig. 13 are given typical courses of ground reactions $F_{x1}$, $F_{y1}$ and $M_1$ measured by means of the force plates. The shown relationships were obtained from the program „Force-point-moment" and HLS system.

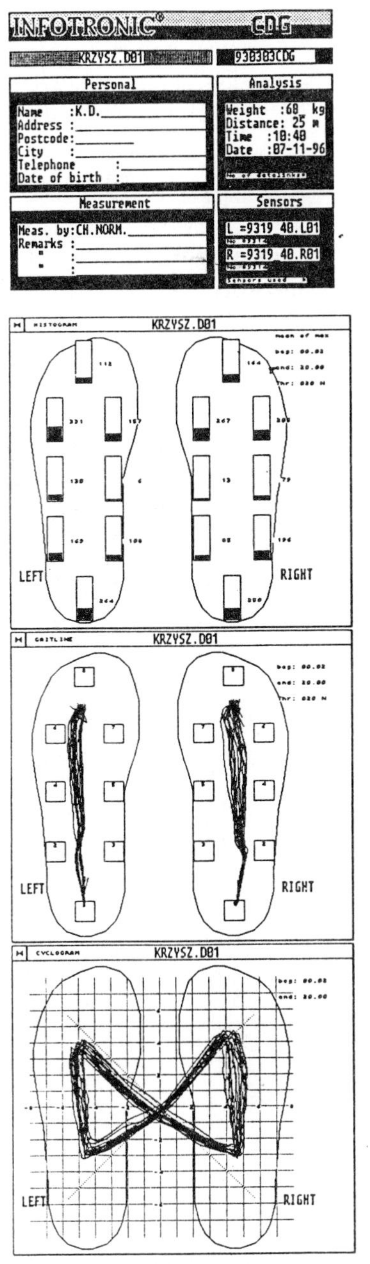

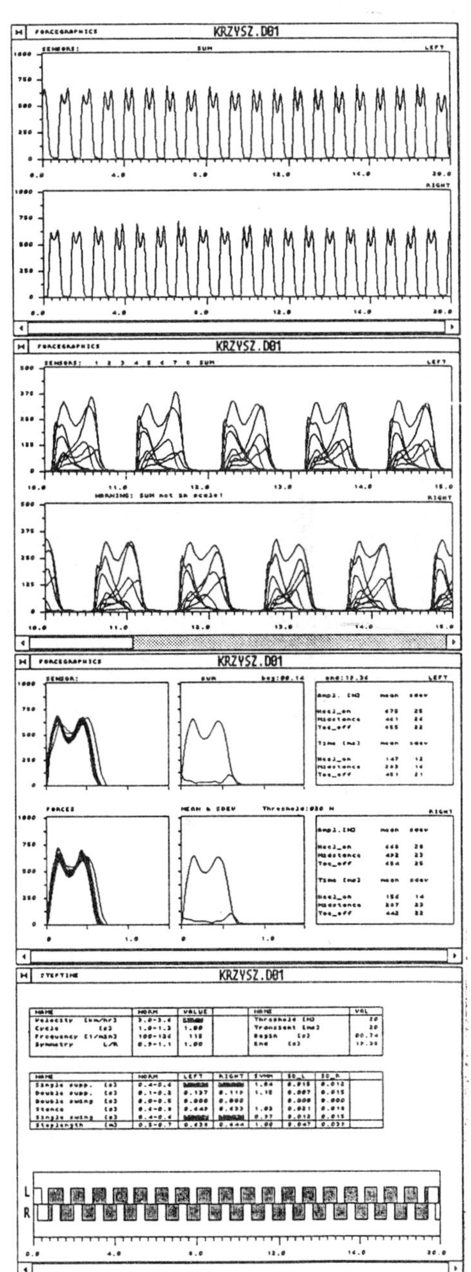

Table 1.

Will shortly described two systems which are used at present namely:
Computer Dyno Graphy (CDG) and Ariel Performance Analysis System (APAS) [37], [38].

Computer Dyno Graphy is used for measurements of vertical component of reaction force as a function of time. It consists of three parts: special shoos equipped with 8 capacities sensors (50 Hz, 0,44 - 111N/cm2, $P_{max}$ = 4000 N) control unit for data collection, computer for data analysis.

This system allow in the some time  four measurements. Each measure takes 20 s. (table 1).

Ariel Performance Analysis System is used for 3-D videographic analysis. It consists from PC 286/25 computer two PANASONIC cameras camcorder PV-910 VHS. The set of six programmes allow co-ordinates measurements and graphical presentation and export in ASC II, LOTUS and DBASE format. Table 1 shows the results in one plane for ankle, knee, hip and shoulder points.

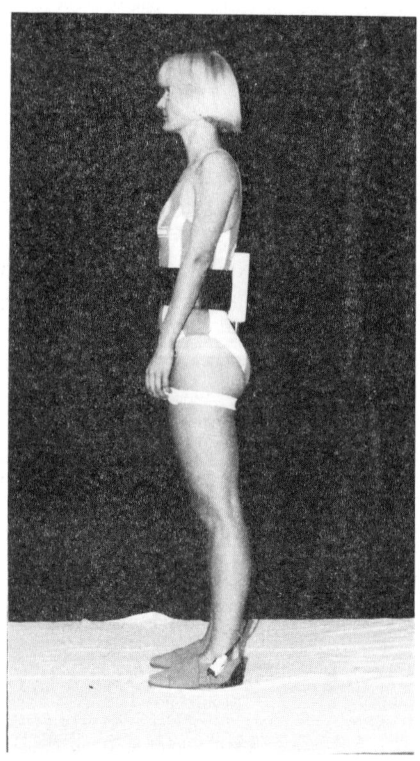
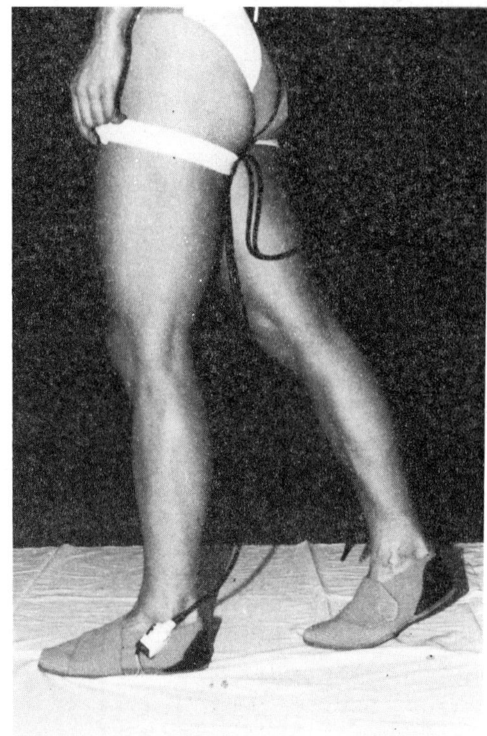

Photo 1. View of the subject during the measurements.

## On-line system using television data.

Beginning in 1972, the group at Ohio State University has been involved in an effort to use television cameras as primary source data for on-line gait analysis [7]. In this approach, a subject is fitted with small incandescent lights attached to anatomical reference points, and walks in a partially darkened room. The brightness of the lights is such that video signal exceeds a preset threshold only in those resolution cells of the image in which the lights appear. The occurrence of such an event triggers the transfer of an eight-b (one part in 256) signal from a horizontal counter and an eight-b vertical counter as a single 16 bit word to the on-line computer (PDP-11/34). While the initial version of this system utilised only camera, work has now progressed to the point that three cameras are used, each fitted with its own microprocessor (Signetics 8x300) for image pre-processing. With such an arrangement, three-dimensional motion of the marker lights can be obtained in external rectangular co-ordinates by means of triangulation calculations performed by the computer.

The television approach has been shown to be very useful for kinematic investigations and one sizeable study involving twenty subjects and concerned with the effects of footwear on gait has been completed. However, if kinematic analysis is attempted by this means, a serious problem arises; namely, normal human gait includes double support phases constituting closed kinematic chains. Since such chains can support internal forces not related to motion, estimation of joint forces and torques is impossible from television data alone unless some assumption is made concerning the co-operation between supporting limbs [7]. Since the Gait Laboratory at Ohio State University is furnished with an accurate force plate (Kistler type 9261-A), which can provide data to the computer synchronised with television measurements, the validity of various assumptions concerning load sharing between limbs can be evaluated. Some results of this type are presented in the following paragraphs.

## Seven Mass Model for Television Data Analysis

The co-ordinate system and general kinematic arrangement of a seven mass model used for television data analysis is shown in Fig. 14. In this model, the pelvic link is considered to be massless and of variable length and orientation.

Its location within the field of view of a television camera therefore requires determination of the co-ordinates of both of its endpoints, $(x_{LH}, y_{LH})$ and $(x_{RH}, y_{RH})$ corresponding to the left and right hip sockets respectively. Once these two point have been located, the position and orientation of all other body segments can be found from simple trigonometric relationships involving the seven angles shown in Fig. 14. If an assumption is made about the way in which forces divide between the right and left limbs during double support, then such position data can be doubly differentiated numerically to obtain estimates of all joint forces and moments without the use of force plate data [7].

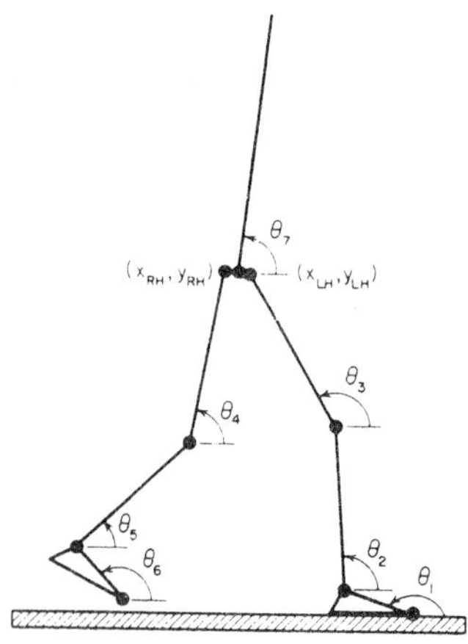

Fig. 14. Stick figure of seven-mass model for analysis of television data.

The method described above begins with consideration of the upper body segment of Fig.14. If $\theta_7$, and $\dot\theta_7$, $\theta_7$ are known along with the corresponding information for the pelvis endpoint co-ordinates, then simple freebody analysis permits calculation of the two forces and the moment acting at the point of attachment of the upper body to the pelvis [7]. During single support phases of gait, the same type of analysis is possible for the swing phase leg, which then allows evaluation of forces and moments on the supporting leg, ending finally in estimates for ground reaction forces and moments. So far as double support phases are concerned, in the hypothesis is advances that ground reaction forces and ankle torques transfer from one foot to the other linearly in time over the duration of double support. Specifically, if $F_y$ is the vertical component of the total ground reaction force, and $F_{yL}$ is the portion of this force exerted by the left foot, then this hypothesis assumes that

$$F_{yL} = q_y F_y, \tag{6}$$

where the partition coefficient $q_y$, is given by

$$q_y = \frac{t - t_{LHS}}{t_{RTO} - t_{LWS}} \qquad t_{LHS} \le t < t_{RTO} \tag{7}$$

$$q_y = 1.0 \qquad t_{RTO} \le t < t_{RHS}. \tag{8}$$

$$q_y = \frac{t_{LTO} - t}{t_{LTO} - t_{RHS}} \qquad t_{RHS} \le t < t_{LTO} \tag{9}$$

$$q_y = 0.0 \qquad t_{LTO} \le t < t_{LHS} + T. \tag{10}$$

In these expressions, HS refers to <u>heel strike</u>, TO refers to <u>toe off</u>, and T is the gait period [12]. Similarly, for the right foot,

$$F_{yR} = p_y F_y \qquad \text{where} \qquad p_y + q_y = 1. \tag{11}$$

## Experimental Results

Fig. 15. shows experimental results obtained from the above model as well as from direct measurements of ground reaction force [7].

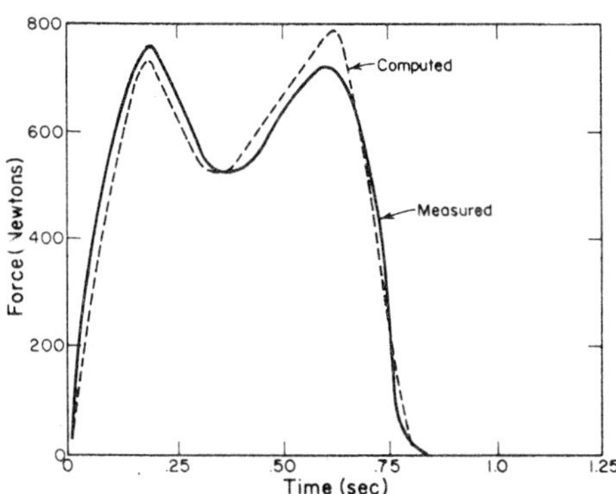

Fig.15. Vertical Ground Reaction Force Associated with Left Leg During One Gait Cycle Obtained by Direct Force Plate Measurement and Computed from Seven-Mass Model

When these results were first obtained, the authors were very encouraged by the rather good agreement between the two curves of this figure and undertook a further investigation of the above hypothesis. Unfortunately, the results of this study showed that horizontal force estimates obtained by this method are entirely wrong for double support phases of gait, even though during single support they are comparably accurate to vertical force estimates. This suggests that the linear transfer hypothesis cannot be applied to the calculation of horizontal forces. To test this conjecture, it was noted that if $G_{xL}$ and $G_{yL}$ are respectively, the horizontal and vertical components of left leg ground reaction directly measured by a force plate, then the true partition coefficients are:

$$\hat{q}_x = \frac{G_{xL}}{\sum_{j=1}^{7} m_j \ddot{x}_j} \qquad \hat{q}_y = \frac{G_{yL}}{\sum_{j=1}^{7} m_j \ddot{y}_j + g} \qquad (12)$$

In paper [ 7] some possible solution of this problem is given.

## 1.4 Muscle drives and control system

After creating a structural model of a man it is necessary to establish a relationship between the number of degrees of freedom number of functions [8].

The force by any given muscles as a function of time is a very important system variable. The direct measurements of this force is not possible in a human subject. The best that can be done is to estimate muscle force using electromyographic data to infer level of activity and muscle cross sectional area to estimates maximum force. Both this estimates are subject to substantial errors. In the human locomotory system in which a large number of muscles are active during the walking cycle, these errors are sufficient to cast doubt on the validity of analysis or simulation results.

The same is concern the control system. As it was mentioned above in order to simulate a multiplay actuated system like the human body it is necessary to postulate algorithms for co-ordination and control. But the co-ordination of human system is not understood. On way to partially circumvent this difficulty is to formulate an hypothesis that an objective function is minimised by the system. A favourite is metabolic energy cost (Capozzo, Leo and Pedotti, 1975, Townsend and Seireg, 1972). The second is minimum of forces (Seireg 1993). However, the viability of this first approach is questionable since there is no accurate model relating energy cost to muscle force and contraction rate. For walking, which is the most commonly modelled activity, the minimum of the objective function is very shallow and such techniques are unable to reliability discriminate between quite large differences in muscular activity programs.

We like also to underline that more effort has been expended to model mathematically the musculoskeletal system and how it participates in multi-muscle motor control than to model how neural networks control movements (F.E. Zając and J.M. Winters, 1990). One major reason is that quantitative data needed to model CNS neutral network control has been quite limited in comparison to musculoskeletal data. CNS data is limited because the experimental techniques available to study single neurones, groups of similar functioning neurones, and the interaction among the different neural groups are at best few, and even than very difficult (Zając and Winter, 1990).

It necessary to say that in the last time engineers and biomathematicians now have renewed interest in neural network modelling. The reason is because of the ability of computers to simulate neural network complex enough. These neural network models are, however, quite „artificial” and must able distinguished from „biological  neural networks” based on biological phenomena (Pellionisz, 1988). Neural controllers are used to control the motion of walking machines. The utilised artificial neural network do not imitate the way that CNS is built. Researchers are trying to utilise the knowledge of the functional structure or neural system. As an example we can mention here the six-legged walking machine neural controller (Berns and other, 1993). The structure of the controller is hierarchical. On the lowest level there are four neural networks two of which control lifting of legs (one for the legs on the left,  the other for the ones on the right), the remaining two control the leg motions in the support phase. One the higher level there are two networks co-ordinating the translocation and support phase of leg motions. The neural network of the highest level transforms information from sensor (the so called reactive element) into signals controlling the functioning of neural networks co-ordinating leg motion.

The conceptual diagram of the neuromusculoskeletal control system  is shown on Fig. 16.

The CNS can be considered here as „the neural network controller" or just „the controller". The musculoskeletal system can be considered „the plant" (Zając and Winters, 1990) [3].

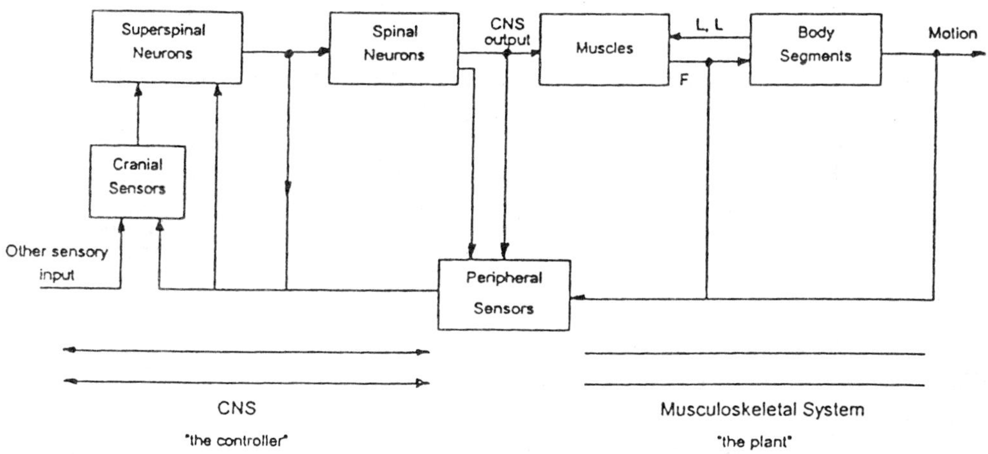


Fig. 16. Conceptual diagram of the neuromusculoskeletal control system [3].

## 1.5. Electromechanical biped

The main goal is here the construction of the mechanism which mimics the human musculoskeletal system as possible with respect to actuator linesaxtion and actuator rate force characteristics. Segments masses and mass distributions will also be simulated as closely as possible. This will provide a system which simulates the human locomotory system but in which all important system variables are fully accessible (Song S.M. and Waldron K.J., 1988). A number of mechanical  biped robots have been constructed and tested in different centres around the world (Takahishi, et. al., 1989, Emura and Arakava, 1989, Raibert, 1986, Grishin A.A., et al., 1991, Bogutsky A.V., 1993).

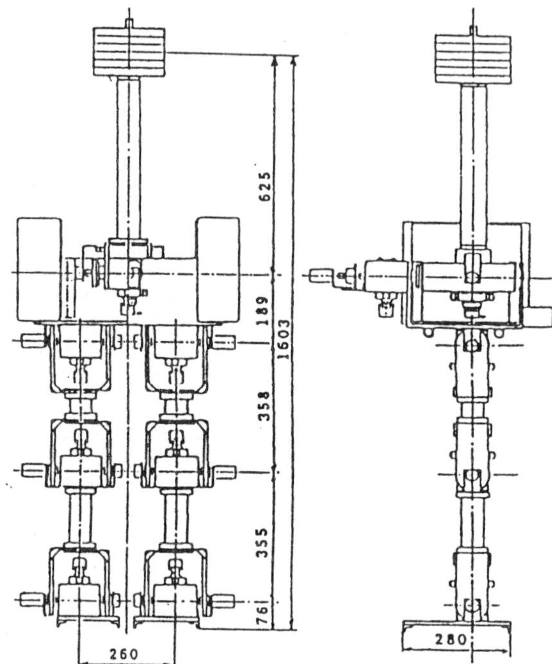

Fig.17. Biped walking robot WL-12B and external force generation system [3]

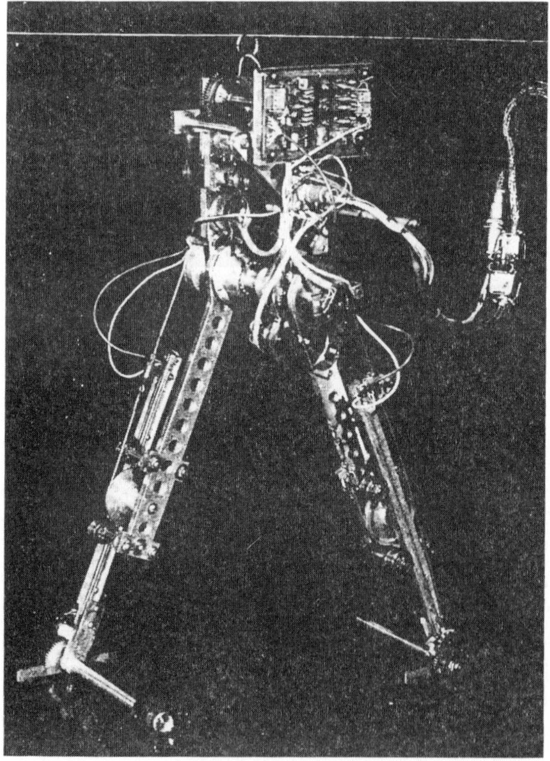

Fig. 18. Biped wehicle with two telescopic legs, controlled by two drives, proposed by Grishin, Formalsky and other [39]

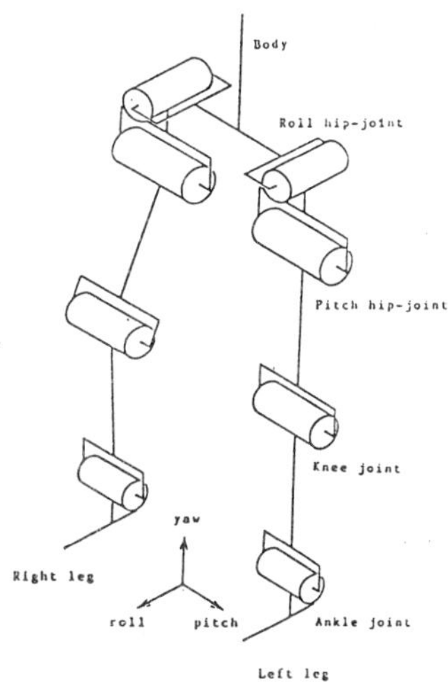


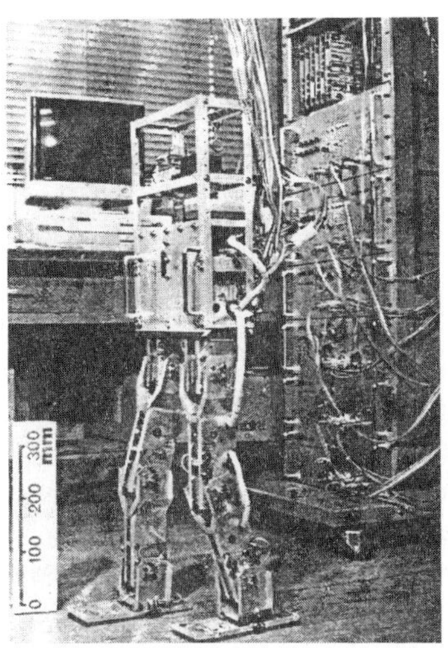

Fig.19. Scheme of the biped robot controlled with 8 motors [3].

Fig.20. A photograph of the biped robot by 8 servomotors [3].

Figure 17 shows assembly drawing of WL-12R. None of these, however, closely mimics the human system. Figure 19 and Fig.20 shows the model of locomotion proposed by Emura and others. Figure 18 shows the prototype of walking biped robot [3].

In the next item we will present our own project concerning the design of an electromechanical model of the biped with the height degree of the anthropomorphism

## 1.6 Design of an own Electromechanical Model

Design of an electrical system ideally necessitates several simultaneous decisions. In order to design a robot manipulator, for example, we need to specify the kinematic parameters, the number of degrees of freedom, the number of joints, the link lengths, the joint displacement ranges, etc.; the dynamic parameters: the masses and the moments of inertia of the links; the actuation system configuration: electric motors, hydraulic or pneumatic actuation; and the sensor system: joint position encoder, velocity, and acceleration sensing etc. Moreover, given the functional objectives of the robot: that is, what exactly we want it to do; its performance: that is, how well it does it depends both on the efficiency of its controller, which is a function both of the raw computing power and the cleverness of the algorithms, and of the kinematic and the dynamic parameters selected earlier. In reality, therefore, the design becomes a highly iterative process, later decisions affecting and modifying the earlier ones. Since very few of the system components may be selected unilaterally without regard to the other components, a tricky question is: „Where to start?" [10]

The investigations started from the computer model of the lower leg of a man.

## 1.6.1 Computer Model of a Human Limb Musculo-Skeletal Model

A computer model of a human limb musculo-skeletal system has been developed. The mathematical model is based on the finite element method and is suitable for ergonomic applications and gait analysis. The mathematical model was coded into a computer package in order to make calculations possible.

The model consists of rigid bodies, flexible elements and actuators. Bones are modelled as rigid bodies. Joints are modelled as flexible elements. Every flexible element consists of six springs; three for translations and three for rotations. If a movement in the biological joint is small or impossible, then the stiffens of the spring for this direction of this movement in the model is made large. For directions of movement, which are allowed by the biological joint, the stiffens of the spring in the model is small. Muscles are modelled as actuators which act along geometrically defined lines of action. The lines of action are obtained by connecting the point of origin of the muscle with the point at which the muscle inserts onto a bone. Some of the muscles are modelled by two lines: the first being the line from the muscle origin to a point, at which the muscle starts to wrap around a bone. The second line is from the point at which the muscle unwraps from the bone to the point of insertion. The force exerted by a muscle is a function of three parameters: its excitation, its instantaneous length, and the velocity with which it is contracting. The muscle force is modelled as a function of muscle excitation, expressed as a number between 0 and 1, and time. The problem of muscle recruitment, or apportionment of force among several available muscles, is solved by an optimisation procedure. Several non-linear merit criteria were tested, such as the soft saturation criterion, and energy criterion. The model consists of 32 muscles for each lower extremity and 64 muscles for each upper extremity (including half of the shoulder girdle) [11].

Many tests were made in order to validate the model parameters. The parameters were obtained from published measurements of human body mass and geometric properties. It was shown that using a model of the human lower extremity it is possible to simulate free motion of the leg (flexion and extension), squats, and gait without raising the feet. Simulation of typical human gaits is planned for the future. The model is a unique model which fully describes the dynamics of phenomena occurring during the working of the human musculoskeletal system.

On the Fig.21 the right leg model is shown. This model is operated by 31 muscles. Some properties of this model will be used by designing of the anthropomorphic biped model.

1 gracilis
2 adductor longus
3 adductor magnus (extensor)
4 adductor magnus (adductor)
5 adductor brevis
6 semitendinosus
7 semimembranosus
8 biceps femoris long
9 rectus femoris
10 sartorius
11 tensor fasciae latae
12 gluteus maximus
13 iliopsoas
14 biceps femoris short
15 vastus medialis
16 vastus intermedius
17 vastus lateralis
18 gatrocnemius medialis
19 gastrocnemius lateralis
20 soleus
21 tibialis anterior
22 tibialis posterior
23 extensor digitorum longus
24 extensor hallucis longus
25 flexor digitorum longus
26 flexor hallucis longus
27 peroneus longus
28 peroneus brevis
29 peroneus tertius
30 gluteus medius
31 gluteus minimus

A - pelvis and torso
B - femur
C - lower leg
D - foot

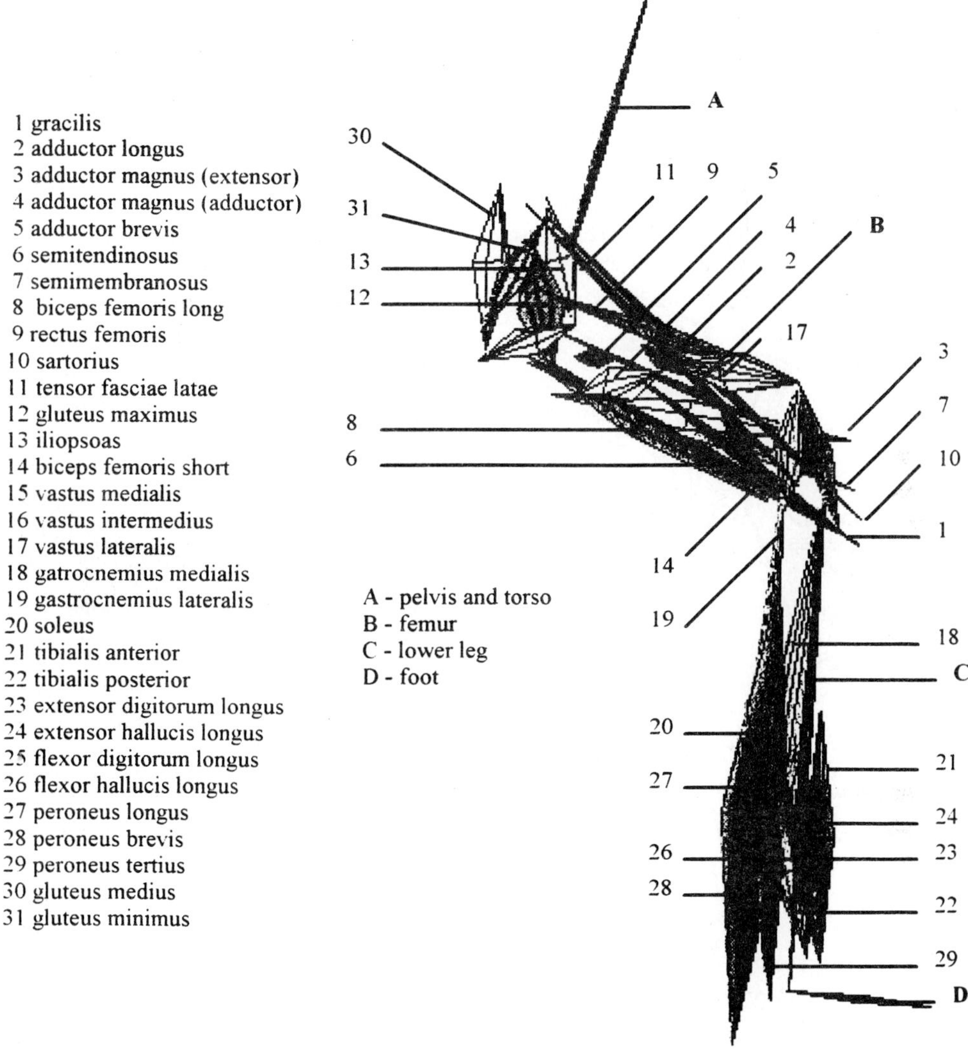


Fig.21. The right leg model

## 1.6.2 Anthropomorphic biped robot

One philosophy, that followed here, is to start designing those components on which we have the least amount of initial information. Recalling that the choice of one component depends on the selection of the others, selecting the least known components, first is the most efficient procedure in terms of minimising the changes that have to be made throughout the design. This is thus a reasonable approach to adopt.

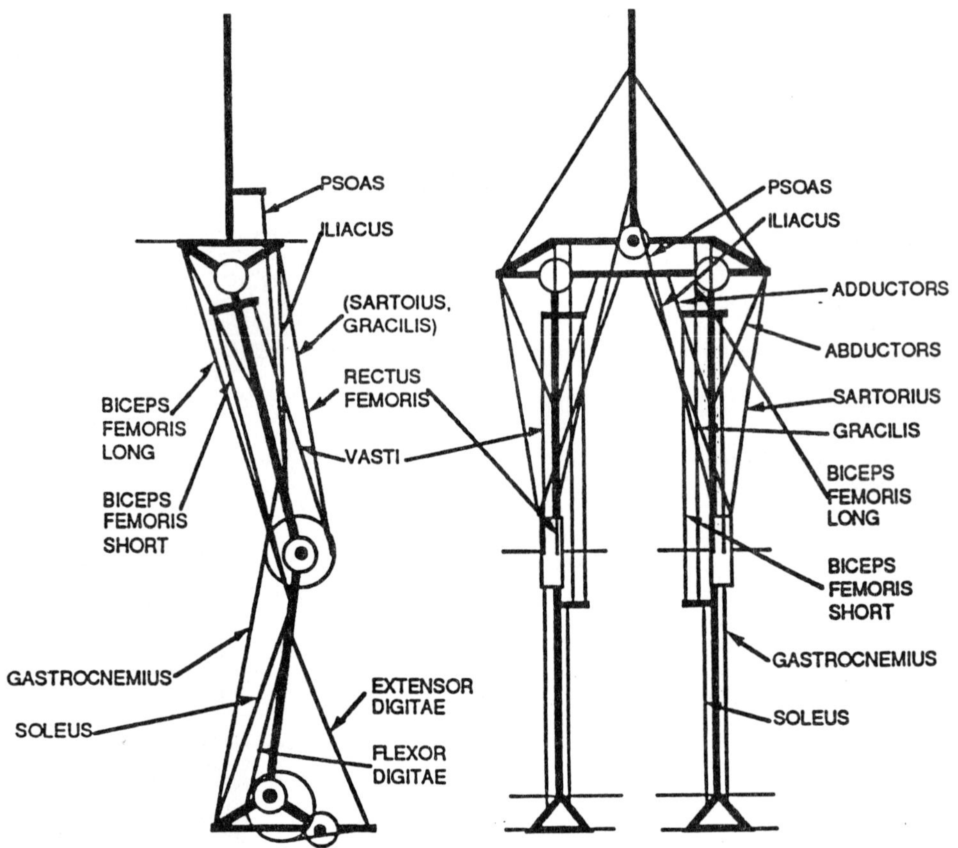


Fig.22. General schematic view of anthropomorphic biped robot

For an anthropomorphic biped robot such as the one we set out to design here, many of the above-mentioned decisions have, fortunately, already been implicity made. The very inclusion of the word „anthropomorphic" in the description of the robot gives us some clear direction as to what the geometric dimensions, the kinematic structure, and the inertial parameters of the machine are going to be [12], Figure 22.

We will shortly discuss typical dimensions and mass properties of the leg. We will attempt to minimise the number of parameters to be included using as a guideline the geometric and inertial properties of a 2 m tall person. The lengths and weights of different leg links of a typical human being with height H and weight W are as followed [13]:

<u>Thigh</u>: 0.24 H, 0.10 W, centre of mass at 0.567 T up from knee joint. Thigh length: T = 0.489 m

<u>Shank</u>:0.24 H, 0.045 W, centre of mass at 0.567 S up from ankle joint. Shank length: S = 0.448 m

<u>Foot</u>: 0.04 H (from ankle joint to centre of mass), 0.15 M (from heel to toe), 0.0015 W, centre of mass at 0.571 F back from the toe tip. Foot length: F = 0.29 m.

<u>Pelvis breadth</u>: 0.28 m.

The natural leg has 30 degrees of freedom and is operated by 66 muscle actons. It is necessary to simplify this model. Let us assume the following numbers of degrees of freedom:

- torso: rotation in the suggested plane (6 degrees of freedom)

- hip: extension/flexion,  adduction/abduction (2 degrees of freedom)

- knee: extension/flexion (6 degrees of freedom)

- ankle plantarflexion/dorsiflexion (6 degrees of freedom) passive spring restraining

- toe rotation (6 degrees of freedom).

Thus for each leg we will have a total of 4 active degrees of freedom. In addition, the torso has one active degree of freedom with respect to the pelvis. For the whole model we have 9 degrees of freedom plus 1 passive degree of freedom. A list of the main leg muscles is as follows: Hip (11 muscles), thigh rotation (1 muscle), knee (10 muscles), ankle (4 muscles), foot (2 muscles), toe (4 muscles): a total of 32 muscles.

In order to mimic the behaviour of human joints we decided to employ tendon driven joints in our robot. Also the agonist - antagonist feature of the human muscle system will be emulated as far as is possible. A third aspect of the human muscle system that we intend to include in our design in the presence  of multi-joint muscles, particularly two-joint muscles. The advantage of two-joint muscles is clearly to facilitate the transfer  of energy from one joint of the system to another. Assuming up to a two function level of interconnection of the muscles, a full set of tendons will have the ability to move every joint, in both the positive and the negative directions, independently as well as having the ability to control all possible combinations of movements between a joint and its adjacent joints. We need two tendons on the agonist and antagonist sides of a joint to fully control it. The problem arises of how many actuation tendons should be included in the machine. Because we will have 9 active degrees of freedom: 1 at torso, 2 x (2 at the hip, 1 at the knee, 1 at the ankle). Actuation of these degrees of freedom in the robot requires 18 tendons. So far we have only accounted for the one-joint muscles. There are three two-joint muscles in the model. Two of them involve both the hip and the knee. For two legs we need four more tendons. Also each leg has one two-joint muscle connecting the knee and the ankle. Two more tendons are therefore needed for the two legs. In summary, we will need 24 active tendons for the anthropomorphic biped robot. We have not included in our model a two-joint tendon performing knee extension and ankle dorsiflexion.

If we take a close look at the human anatomy we find that most muscles actuate limb motion in several directions. For example, a shortening of the sartorius muscle will cause both hip flexion and medial/lateral thigh rotation. Each joint is acted upon by several muscles which act in synergy. Obviously, the most drastic functional simplification would be to ignore how the joints are actuated in the biological system, except that one should be able to actuate them in any direction typically by using actuators, such as electric motors, acting directly on the joints. In this case there is a synergy between the electric motors since they do not act against each other. Our approach lies somewhere in between. We will have several tendons acting on a single joint but not as many as we see in a human leg. Based on this short discussion the following list of actively driven tendons was assumed.:

1. Pelvis forward tilt

2. Pelvis backward tilt

3. Hip extension: *Gluteus Maximus*

4. Hip flexion: *Iliopsoas*

5. Hip abduction: *Gluteus Medius, Gluteus Minimus*

6. Hip adduction: *Adductor Longus, Adductor Brevis, Adductor Magnus*

7. Knee extension: *Vastus Lateralis, Vastus Medialis, Vastus Intermedius*

8. Knee flexion: *Biceps Femoris (short head), Semitendinosus, Semimembranosus*

9. Ankle plantarflexion: *Soleus, Tibialis Posterior*

10. Ankle dorsiflexion: *Tibialis Anterior*

11. Hip extension/knee flexion: *Rectus Femoris*

12. Hip flexion/knee extension: *Biceps Femoris (long head)*

13. Knee flexion/ankle plantarflexion: *Gastrocnemius*

Total:   11 x 2 + 2 = 24 driven tendons plus unactuated Spring/Tendons:

1. Hip medial/lateral rotation

2. Toe extension/flexion: Extension (*Extensor Hallucis Longus, Extensor Digitorum Longus*), and flexion (*Flexor Hallucis Longus, Flexor Digitorum Longus*)

We will now discuss the problem of motor selection. An important design goal is to configure the actuation system so that digital control technique can be used to faithfully mimic the actuation characteristics of the muscles, even though the tendon geometry, and certainly the actuator mechanics, may be somewhat different. This requires a system adapted to precise control with relatively bandwidth, and easily interfaced to a digital system.

We may consider the following actuation options:

A.        Electric Motors

1. Brushless DC: Direct drive, tendon drive or compliant tendon.

2. Commutated DC: Direct drive, tendon drive or compliant tendon.

3. AC Induction motor: Direct drive, tendon drive or compliant tendon.

4. Stepping motor: Direct drive, tendon drive or compliant tendon.

The advantages of electric actuation are flexibility in application together with a clean system with a compact power supply and moderate maintenance. Use of an electric motor in combination with a ball-screw produces a stiff and efficient linear actuator.

The disadvantages are poor force to weight ratio making it necessary to run at a high speed to generate the required power. For this reason speed reducers are usually necessary. The side effects of use of speed reducers include increased complexity and weight, compliance and backlash.

B.        Hydraulic Actuation

1. Linear actuator with direct drive, tendon drive or compliant tendon.

2. Rotary actuator with direct drive, tendon drive or compliant tendon.

Advantages include the highest force/weight ratio available. There is no need for speed reducers, hydraulic actuation is suitable for heavy-duty applications.

Disadvantages include the potential for fluid leakage, difficult maintenance, and usually a bulky power supply.

C.        Pneumatic Actuation

1. Linear actuator with direct drive, or tendon drive.

2. Air motor with direct drive, tendon drive or compliant tendon.

Advantages include inexpensive components and a convenient power supply requiring only a compressor or compressed air supply.

Disadvantages of pneumatic cylinders include very low force/weight ratio and high inherent compliance in the system. The characteristics of air motors are much like electric motors in requiring high operating speed to produce effective power, and hence needing speed reducers.

One choice that is popular among the robotics community is the use of brushless DC motors. The main advantages of the brushless motors over commutated motors are lower rotor inertia, lower friction, higher output torque for equal motor volume, and reliability and long life due to the absence of brush wear. The principle disadvantage is the complex electronics necessary for commutation using rotor position feedback to control currents in the coils. Another disadvantage is lower torque for equal motor volume. Also brushless motors exhibit reluctance cogging [9].

The next problem to be discussed is that of how to arrange so many actuators on the legs? The objective is to find whether an actuation system capable of delivering sufficient power  in order to produce human like motion to a biped robot with human-like geometric and dynamic properties can be configured. While considering this question it should be kept in mind that the actuators may need to carry their own weights, and that the inertial properties of the biped will be closely related to the placement of the actuators.

After selecting the types of joints and the type of actuators we face the problem of the actual physical placement of the actuators. This is guided by our objective that the inertial properties of the robot should resemble, as much as possible, those of human leg. The first principle is perhaps to position an actuator to be as close as possible to the joint (joints for multi-joint tendons) which it is driving. This objective may not always be realisable since the total weight of the actuators responsible for a joint may exceed the anthropomorphic weight of the adjacent limb. In this case we may need to collect the actuators in the pelvis level so that the weight is counted as part of the trunk. This strategy is, in fact, present in the biological system since the important foot actuators are all on the shank, and many of the major hip actuators are in the trunk. This preserves the passive mechanical properties (such as the period of oscillation) of the legs taken separately. In case the total structural weight of a limb and the associated actuators becomes less than the anthropomorphic weight of the limb, extra weight can be added to the limb to compensate for the difference.

It is not easy to quantify the departure of the robot dynamic model from the human model as caused by the heavier actuators. In order for us to gain some insight into human locomotion from experiments performed on an electro-mechanical simulacrum we should be  able to quantify or estimate the expected departure of the dynamic behaviour of the machine from that of a perfect human-like model. We intend to „pack” all the motors together   at   the   torso,   this   being   the   position   with   the   best   choice   of   displacement/velocity/acceleration.

*Displacement*: The heaviest portion of the robot should be, in general, located as centrally as possible. Displacements away from the joint would cause large moments about them. The maximum inertial moment should happen around the front leg ankle at the beginning of the single support phase, since in this configuration the torso is farthest from the ankle. However, the ankles don't need to support the moment. The robot moves on to the next phase due to its inertia (this resolves the apparent contradiction that the base motor of an arm manipulator is the largest of all joints but the „base” motor of a walking robot and a human being is not).

*Velocity*: A significant part of the mechanical energy expenditure of the robot is due to its kinetic energy. The forward velocity is not a concern in itself in the placement of the motors. The change in its magnitude, i.e., the forward acceleration is.

*Acceleration:* The forward and vertical acceleration of the centre of mass are closely related to the amount of power spent by the machine. It turns out that in a single gait cycle the body accelerates and decelerates and this effect diminishes as we go higher up on the body with the eyes having the lowest displacements and velocity fluctuations (this has been transformed to an optimality criterion for the human locomotion).

The mechanical structure of the hip joint could be a ball rod end (similar to a spherical joint or a spherical bearing). The „collar" under the hip joint in Figure 22 is simply a means to provide the correct anthropomorphic moment arms to the muscles activating the joints. The knee joint should be a revolute, or better a linkage to simulate the migration of the joint axis and the ankle joint might be a revolute, or perhaps a flexure. Options for the structural material include aluminium, steel, and composites: either glass epoxy or graphite epoxy. Configuration options that might be explored include a rigid torso, a compliant foot, a metatarsal joint, a movable head, and a mechanically sound one, there is a strong argument for a more distributed motor placement. Let's review the relative pros and cons.

Each leg mass is about 15% of the total body mass. The HAT (head, arms, trunk) of a person is about 70% of the total body mass. Each leg of a 80 kg person will have mass about 12 kg with the thigh mass being 8 kg, the shank mass 4 kg and the foot mass 0,4 kg. For our robot the total motor mass is about 50 kg (about 22 kg per leg plus two 3 kg motors for pelvic tilt). Therefore if we put all the motors in the trunk 50 kg = 70% of body mass. Each leg should therefore have mass about (50 / 0.7) x 0.15 = 11 kg (approximately). Given our selection of material (square cross-section aluminium tubing with 7 mm side and 2 mm thickness) each leg has mass about 2 kg (0.78 kg for each of the thigh and shank, and 0.47 kg for the foot).

Now in order to make the inertia properties of the robot resemble that of a human being, we would need to put extra mass into the thigh, shank, and foot. Therefore, why not remove some of the motors from the trunk and place them in the limbs? The robot will be carrying more useful mass in that case.

However, it should be noted that there are wiring and cable routing problems to be encountered in such a modified system. The thigh contains the knee extensor, and knee flexor/extensor actuators (3.3 + 1.8 = 5.1 kg). The shank contains the knee flexor and ankle extensor actuators (0.3 + 2.2 = 2.5 kg). The robot should be equipped also with necessary sensors such as position sensors (potentiometers, resolvers, incremental encoders, absolute encoders), velocity sensors (tachometers), force sensors (load cells, strain gauges, capacitive sensors) as well as attitude sensors (inclinometers, directional gyros), angular rate sensors (rate gyros), acceleration sensors (accelerometers) and exteroceptive sensors to model the environment in which it is operating.

### 1.6.3 A Method Of Reference Trajectory Generation

Movement of an anthropomorphic biped should be similar to that of a human. The structure of its control system should include trajectories will result in a humanoid gait. We propose to use an Artificial Neural Network to generate reference trajectories. We recognise that the functioning of the neural network should imitate the Central Pattern Generator located in the spinal cord  (T. Zielińska [9]).

In the work presented here a recurrent back propagation neural network was chosen for gait pattern generation. The learning algorithms for such a network use least square error optimisation methods. Errors detected in the outputs of the network are used to adjust the neural network parameters, specifically the weights and activation functions.

The Central Pattern Generator of a living organism is developed while to organism is growing. The performance of the generator depends on the dimensions and mass parameters of the organism. It is assumed that information about the difference between the generated signal and the realised movement is utilised for learning in the networks generating these patterns in nature. The memory in these neural networks is believed to be built via network feedback.

A three layer recurrent back propagation neural network was used in our work. The input layer contains 5 neurones, one for each knee and hip angle, and the fifth one for the time information. Note that only motion in the saggital plane has been modelled at the present time.  The hidden layer contains 5 neurones, and the output layer contains 4 neurones, one for each knee and hip joint angle at the next time step. The input neurones are straight feed-forward neurones.

The neurones of the hidden and output layers have sigimoidal activation functions. The input training data that was used was the image of a real gait. The outputs from the output layer were connected back to the input layer as is shown in Figure 23.

The inputs to the back propagation network were discrete value of 2 knee angles, 2 hip joint angles (left and right) at time j and the time value j (Figure 23). Whereas the outputs are the subsequent knee and hip angles at the next time step in the gait. These values are feedback to the input.

The network was considered to be trained when the average error declined to less than 0.0001 and the maximum error did not exceed 0.04. (All the input-output values were normalised to values between 0 and 1).

Once trained, the neural network generated a gait pattern by receiving the initial 5 input values from the biped's environment. The network based on its stored (during training) patterns generated angle values for the next time step. These values, together with the discreet value of the next time step, were treated as the imputes for the following time step. In Figure 24 the training pattern (human), and gait image generated by the system is displayed.

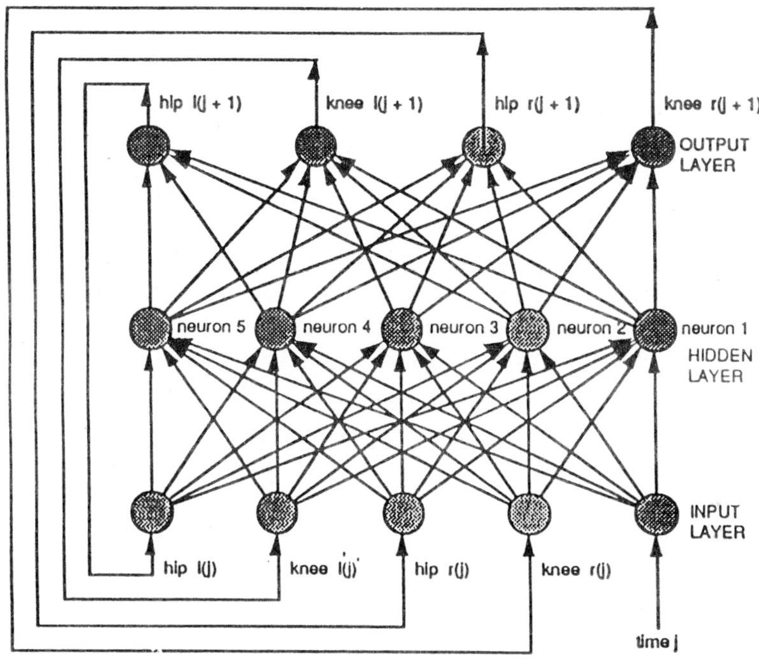


Fig. 23. The structure used for the neural network. The notation „knee r/l)j)" denotes the knee joint angle of the right/left leg at time interval j. Similarly „hip r/l(j)" denotes hip joint angle of the right/left leg at time step j.

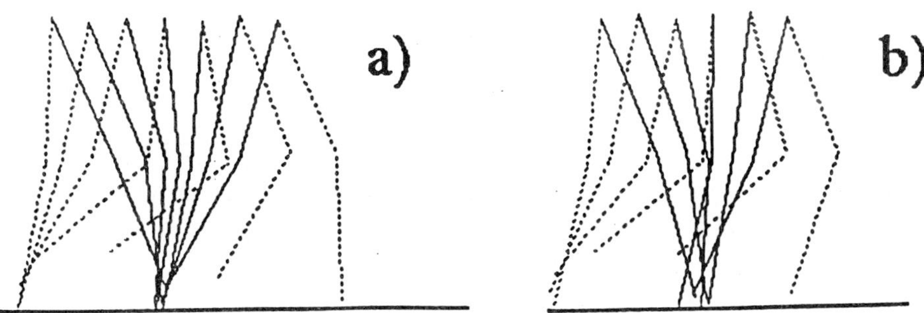


Fig. 24. Gait images:   a) natural (human) gait,  b) gait generated by the network.

# 2. MULTI - LEGGED WALKING ROBOTS

## 2.1 Old walking machines

The history of the use of land transportation by human being is rather old [14].

In the earliest days, man depended on his own legs  for transportation. Some time later, animals were trained by men to curry  people or cargo. The invention of the wheel, which is rightly regarded of the greatest invention in the history of human transportation, greatly improved the efficiency of transportation. Vehicles built on wheels and pulled by man or animal become the most effective means of transportation on land. Next animal or human powered vehicles were, in time replaced by engine powered vehicles.

At the present time, nearly all terrestrial vehicles are based on wheeled locomotion.

But on the other hand the animal can adjust the length and height of its steps to met irregularities of the ground and to break shock of  impact with the ground. The limb is equivalent to a wheel whose diameter can be varied and  where the vehicle is fitted with very powerful shock absorber.

The feasibility of applying the principle of jointed limbs for the propulsion of land vehicles over rough country has been discussed by Shigley (1961), who concluded that each wheel of a self-propelled vehicle can be replaced by four „feet" placed on the ground in sequence with one-quarter of a cycle difference in phase between each „foot"; to replace four wheels, four groups each with four feet would be required , and the timing of a hind group would have to be co-ordinated with that of a front group (Fig. 25). The energy required for vertebrate locomotion is received from striated muscle fibres. The output of mechanical  power depends of the rate (v) of which a fibre shortens against a given load (P). The conditions under which a muscle yields a maximum of mechanical  power have been early defined by Hill (1950). Those problem were developed next by Wilkie (1960).

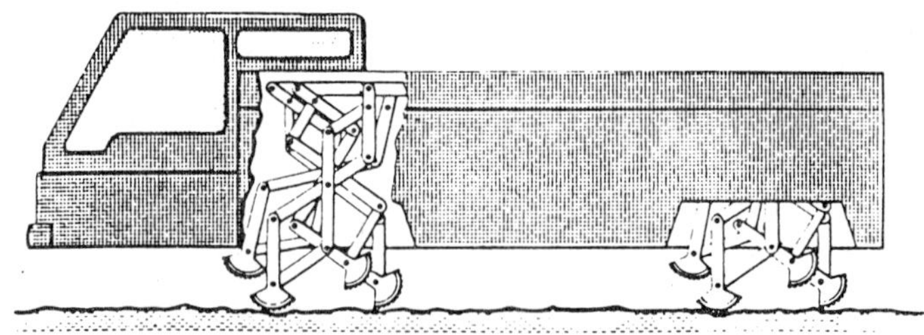

Fig.25 Drawing of a pantograph-legged vehicle using hydraulic power

Comfort in transportation, or isolation from terrain irregularities, in irregular terrain also favours legged locomotion. According to the experience and observation, above a certain level of terrain roughness it is more comfortable to ride on horseback, than to sit in a vibrating wheeled or tracked vehicle while both are travelling at the same speed. This is also important in autonomous vehicles which must function as instrument platforms.

Wheeled or tracked vehicles substantially damage natural terrain by creating continuous ruts. Walking machines leave only discrete footprints [14].

Hence, at least five potential advantages of legged vehicles over wheeled or tracked vehicles in rough terrain can be concluded from the above discussion. These advantages are:

1. Higher speed,

2. Better fuel economy,

3. Greater mobility,

4. Better isolation from terrain irregularities,

5. Less environmental damage.

In addition to these potential advantages as incentives to develop a legged locomotion machine, as mentioned above roughly fifty percent of the land surface Earth is not accessible to conventional wheeled or tracked vehicles (Anon 1967). A walking machine which can travel where terrain difficulties make wheeled or tracked vehicles ineffective will be very useful in terrestrial applications in commerce, science, agriculture, military ... etc., and as a planetary rover [14].

Even before the potential advantages cited above were understood, inventors attempted to design walking machines. Two examples of many such attempts are discussed here.

P.L.Tschebysev (1821-1894) design so called walking mechanism and built its model [15]

Kinematic diagram of this mechanism is shown on Fig.26. The Platform $CC'C_1'C_1$ by moving ahead supports one after another on the pair of the legs land 4 and next 2 and 3.

$$A_1B_1 = B_1C = B_1M_1 = A_2B_2 = B_2C = B_2M_2 = A_3B_3 = B_3C_1 = B_3M_3 =$$

$$= A_4B_4 = B_4C_1 = B_4M_4 = 1,$$

$$A_1C' = A_2C' = AC_1' = A_3C_1' = A_4C_1' = A_4C_1' = 0{,}355$$

$$CC' = C_1C_1' = 0{,}785$$

$$A_2A_4 = A_1A_3 = C'C_1' = 0{,}634$$

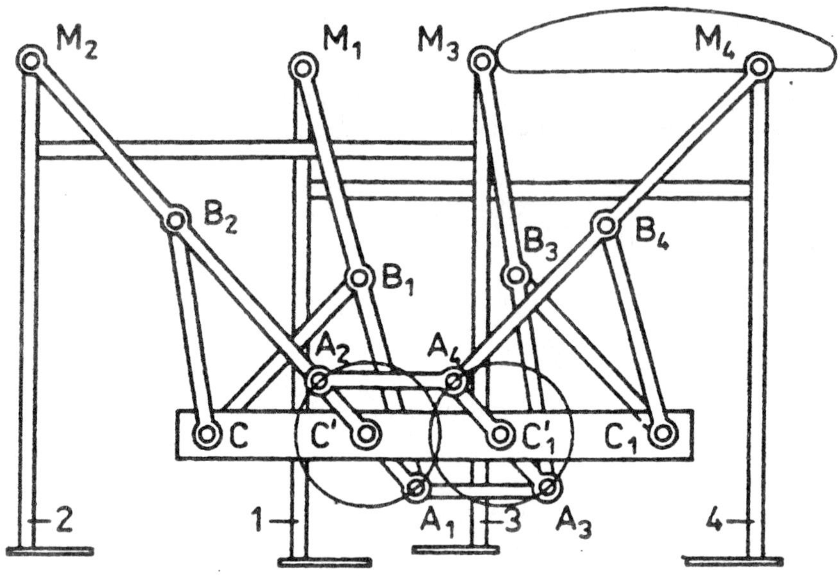


Fig. 26. Structural scheme of „feet - walking" Tschebyshev Machine.

By these dimension of links four rectifies were connected on such a way that its crank form on parallelogram $A_1$ $A_2$ $A_3$ $A_4$ (link $A_1 C'$ is rigidly connected with the link $A_2 C'_1$). On Fig.26 the trajectories of the points and $M_3$ and $M_4$ in the relative motion according to the platform $CC'C'_1C_1$ are shown. The trajectory is similar to these which is made by the end of the lover limb of a walking man.

If the points $M_2$ and $M_4$ are on the linear part of the relative trajectories the mechanism stand on the legs 1 and 4 and legs 2 and 3 are in the air and more to the forwards. If the points $M_1$ and $M_4$ finishes its straight motion and feets 2 and 3 come to the contact with the ground. The mechanism by following motion stand on the feets 2 and 3 and the legs 1 and 4 more upstairs and starts to more ahead according to the hot form motion.

In 1893, Rygg obtained a patent for the design of a mechanical horse (see Figure 27) There is no evidence to prove that he actually built this machine [14].

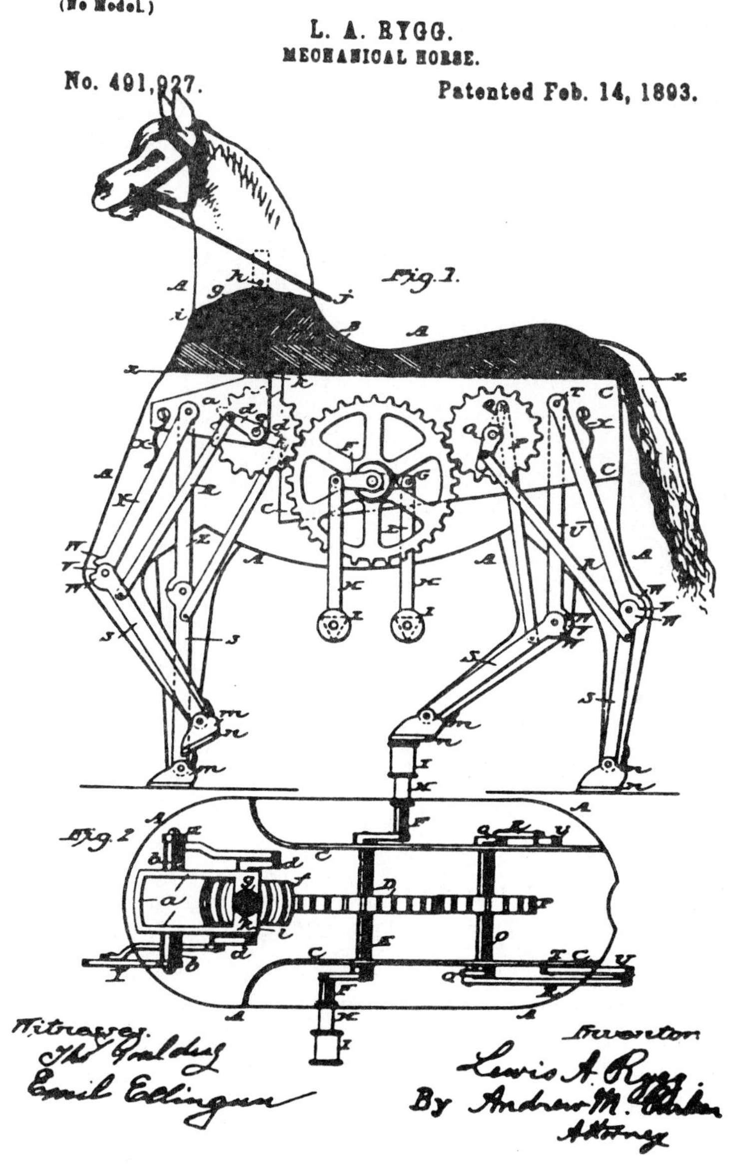


Fig. 27. Patent drawing of a mechanical horse in 1893 [14].

## 2.2 Old Chinese machine

Till 1986 I was thinking that the oldest fourlegged machines arrived in 19th century. In the year 231 a famous Chinese commander Zhu Ge-Liang used the quadruped walking machines for food transportation after the army. The machine was like artificial cow and was able to carry 200 - 250 kg with the speed 10 km a day. A few years ago a young Chinese engineer Wan Ljan has built a model of such a machine in the scale 1:4. This machine was presented during my lectures at the technical University of Tianjin in 1986. The general view of this machine and short description (in Chinese and English is  given below (Fig. 28). The structural diagram which we prepared together is shown on Fig. 29 (one side of the machine).

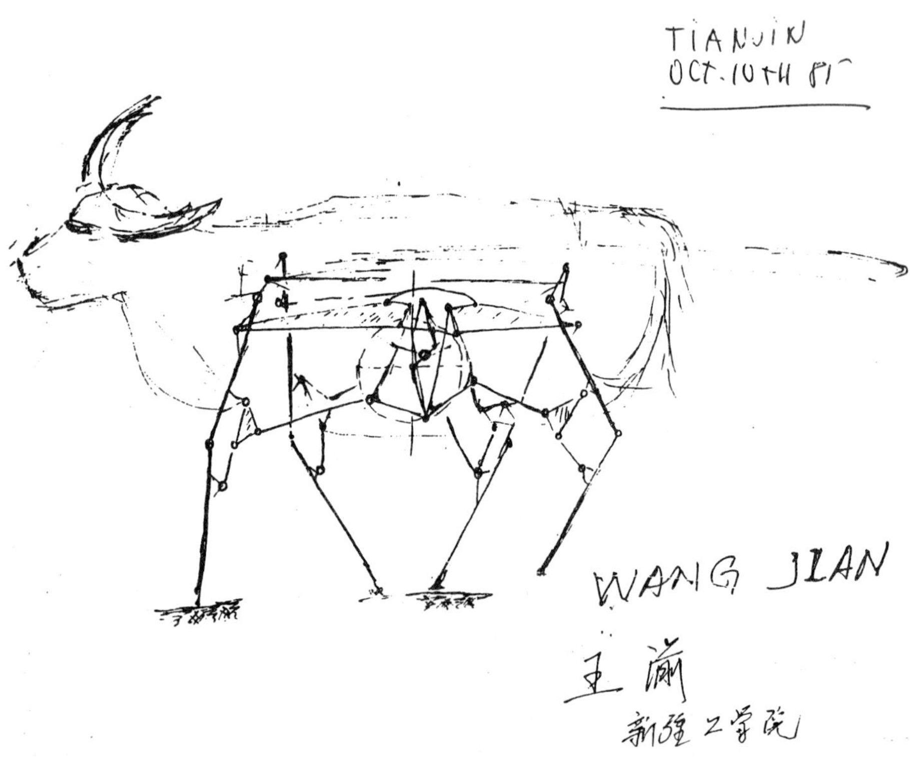


Fig.28. General view of old Chinese machine

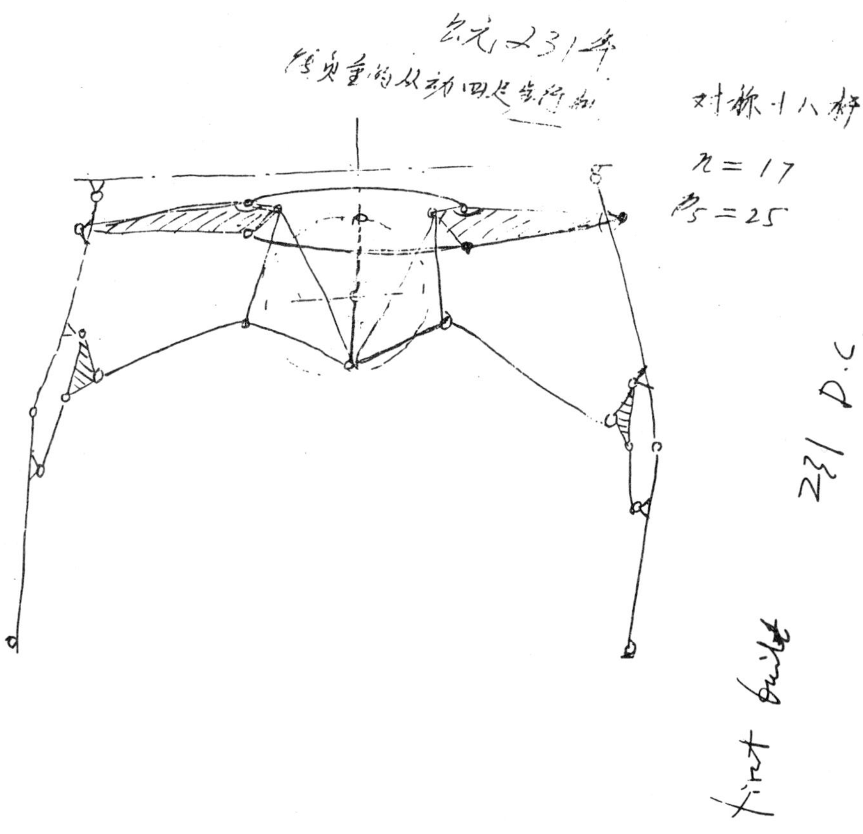

Fig.29. Structural diagram of the machine.

If we treat this mechanisms as a plane one we can calculate the mobility from the formula

$$w = 3n - 2p_5 = 3 \times 17 \times 2 \times 25 = 1. \tag{13}$$

The same result we obtain for whole machine. Fig. 30 shows the classification of the mechanisms. A special method to calculate the displacements, velocities and accelerations was elaborated by Dr. Młynarski [17]. After classification we obtained four groups of second class and one group of fourth class (Fig. 30). The proposed method allow to modified this last group and transform it to the group of second class.

中国古代成功地大批使用过步行机

据中国古籍《三国志·诸葛亮传》载：建兴九年（公元231年）亮复出祁山，以木牛运（粮）。《诸葛亮集》中有"作木牛流马法"，其外形用了牛的典型特征——牛头牛角，前后四足，可以象马一样轻快地迈步行走，所以称为流马，而流马的关键是内部结构的尺寸之数。木牛有两条辕杆，由人推着，人行六尺，马行四步，装载200~250斤行军粮，每天走二十里，一说千里，较闲者不会太劳累。由于它迈步行走很逼真，使人觉得木牛复活了，会自动行走。古籍记载了许多杆件和孔位，是典型的低副多杆机构。但记载有些失缺，不久失传了，约二百年后，大数学家祖冲之又重新发明出来，再次失传，一千余来，人们一直津津乐道。1985年4月，新疆工学院机械系王湔（工程师）完成了木牛流马内部传动机构的设计，复制成运动实物模型，为历史研究提供了重要佐证。

In the Old China, walking machines were used successively. According to history, in 231 A.D., the then famous army leader Zhu Ge-liang made use of wooden Cows to transport grains. The configuration is similar to that of cow. It had four legs and could run and walk as real horses. hence the name "flying horse". The key problem of this wooden horse (cow) is the dimensions of the internal mechanism. It had two bars pushed by man. It could carry 200 – 250 kg of food supply moving 10 km a day. Because of its real marching activity, man feels it became alive and can walk automatically.

It was a typical mechanism with more than 2 constraint. But unfortunately, the details of its structure were lost. It's only 600 years later that our greatest mathematician Zu Chong-zi invented it again, nevertheless it was lost again, and the Chinese are always talking about this cow with pleasure. at last in April 18 an engineer Mr. Wang completed the design of its internal structure and its whole body providing important evidence for scientific research. End—

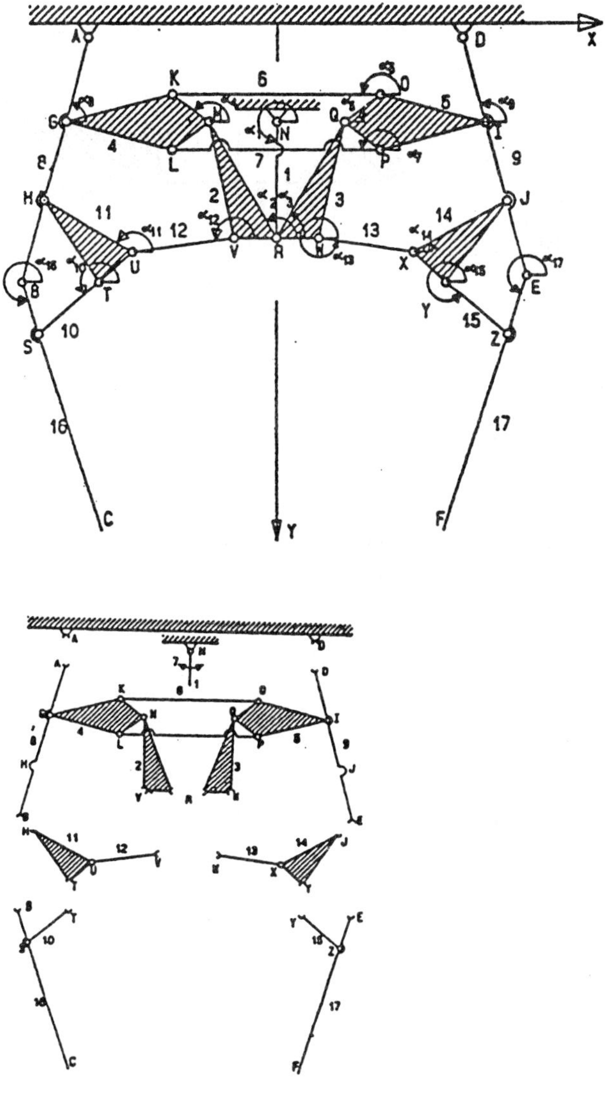

Fig.30. Classification of the mechanisms

Let assume two decision variables $\alpha_2$ and $\alpha_3$ and lengths of the links and position of the link 1 - $\alpha_1$ (Fig.31).

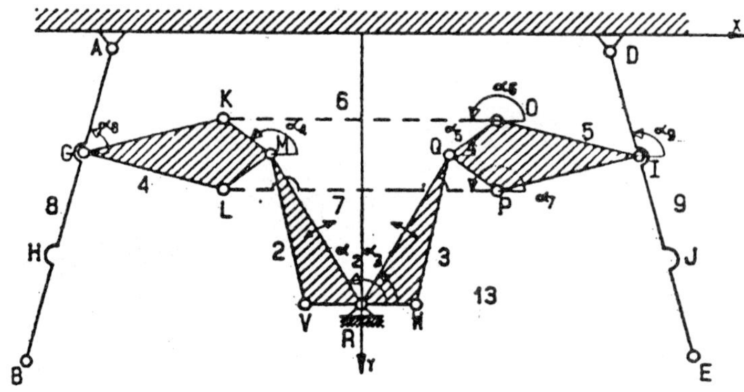

Fig.31. The mechanisms after modification

At the beginning we determine the co-ordinates of the point R

$$X_R = X_N + l_1 \cos\alpha_1 \quad \text{and} \quad y_R = y_N + l_1\sin\alpha_1 \tag{14}$$

Taking into account variable $\alpha_2$ we obtain.

$$X_M = X_R + l_{RM}\cos\alpha_2 \quad \text{and} \quad y_M = y_R + l_{RM}\sin\alpha_2 \tag{15}$$

Solving the set of equations for vector contour MGA we obtain.

$$X_M + l_{MG}\cos(\alpha_4 + x^1_{4M}) + l_{GA}\cos\alpha_3 - x_A = 0, \tag{16}$$

$$Y_M + l_{MG}\sin(\alpha_4 + x^1_{4M}) + l_{GA}\sin\alpha_3 - y_A = 0,$$

and $\alpha_4$ and $\alpha_3$ as a function of $\alpha_2$. Next we determine the co-ordinates of the points K and L

$$X_K = x_K + l\cos\alpha_4, \qquad x_L = x_M + l_{ML}\cos(\alpha_4 + x_{4M}), \tag{17}$$

$$Y_K = y_M \, l_{MK}\sin\alpha_4 , \qquad y_L = y_M + l_{ML}\sin(\alpha_4 + x_{4M}).$$

Assuming $\alpha_3$ as a second decission variable we hare

$$x_Q = x_R + l_{RQ}\cos\alpha_3, \tag{18}$$

$$y_Q = y_R + l_{RQ}\sin\alpha_3.$$

After solving the set of equations of contour QID:

$$x_Q + l_{Qr}\cos(\alpha_5 + x_{5Q}) + l_D\cos\alpha_9 - x_D = 0,$$

$$y_Q + l_{Qr}\cos(\alpha_5 + x_{5Q}) + l_D\sin\alpha_9 - y_D = 0, \tag{19}$$

we obtain $\alpha_5$ and $\alpha_9$ as a function of $\alpha_3$ and next we calculate the co-ordinates of the points 0 and P:

$$x_0 = x_Q + l_{QO}\cos\alpha_5, \quad x_p = x_Q + l_{Qp}\cos(\alpha_5 - x_{5Q}),$$

$$\tag{20}$$

$$y_0 = y_Q + l_{QO}\sin\alpha_5, \quad y_p = y_Q + l_{Qp}\sin(\alpha_5 - x_{5Q}).$$

On the basis of the determined co-ordinates of the points K, L, 0 and P we calculate the differences of lengths between joints K and 0 and link 6:

$$\Delta\ell_6 = \sqrt{(\chi_k - \chi_0)^2 + (y_k - y_0)^2}\,\ell_6, \tag{21}$$

distance between L and P, and lengths of the link 7,

$$\Delta\ell_7 = \sqrt{(\chi_L - \chi_p)^2 + (y_L - y_p)^2}\,\ell_7. \tag{22}$$

The goal function in the process of finding the real position of the links 2 ans 3 will be

$$f_c = \left|\Delta\ell_6\right| + \left|\Delta\ell_7\right| \to 0. \tag{23}$$

After solving (23) we get the real values of the angles $\alpha_2$ and $\alpha_3$ and next $\alpha_4$, $\alpha_5$, $\alpha_8$, and $\alpha_9$. The some procedure can be applied for the other groups, which allow us to determine the angles $\alpha_{10} \div \alpha_{17}$. Finally we get the co-ordinates for point F (link 17) in a form

$$x_F = x_E + \ell_{EF}\cos\alpha_{17}, \tag{24}$$

$$y_F = x_E + \ell_{EF}\sin\alpha_{17}.$$

The velocities and accelerations can be obtained on usual way [17].


## 2.3 Contemporary for legged machines

In the mid 1950's, a number of research groups started to study and develop walking machines in a systematic way. About a decade later, walking machines began to be designed and built by different groups in laboratories. Up to the present time, according to our knowledge, several tens of experimental walking machines have been built. Some important examples are Shigley 1960, McKenney 1961, Baldwin and Miller 1966, McGhene 1966, Cox 1970, Vucobratovic et al. 1972, Mocci et al. 1972, Kato and Tsuiki 1972, Schneider et al. 1974, Okhotsimski et al 1977, McGhee and Iswandhi 1979, Hirose and Umetani 1980, Kessis at al. 1981, Raibert and Sutherland 1983, Russel 1983, Morecki et al. 1985. Although some of these machines were able to walk in laboratories and demonstrate some mobility in controlled conditions, none exhibits any of the advantages mentioned above in a practical sense.

The reasons for this slow progress mainly arise from the complexity of leg co-ordination control, the limited understanding of walking gaits and the lack of the development of practical machine legs. However, based on these previous research affords and modern technologies in robotics and in microcomputers, a major improvement in legged walking machines has been accomplished [14, 20].

A new classical example of the walking machine is a system called the quadruped proposed in 1964 by General Electric Corporation, in the United States (Fig. 32), nicknamed the walking truck or horse, its proper name being Cybernetic Anthropomorphic Machine System (CAMS). Each of its four „legs" is a three-link pedipulator, about 2.3 m in length, performing plane movement.

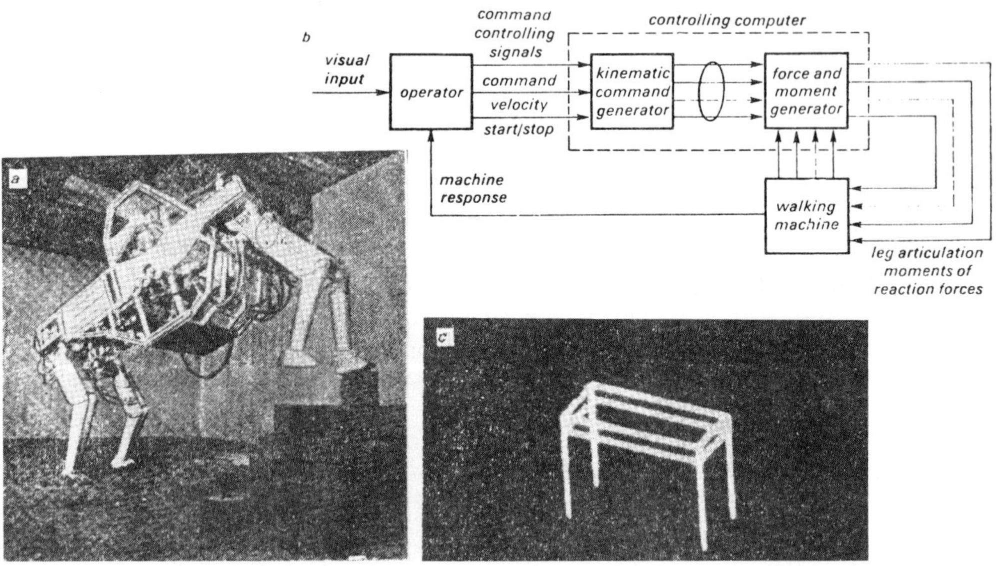


Fig.32. Four-legged walking machine.
a-four-legged walking truck (after [33]); b-block diagram of computer controlled walking machine; c--computer gait simulation of walking machine [34].

The machine weighs 1.5 t, it is 3.5 m long and 3 m high. The operator seated in a special cabin controls simultaneously 12 independent power transmission systems, by movement of his upper extremities he controls the movement of the front extremities of the machine and by movements of his lower extremities he controls the rear extremities of the truck. The operator can adjust both the length and rate of gait of the system with a velocity of about 10 km/h. To control such a system the operator must first train himself in finding an optimum programme for the gait. An additional difficulty is that the operator is seated several meters above the ground, consequently he must make allowance for the scale of movement and for the relief of the area in which he is operating.

An optimum gait programme can be determined on the basis of a study of the gait of the horse or cow. If we denote the left forelimb of the mechanical truck by the symbol 1, the right forelimb, by the symbol 2, the right hind limb, by the symbol 3 and the left hind limb, by the symbol 4, and if, moreover, we assume that only one limb can be up the air at a time (for stability reasons), we obtain six possible types of gait, namely:

$$1\text{-}2\text{-}3\text{-}4, \qquad 1\text{-}3\text{-}2\text{-}4, \qquad 1\text{-}4\text{-}3\text{-}2,$$
$$1\text{-}2\text{-}4\text{-}3, \qquad 1\text{-}3\text{-}4\text{-}2, \qquad 1\text{-}4\text{-}2\text{-}3.$$

A slowly moving horse or cow (for example, when grazing) chooses, as shown by experience, gait type 1-3-2-4, which guarantees maximum stability.

In spite of the problems arising from the very construction of the „truck" the operator, as its designers report, can control the machine and perform various operations[1].

Another walking-machine system, likewise four-legged, was proposed by R.R. McGhee of Ohio State University [34]. It is a walking horse model, in which a computer acts in place of the walking horse model, in which a computer acts in place of the human operator (Fig.32, b, c) [35].

One of the latest design of quadruped robot is shown on Fig.33 [18]

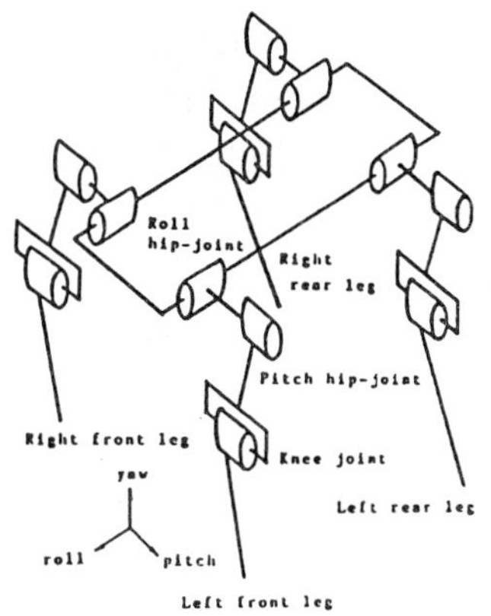


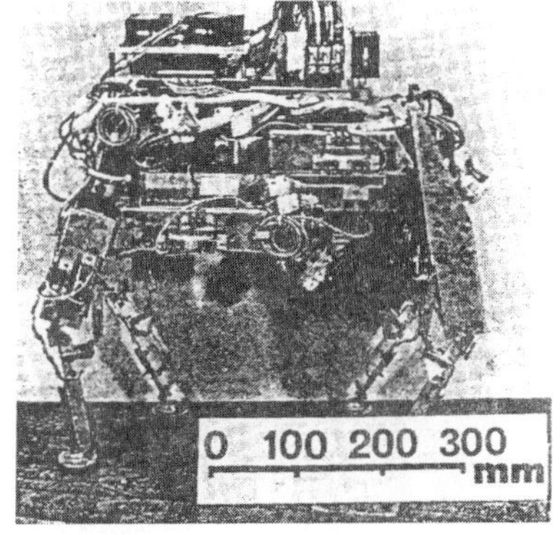


Fig.33  Quadruped robot [18]

a) scheme of quadruped robot controlled by 12 servomotors.

b) A photograph of the quadruped robot.

## 2.4 Design and testing of MK-4 walking machine

Will shortly described the  MK-4 walking machine, which was design and tested by the team for Robotics and Biomechanics of Engineering, Warsaw University of Technology [19, 20]. A method  of gait modelling - creation of the model (template) of motion - for a quadruped walking machine with construction of its legs imitating the limbs of digitigrade mammals (horse, rabbit) will be described (Fig.34).

Only slow motion are considered (statically stable motion). Two kinds of motion are discussed, namely: a gait consisting of a fixed sequence of leg transfers (crawl), and a so called „free gait". The machine moves with a free gait when there is no possibility of continuing the crawl. Such a situation can be encountered when the displacement of the leg which should be moved to fulfil the sequence of motions of the crawl can result in the loss of static stability (e.g. in motion over a variable slope terrain).

The machine is of static walker type which is to say that in every instant the projection of its centre of gravity onto the ground is inside the support polygon. This way of moving is possible under an assumption that the machine moves slowly (the speed of motion does not exceed 5 km/h) and the rate of change of velocity is not rapid. Such a motion is easy to execute, such that most of the currently constructed machines are of the static walker type.

After the structure of the machine's legs has been assumed (Fig.35), the next task was to find the gait (a fixed sequence of leg transfers) that would assure the static stability of the device.

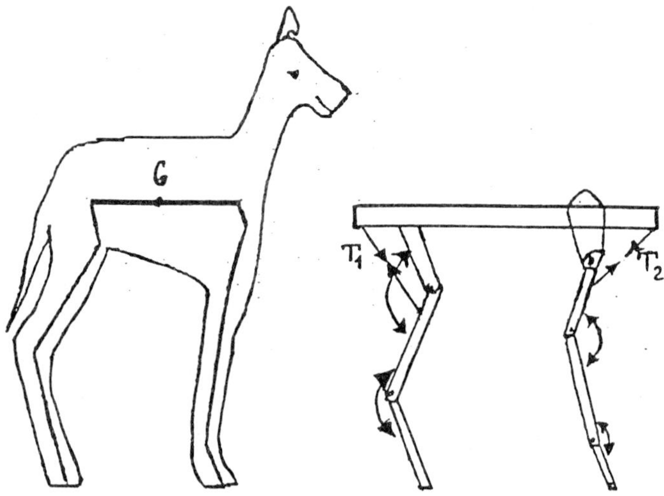


Fig.34. Structure of the animal's legs

G - centre of gravity of the body,  $T_1$, $T_2$ - major muscles driving the leg.

Fig.35 shows the structure and dimensions of the MK-4 machine $\left(\Delta L = \dfrac{L}{12}\right)$. Each leg is on plane mechanisms with two degrees of freedom actuated by hydraulic actuators. The machine is able to move in saggital plane with constant velocity.

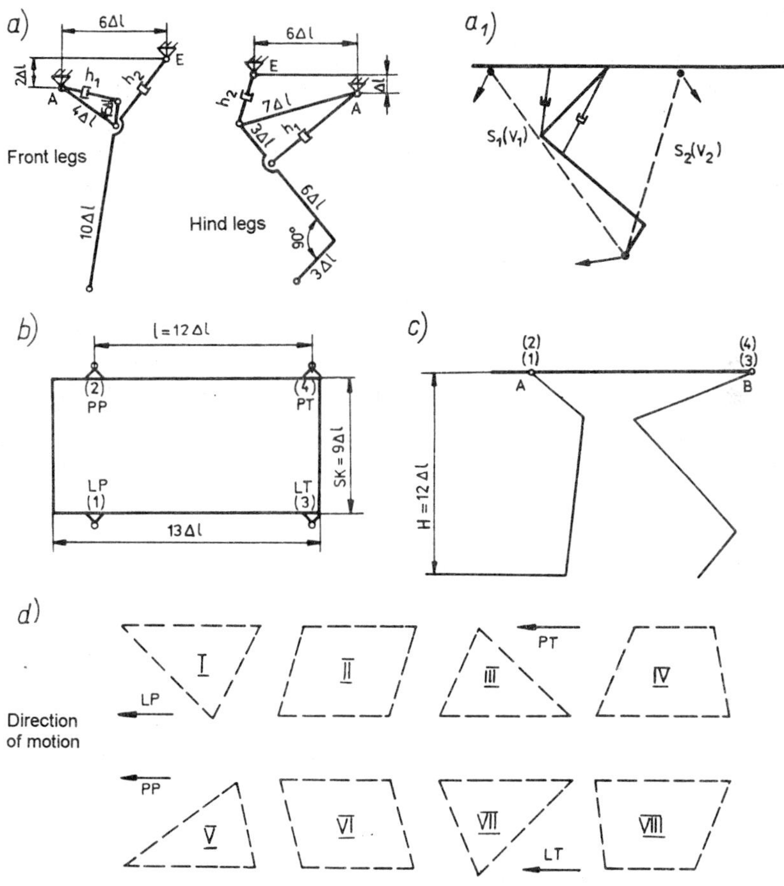

Fig.35. The model of MK-4 walking machine

a) the structure and dimensions of the legs ($\Delta L = H/12$)

$a_1$) the leg equipped with sensors

b) the bottom view

c) the side view:

$S_K$ -wide of the platform

L - length of the platform

H - high of the machine

$\Delta$ - connecting points of the legs: (1), (2), (3), (4) the legs indexes

d) the changes of supporting points

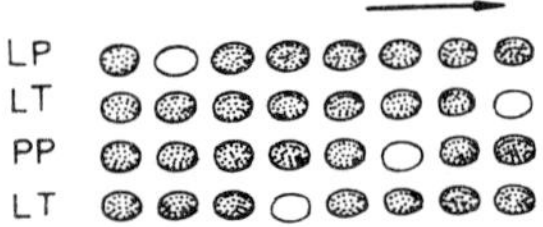

Fig. 36. The sequence of the leg LP, LT, PP, LT

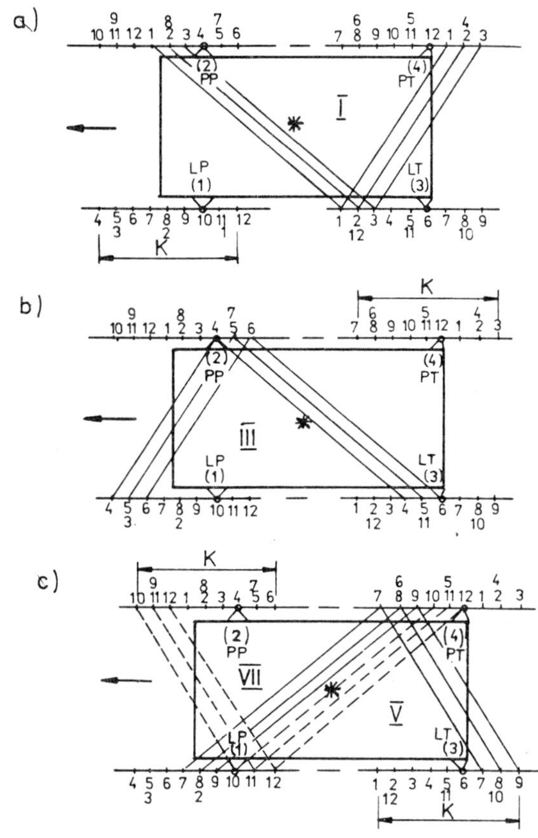

Fig.37. Supporting points during the gait points

a) Three point phase I;

b) three point phase III

c) three point phases V and VII

(1), (2), (3), (4) - leg's indexes,

1,2,3...., 12 the numbers of consecutive positions

k-step length, $\dot{\Delta}$ - connecting points

x- centre of gravity

For the analysis the following assumptions have made:

– the model describes a machine of the static crawler type [21] (or in other words: the described machine moves with statically stable gaits:

– the machine's model is divided into:

- mechanical part: legs, body, actuators, sensors

- control part,

- interface between the mechanical part and the control part,

– the mechanical part realises the gait whereas the control part organises the functioning of the mechanical part, so that the realisation of the gait would be possible,

– the control system sends the control signals in discrete instants of time,

– digital model reference control is used - the control of motion is realised without feedback (in the case considered this means that the gait modelling process does not influence the current state of the machine, but takes into account information about the state of the environment).

As it was mentioned the fixed number of legs and actuators (two reciprocating hydraulic actuators causing the planar motion of each leg) has been taken into account - Fig.36 (machine MK-4 [20]). The legs are designed in such a way that for the assumed ranges of motions of actuators the positions of leg ends can be determined unequivocally (see the range finger system, Fig.38). In the case of a different walking machine the proposed model has to be modified adequately.

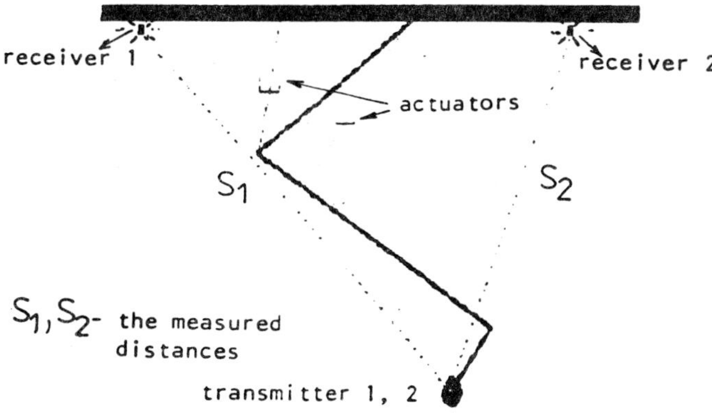


Fig.38. The range finder system

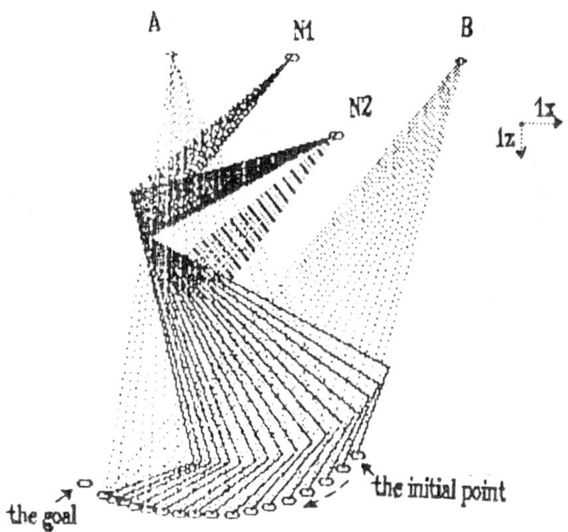


Fig.39. Continuos path motion of the leg.
$1_x$, $1_z$ - units of distance;
A, B - the points at with the ultrasonic transmitters are fixed;
N1, N2 - the points at with the actuators are fixed to the legs;

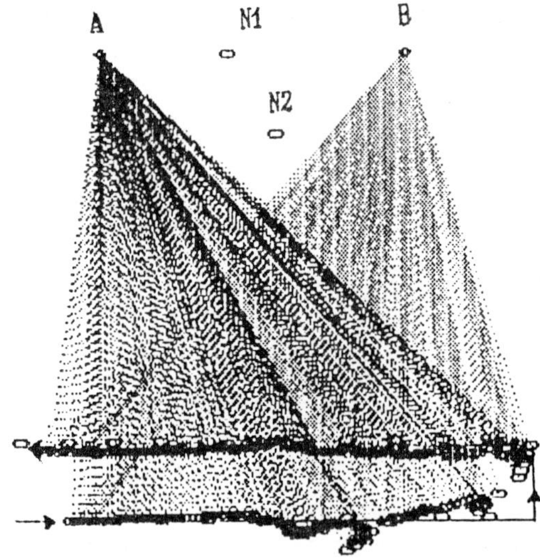


Fig.40. Point to point motion of the leg.
A, B - the points at with the ultrasonic transmitters are fixed
N1, N2 - the points at with the actuators are fixed to the legs

Taking into account these assumptions the machine is treated as an object which puts before itself a goal consisting in the realisation of the process of walking (the reproduction of the created gait model). The description of the mechanical part of the machine can be treated as a symbolic representation of relationship taking place during the motion of the real device. This is the reason why the relationships described are not identified (at the most we could have modelled them). The description of the mechanical part below is only necessary for a better understanding of the gait model and for pointing out the difference between the model (template) of motion and the real motion.

In the paper [21] the description of the proposed machine, the gait model, the form of function F in the gait parameters, the modelling of the free gait and the generation of theoretical values of control signals are given. Some of the computer simulation results will be discussed.

The correctness of the relationships describing the gait model (quadruped crawl) was tested using computer simulation methods. In a similar way the method of modelling the free was tested. We have ascertained that the possible  motion tree  (Fig.38) search is effective with respect to the speed of data processing. No flaws have been found in the method (for all of the tested situations the method found a satisfactory solutions). The simulation programs were coded in FORTRAN and executed on a IBM 360/370 computer.

The program modelling the gait of the machine was coded in Pascal and executed on an IBM PC microcomputer. Using computer simulation the correctness of the proposed method of control on an executive level was tested. Fig.39 shows the „history" of a leg's motion obtained as a results of the simulation of the functioning of the control system. The above mentioned simulations enabled us to ascertain that the control point-to-point process utilising relationship is much more effective (taking into account the processing time) than when using  a given relationship[20]. In the case of the trajectory following process the processing time is shorter when using  but the trajectory is not followed accurately (Fig.40).

## 2.5 New design of four-legged machine

On Fig.41 top view (a) flank view (b) and front view (c) of quadruped, which is now under preparation are shown.

Both the body and the legs can operate in a few possible configurations. The change of a body configuration is possible through two direct drive joints mounted in the body's axles. The four elements of the body (4) are simultaneously containers for the electronic systems of control, drive and for electric batteries.

The joints allow for the change of the position of the machine's centre of gravity and, consequently, for the change of its geometry and dynamic and static properties.

Each leg of the machine is suspended from the direct drive joint with two degrees of freedom which allows it to rotate in relation to horizontal and vertical axes. The drive for leg's rotation is provided through indirect belt transmission with positive drive. The movability of a leg in a knee joint and in an ankle joint is achieved by the so called kinematic pair of the 5th class (one degree of freedom). The drive can be achieved with the use of direct drive step motors or belt transmission. The drives should be placed inside the elements of leg (3) and (7). The foot of leg (8), owing to its size, provides for good interaction with ground and minimises pressure. It can have self-aligning connection and can be driven from a drive placed in an ankle joint.

Walking machine should be made of light welted alloys. The elements of legs will be best manufactured from light sections.

- The machine has two interesting possibilities. The possibility to change the configuration and kind of the movement.

- The possibility to change dynamic properties of the main body of the machine: polar moment of inertial and the position of gravity centre owing to flexibility in joints (5) and (8).

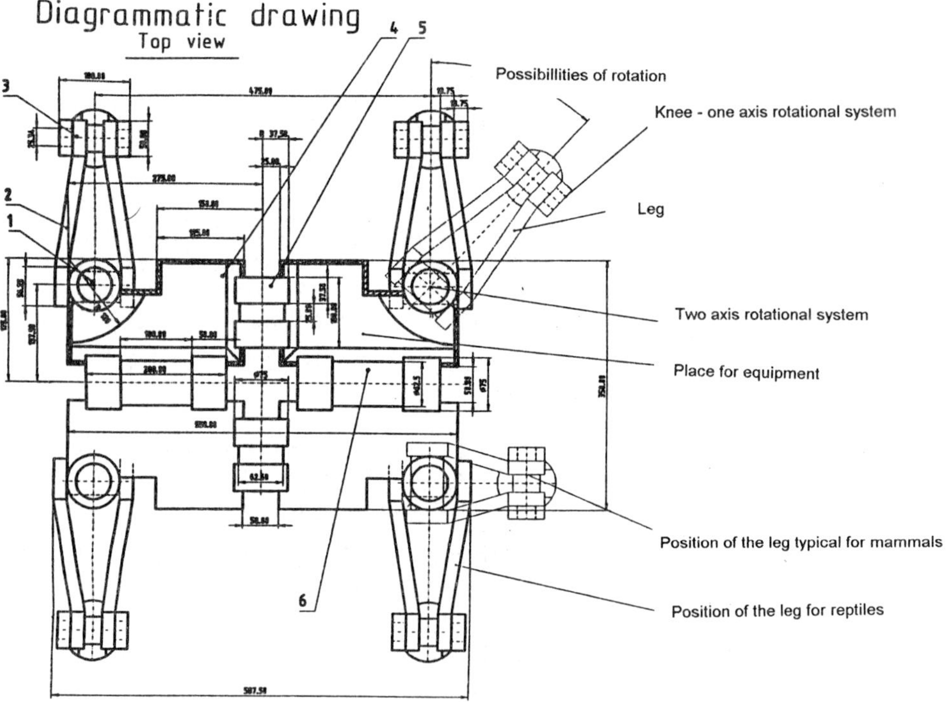


Fig.41. The quadruped walking machine: a) top view.

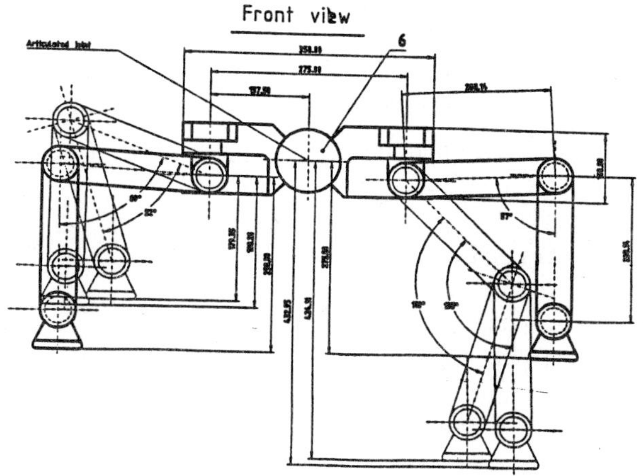


b)

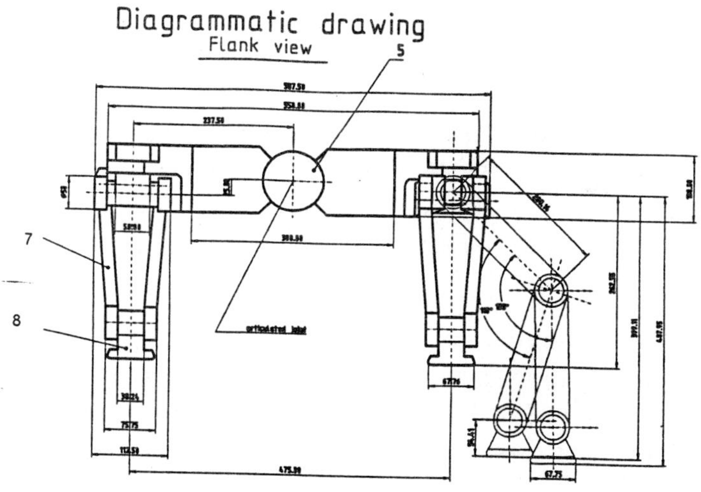


c)

Fig.41. The quadruped walking machine: b) flank view; c) front view.

## 2.6 Six-legged walking machines

In the last years several six-legged machines were design, built and tested.

The designers of six-legged machines usually use the principles of insects locomotion.

Will shortly described these principles [1].

## 2.6.1 Insect locomotion.

Insects move by means of limb, their rigid trunk (chitonous armature) being hardly involved at an. This situation greatly facilitates control of locomotion movements. According to D.N. Wilson and other investigators, the locomotion of insects proceeds by the following principles:

(1) The limbs move in a „wavy" fashion, i.e., the movement starts from a forward push of the posterior limbs, the others following suit successively.

(2) The limbs on the opposite side move in counterphase.

(3) The time of forward push of the limbs is constant.

(4) The rate of movement is being increased by shortening the phase of limb withdrawal to the rear, relative to the trunk (the repulsion phases).

(5) The time intervals between steps of the posterior and central limbs and between the central and anterior limbs are constant but the time intervals between the   step of the anterior and posterior limbs vary in inverse proportion with velocity.

Denoting the right limbs by the symbols $R_1$, $R_2$ and $R_3$ and the left one by the symbols $L_1$, $L_2$ and $L_3$ we can present in keeping with these principles the following diagrams of locomotion (Fig.42 ). The diagram in Fig.42a shows very slow movement. In this case, the right limb are the first to move and once this movement ends, the left ones start moving, and so fort. As the locomotive velocity increases, the limbs on the other side  start moving ever sooner. Thus, a simultaneous transfer of limbs. $R_1$ and $L_3$  and $R_3$ and $L_1$  (Fig.42b) or $R_3$, $R_1$ and $L_2$  and $R_2 L_3$ and $L_1$ (Fig.42c) eventually takes place and so forth.

The principles just presented have been confirmed in many six-legged insects although, some investigators have found departures from the above diagrams. The locomotion of insects with more than six legs, e.g. the tarantulas (eight plus two subsidiary limbs) only partially confirms to the principles worked out for six-legged insects (Fig. 42d).

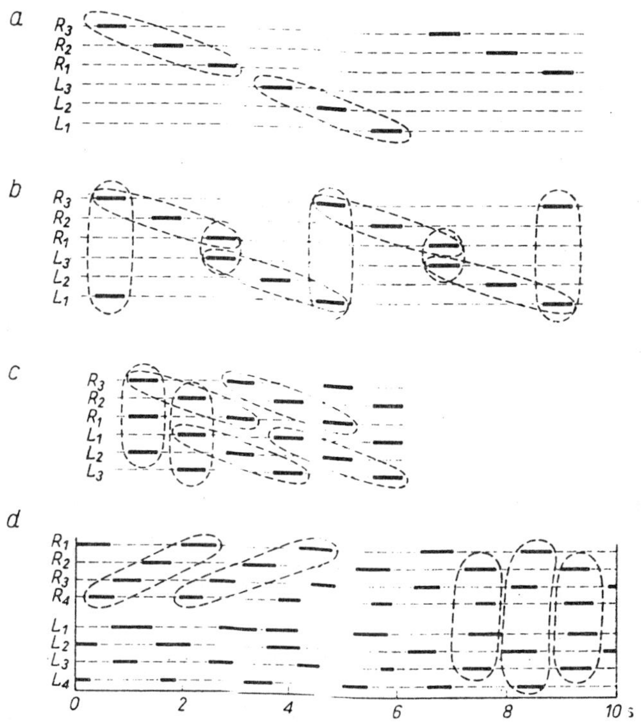



Fig.42. Diagram of locomotion of insects (after [1]).
a, b, c - with six limbs,  d- with eight limbs.
The horizontal axis is the time axis, heavy dash denotes time of the phase of limbs forward
move, one-sided limbs surrounded by dotted slant lines, limbs simultaneously in free phase
surrounded by dashed vertical lines.

## 2.6.2 Description of selected machines

In my opinion only very few machines found a real technical applications. We like to
mention a few of it.

The machine built at the Ohio State University [14] (Fig.43a, b, c) walking machine
built in Robotics Laboratory, Machinery Division Port and Harbour Research Institute
Ministry, of Transport Japan [22] Fig.44 and Dante II a walking a rappelling robot system
[23] Fig.45 and Fig.46.

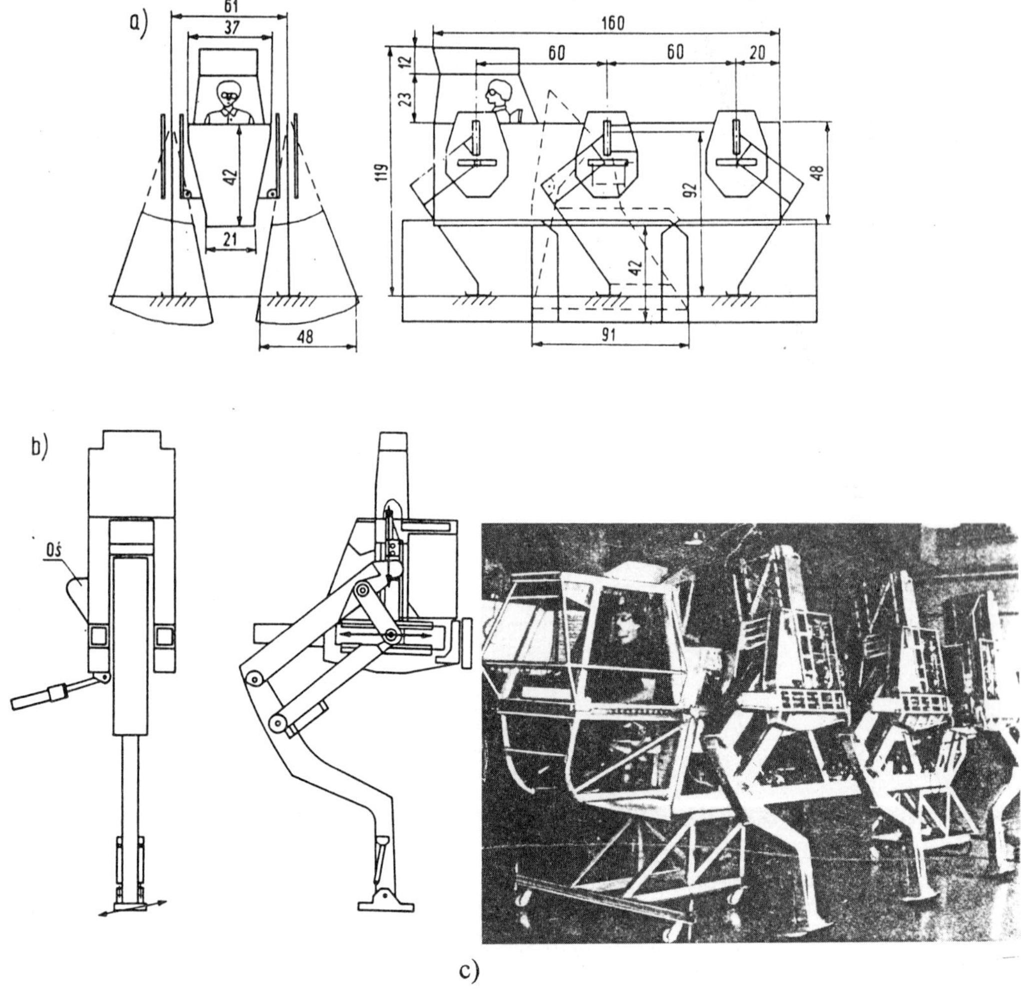

Fig.43. The ASV Machine

a) View of the machine

b) The front and side view of the leg

c) General view of the machine

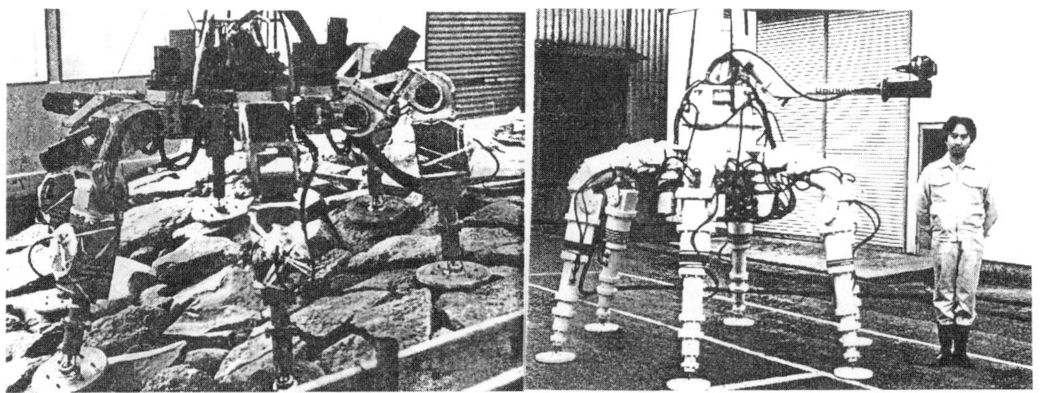

Fig.44. Six-legged walking machine
design of the Robotics Laboratory, Machinery Division.
Port and Harbour Research Institute, Ministry of Transport Japan [22].

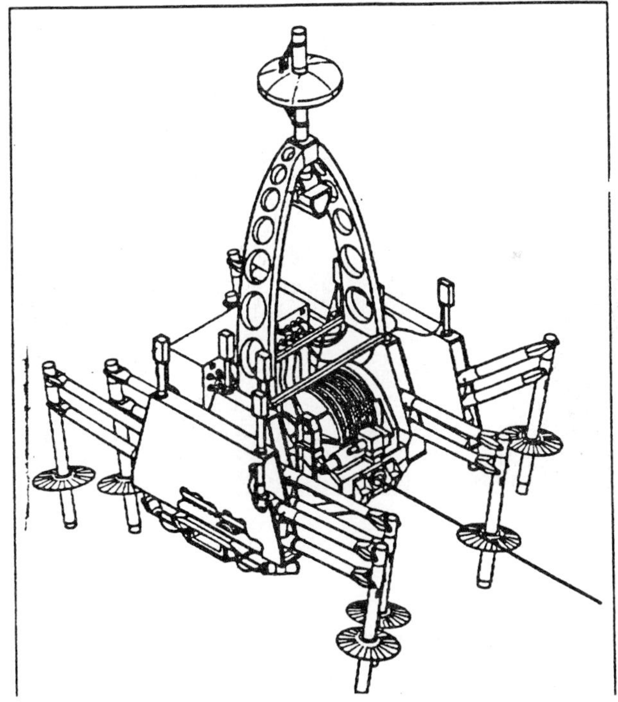

Fig.45. Dante Rappelling Robot.
Dante is about 2,5 m wide, 3,5 m long and 4 m tall. The robot's mass is 770 kg [23].

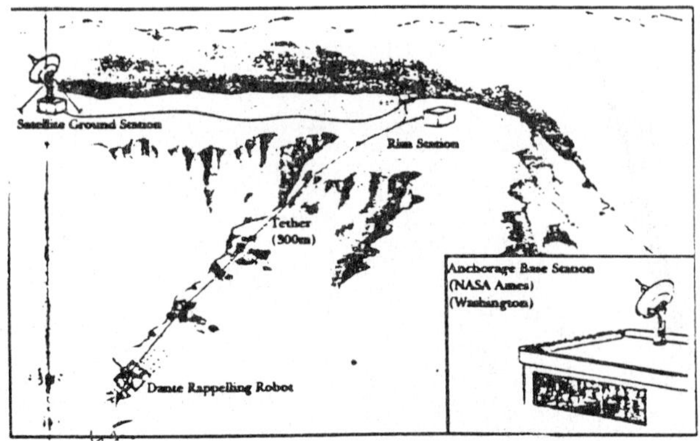

a) Dante mission scenario in Mt.Spurr.
During the mission, Dante rapelled 165 m into the crater.

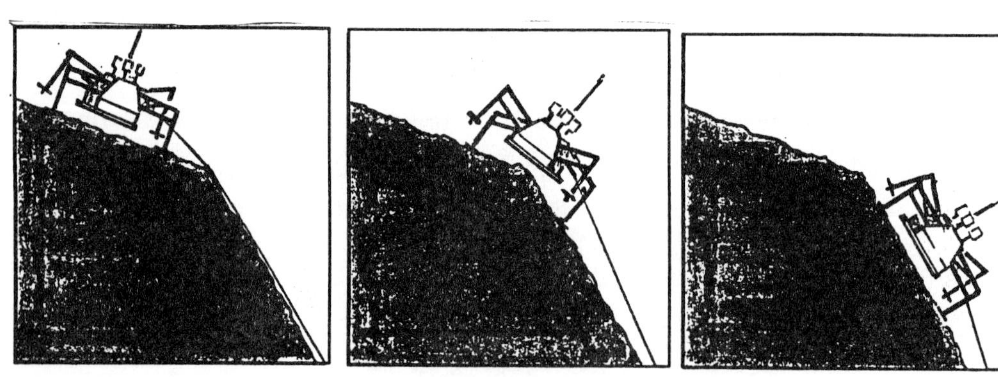

b) The sequence of positions.

Fig. 46. Rappelling sequence: tether tension is increased with slope so that transverse forces acting on the feet are essentially eliminated.

In the last time a new machine for forest activity arrived  (Fig.47) [36]

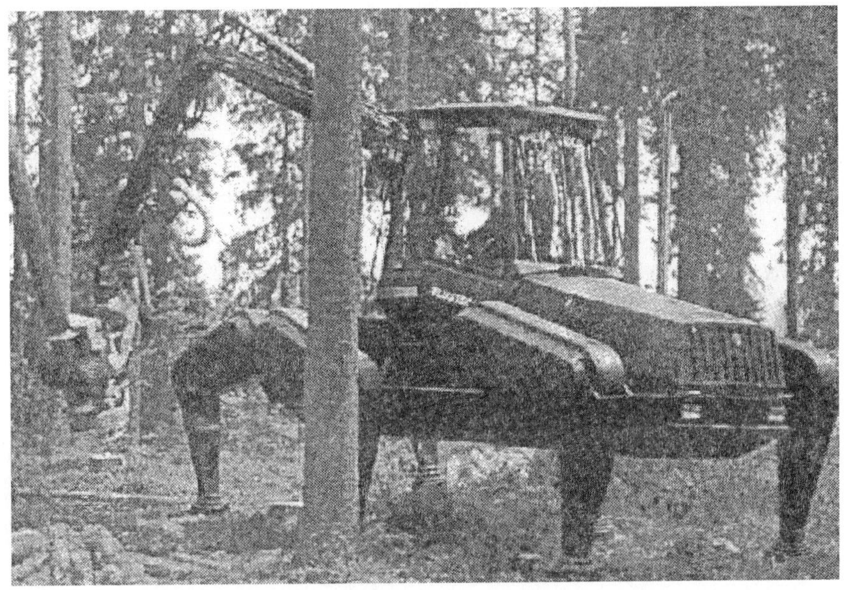

Fig.47. General view of the finish walking robot [36]


## 2.7 Six-legged walking mili-robot - HERMES

Will described the six-legged mili walking machine, which is now under investigations.

### Robot history

The Hermes robot is most recent of a long line of walking robots offered by ISIR[x/]. It was developed as a robot for a museum display to show case of unique insectoid micro-rovers. Building on ISIR's experience prototyping rovers for planetary missions, Hermes was designed to be a small, rugged and powerful robotics exploring tool [24].

### General Description

Hermes is a six-legged walking robot which incorporates high powered processing, rich sensing, and high mobility into a compact body. These features make it ideal for supporting research into high degree-of-freedom systems and co-operative behaviour. The compact body makes it suitable to be used as an extension vehicle deployed from a mother craft or for tasks that require mobility in tight spaces. This, and its ability to carry a video camera, make it a useful tool for remote inspection tasks.

---

[x/] IS Robotics was founded by leading scientists from mobile robotics laboratories at MIT and JPL

Walking with six-two-degree-of-freedom legs, Hermes easily scrambles over rough terrain. Force sensing in each leg, bump sensors, and IR proximity sensors provide information that the robot can use to negotiate around obstacles. A pitch and roll inclinometer allows the robot to adjust to uneven terrain. The robot is supplied with code which utilizes all these sensors during an exploring demonstration. With a serial cable attached, the robot can be directed by supervisory commands from a host computer. A detachable LCD display can be used to monitor the state of the robot during programming. As an option we can mount a colour video system that transmits a robot's eye view of the world.

Fig.48 a, b shows the general view of the Hermes machine

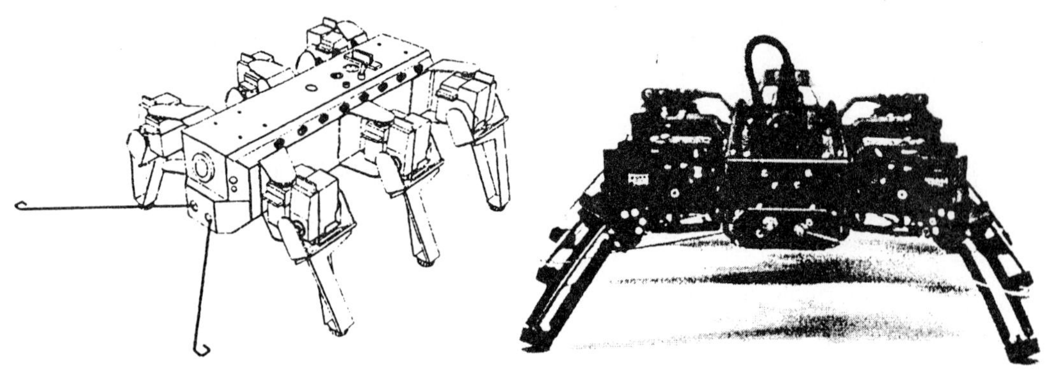

a- schematic diagram,                                   b- a photograph

Fig.48. General view of Hermes machine.

The machine consists of mechanical part, actuators, sensors, input/output devices, supply system.

Will shortly described some parameters of the machine.

The dimensions of the machine are: length: 0,39 m, width - 0,26 m, height - 0,14 m. The weight is 2,5 kg.

Each leg (Fig.49) has two degrees of freedom. The legs are operated  by 12 small high-torque (0,72 N·m) bearing servo-motors. Each leg lift up to 5 cm vertically.

The machine is equipped with 6th easy-to replace leg modules.

The machine is equipped by following sensors: collision detection on each leg, two forward-mounted whiskers for obstacle detections, 3-bit support force detection on each leg, four element inboard IR proximity sensors and pitch and roll inclinometers.

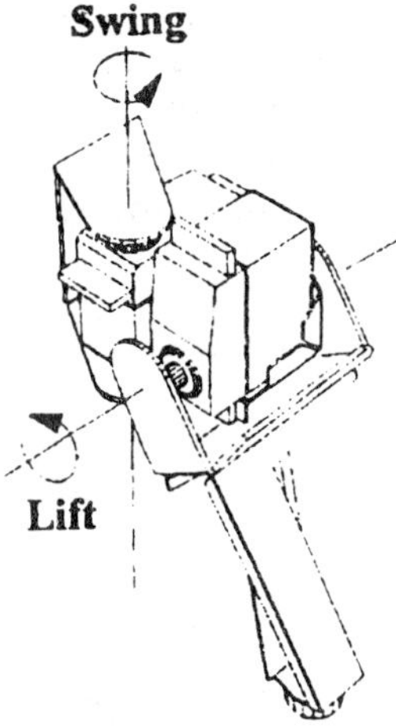


Fig. 49. The leg of the machine.

The control system consists from Motorola 68322 microprocessor 16.78 MHz with 1 MB of battery-backed SRAM and 64KB EPROM with operating system, diagnostic and demo programme.

Programming environment consists of: Behaviour Language/subsumption compiler supplied. LISP- like AI language allows user to add and modify the behaviours, graphical based monitoring interface.

The input/output Devices consists of: colour CCD video 66 camera + video transmission system, 16 large red LEDs (8 per side), detachable monitoring unit with LCD display, programmable tone and duration piezo buzzer, serial line communications with hook-up to a Macintosh computer. (Host computer: Power Macintosh 7500/100, 16 MB RAM, 1000 MB HD, CD 4xdrive, video card on board „14" monitor, keyboard).

Configurations:
        autonomous operation - internal NiCd batteries (rechargeable),
        duration: 15-20 minutes with video system switched on,
        tethered - external 5V
        DC power supply, direct serial communication with host computer  for
        continuos robot use.
The identification of the locomotion possibilities of Hermes machine was the subject of Mr. Szabelak Msc. thesis [25].

The machine gait is similar to insects wave gait. Always four or five legs are in support phase, one stepping pattern, static stability (static crawler). The diagram is shown on Fig.50.

Diagrams:

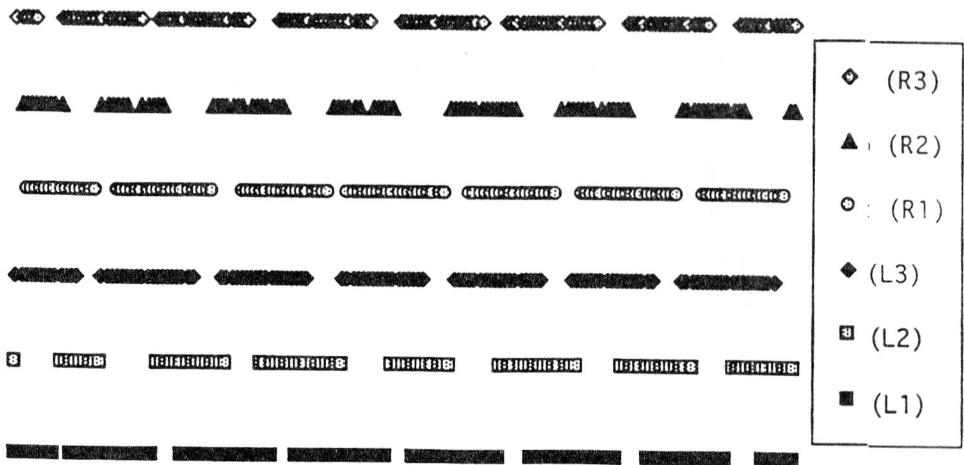


Fig. 50. Gait diagram.

On Fig.51 the sequence of legs motion and path prints are shown. Fig.52 shows the changes of support polygon. The constant velocity of gait is 0,028 m/s.

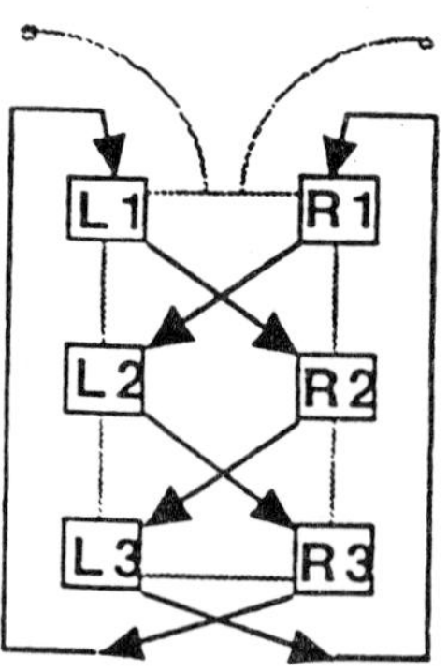


Fig.51. The sequence of legs motion

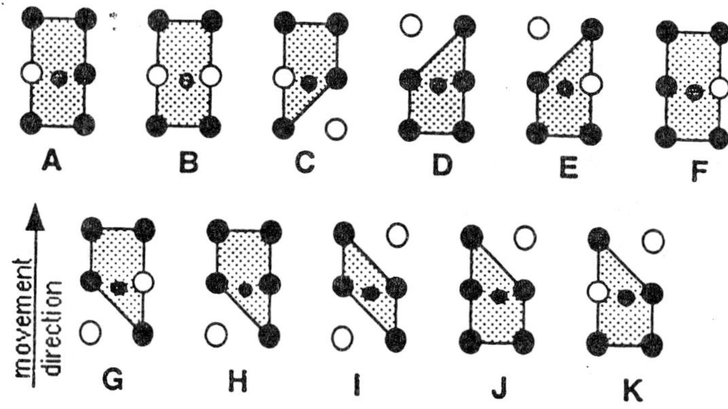


Fig.52. The changes of support polygon

Kinematical analysis of the machine was performed. The kinematical model of the leg is shown on Fig.53. For analysis following parameters were used: $L_1 = 0,021$ m, $L_2 = 0,105$ m, $d = 0,04$ m. The variable internal angles $\alpha$ and $\beta$ of angular position of motor axis, $P(x_p, y_p, z_p)$ - the Cartesian co-ordinates of the leg's end. The workspace is: a part of the torus.

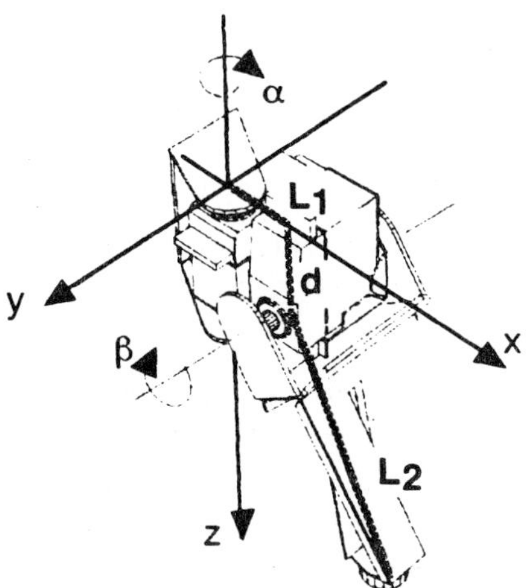


Fig.53. Kinematical model of the leg.

Direct problem of kinematics is described by (25)

$$\begin{cases} x_p = (L_1 + L_2 \cos\beta)\cos\alpha, \\ y_p = (L_1 + l_2 \cos\beta)\sin\alpha, \\ z_p = (d + L_2 \cos\alpha)\sin\beta. \end{cases} \tag{25}$$

Inverse problem is described by (26)

$$\begin{aligned} \alpha &= \operatorname{arctg}\frac{y_p}{x_p}, \\ \beta &= \arcsin\left(\frac{z_p - d}{L_2 \cos\alpha}\right). \end{aligned} \tag{26}$$

IR sensors were tested and some characteristics were obtained.

Three kind of experiments were performed

- determinations of sensivity cone,

- sensivity as a function of the distance and object dimensions,

- influation on perturbations of: colour, fracture, object position [25].

## 2.8 Micromechanisms and Microwalking Robots

### 2.8.1 Basic terms and definitions

Micromechanism is a device handling micro objects and as a device itself being micro sized. By interpreting „micro" as smaller than the size of ordinary machines, we understand everything that involves a smaller size than existing machine [26].

MM consists of a man-operated control (c), drive source (s), actuator for positioning ($A_p$) and actuator for main operation ($A_w$) (Fig. 54).

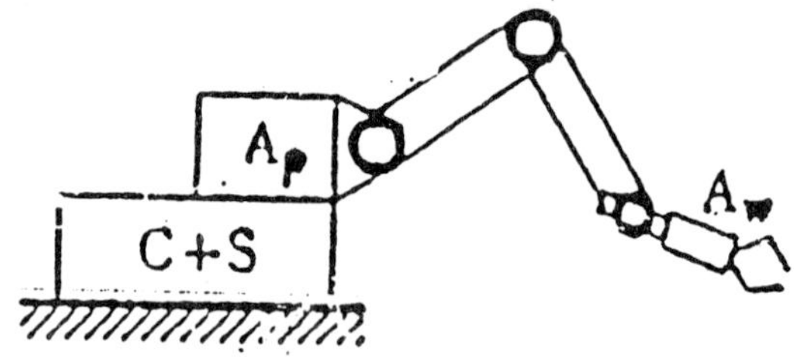


Fig.54. Basic micromechanism [26].

We can distinguish different classes of micromechanism namely: fixed MM, floating MM, self-running MM.

Present state of development of MM is shown in Fig. 55. Three generations of MM can be distinguished, namely.

- First generation including MM having dimensions from several mm to one mm. Here belong such devices like wrist watch, which contain the motor and gears of outer dimensions of 0.5 mm.
  The devices belonging to this generations are based on conventional technology of precision mechanisms.

- Second generation includes devices having dimensions from 1 mm to several μm. The development of this generation is based on technology of semiconductor materials.

- Third generation are of dimensions from several μm until bacteria dimensions. The further development of this generation depends strongly on investigations of living organisms.. It is expected that development of the MM in the future will be based on molecular technology. According to the opinion of Japanese researchers all machines of size less than few mm should be investigated to make them smaller.

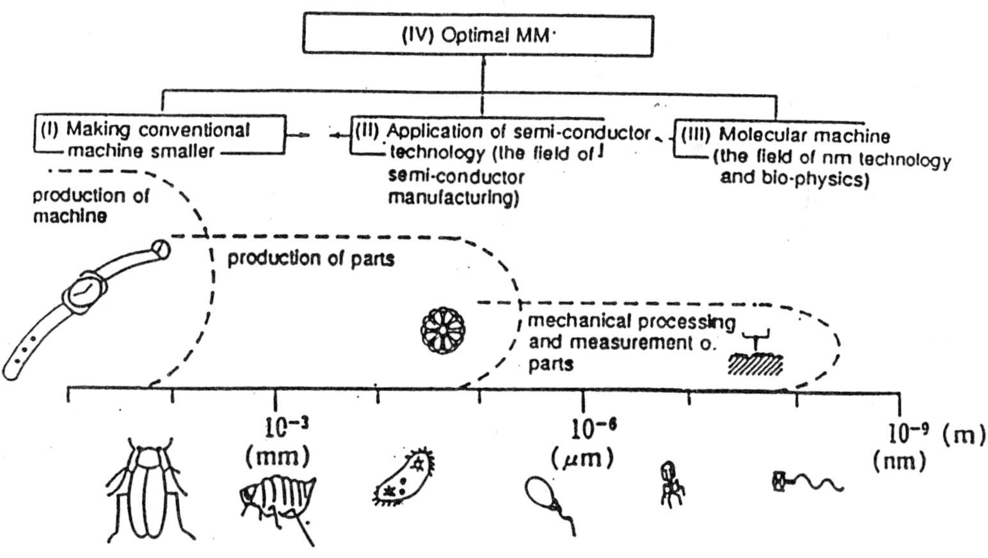


Fig.55. Present state and fields of research in MM [26]

### 2.8.2 Present state of research

The dimensions shown on Fig. 55 change from $10^{-3}$ to $10^{-9}$ m.

The principles of their functioning and research methods change from size to size.

The middle level on Fig. 55 shows the present situation of MM as a function of dimensions. The wrist watch belongs now to the smallest machines of every day using.

In the case of bearing of the electrostatic motor on silicon wafer the minimal size is tenth of the mm. The mechanical transformation and measurements of parameters of size of tenth μm is also possible.

The field marked (I) in the upper part of Fig.55 is dealing with further development of MM based on conventional technology.

To this fields belongs also stepping motor and micro air turbine with outer diameter 2 mm.

Next examples are sphere shells produced from different materials with diameter of several μm used in chemical industry, 1 to 2 μm amorphic foil used in the metal industries.

It is planed that the first generation of MM will be realised in this way. Field (II) is developed based on semiconductor technology such as lithography, etching, vacuum evaporation etc.

As a technical examples we can present here accelerometer oscillator of several dozen μm placed on an As wafer, liquid element and biochamber for cell fusion, which are now realised.

The third field (III) is dealing with molecular machines. In this area molecular machines of bioactuators have been gradually made clearer. An experimental production of an enlarged model simulated bacteria was recently reported. Still the major difficulties in entering into the nano scale of molecule exist.

The fourth (IV) area is dealing with so-called optimal mechanisms. The main goal of the investigations to recognise the possibility of the components of MM and possible production. A progress in the field of micro materials and micro-trybology is expected.


### 2.8.3 Systematics of the mobile micromachines.

To this class of micromachine the following machines belongs:

- walking machines,
- mobile machines,
- running machines,

- floating machines,
- flying machines.

We will concentrate on the first and second class of these machines.

### 2.8.4 Microwalking machines with two and four legs.

On Fig.56 two kinds of walking machines are shown: biped robot and quadruped machine. (Miura 1995) [28]. These machines are built for dynamic motion.

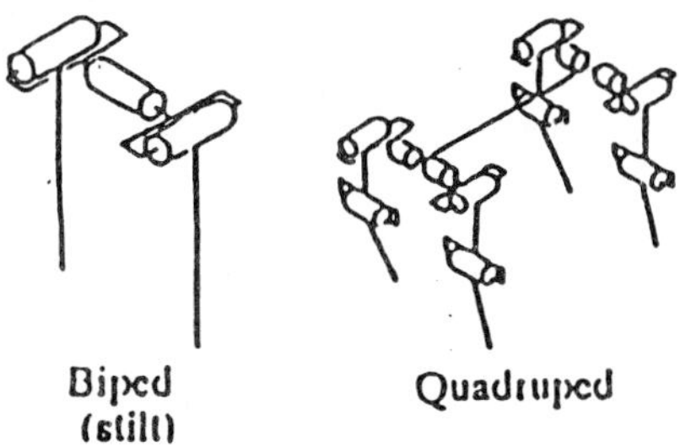


Fig.56. Microwalking machine
a - biped machine
b - quadruped machine

Fourlegged Microwalking Machine Driven By Electromagnetic Force[1] was built and tested.

The drive of micro walking machine in this case is based on mutual interaction between constant magnet field, magnetic field produced by the electromagnet, and force of the spring. On Fig. 57 a the diagram of the micromachine is shown. It consists from the two independent parts connected by the coupling.

Each part of the machine can move independently. To the left part of the body the constant magnet is connected and to the right part the coil, which creates electromagnet.

The distance between the two parts of the body is fixed by the coil spring surrounding the magnet and electromagnet.

There are two possible kind of movement. The first case take place if $F_s > F_m$ which means that spring force dominated. If $F_m > F_s$, magnet is dominated.

We will discuses the second case. If the electrical current is off the foreleg and handle are stationary and the interval between them is minimum because the repulsion force from the spring $F_s$ is smaller then magnetic force $F_m$ (Fig. 57.1) When electrical courrent is switch on the sum of forces $F_{em} + F_s > F_m$ becomes, greater than the force $F_m$, and the foreleg and hindleg move in the direction of force $F_s$.

Since the friction force of the handle $N_b$ is greater, than that of the foreleg $N_a$ ($F_s + F_m > F_m + N_b$) the foreleg moves from $B_1$ to $B_2$ (Fig.57.2). The other part is fixed.

When the electrical current is cut off, the foreleg and the handle contract towards the centre of the machine (Fig. 57.3). Since friction force $N_b$ is now smaller than $N_a$ ($N_b < N_a$) the hindleg moves from $A_1$ to $A_2$.

---

[1] This part was topic of M.Sc. dissertation of Mr J. Niećko under supervision of Prof. A. Morecki (Dec.94)

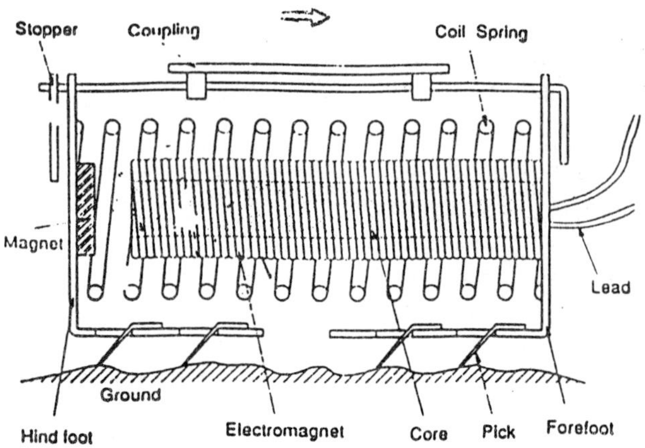


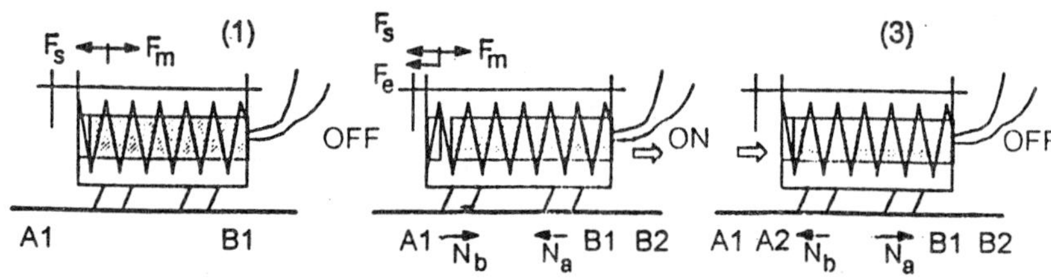


Fig.57. Four legged machine driven by electromagnetic force [29,30,31]
a - schematic diagram,　b - principle of walking.

These three phases of motion described above create so called single step of the machine.

By repeating these steps the machine is able to move in one direction.

During the design process one of the most critical problem was to select a proper servoactuator. Finally the dimensions of electromagnet were: length - 10 mm, diameter - 10 mm. The second problem deals with the design of the  legs. Additionally during the movement the torsion motions of the two parts of the machine were observed. They were eliminated by special  connections. The supply of the machine with energy created also a problem. The  special experimental rig was built and used for experiments. The influence of the surface on the machine motion and influence of wires were tested also.

The possibility of moving the machine on slope was not investigated.

### 2.8.5 Microwalking machines with six legs

The legs of six legged walking machine are similar to mammal leg's and the gait is realised in the way of control of „flexion" movements of elastic „leg". By the elastic leg we understand (Fig.58 a) a tube of rubber fibres which deformation can be obtain by controlling the air or liquid flow.

The leg deforms easily in axial direction and not deform in radial one. The deformation can be obtain by independent control of pressure inside the internal chambers. The leg has 3 DOF (flexion, extension and side movements). The diameter of the leg changes from 4-12 mm length from 20-50 mm, mass from 0,3-8g, flexion force is 0,15-1N. On Fig.58 a. the six legged machine, which walks on the finger is shown. The second type of the machine has six legs (Fig.58 b) which are of overhang type. Each leg has diameter of 2 mm and 12 mm length. The dimensions of four legged machine are 12x10x12mm and the six legged machine 12x20x7mm.

The air comes through 18 tubes with internal diameter 0,2 mm each. In general 12 tubes are enough for control (back and fourth rotating movements), the speed of the gait is about 20 cm/min and load 300 mg for fourlegged and 100 mg for six legged machine [29]. To this class of machines belong devices with light drive, electrostatic drive, ultrasonic motor, piesoelectric element, electromagnetic force, air turbine drives.

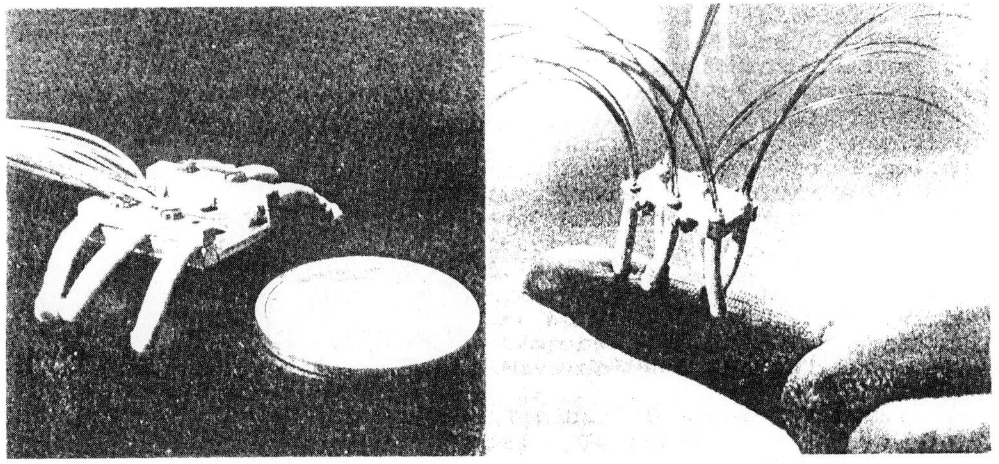

Fig.58. Microwalking machines [27,29].
a) six legged machine with mammals type legs;
b) six legged machine with reptiles type of legs.

## 2.8.6 Micromobile robot driven by gas turbine

The micromobile robot is shown on Fig.59[2]

Two gas turbines (3) are mounted in separate chambers, on left and right side of the machine body (1). The turbines are independently control [30,31]

The driven moment produced by the turbines is transform by  two rollers with borrel on the end (4) (active wheel) trough caterpillar (6) on front wheel (5) (passive). The moment is control by the changes of gas flow transmitted by elastic tubes (11)  to input nozzles (2) (diameter 1 mm).

The dimensions of the robot are the 9,9 x 4,5 x 6,4 mm. During the experiments it was necessary to change some dimensions of the chamber. Three different models were built and tested. On Fig.59 the general view of the whole system is shown.

The results of some experiments are shown on Fig.60.

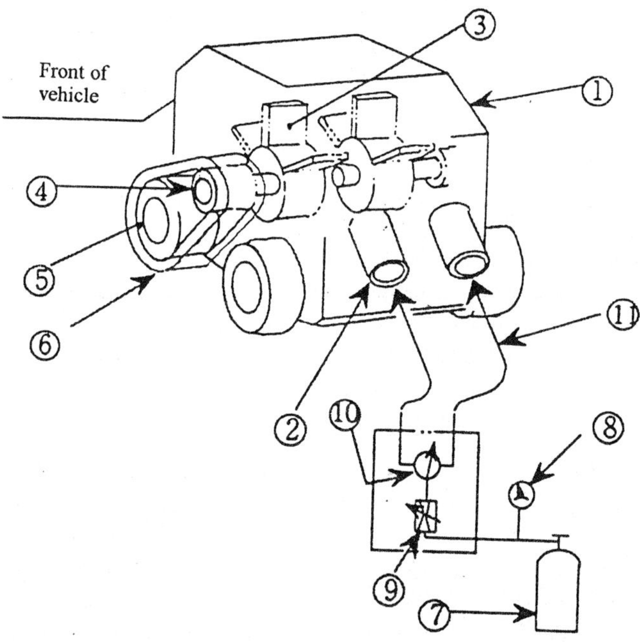


Fig.59 Micromobile robot driven by gas turbines.

---

[2] This machine was a topic of MSc dissertation of Mr Baran under supervision of Prof. A.. Morecki, June 1996

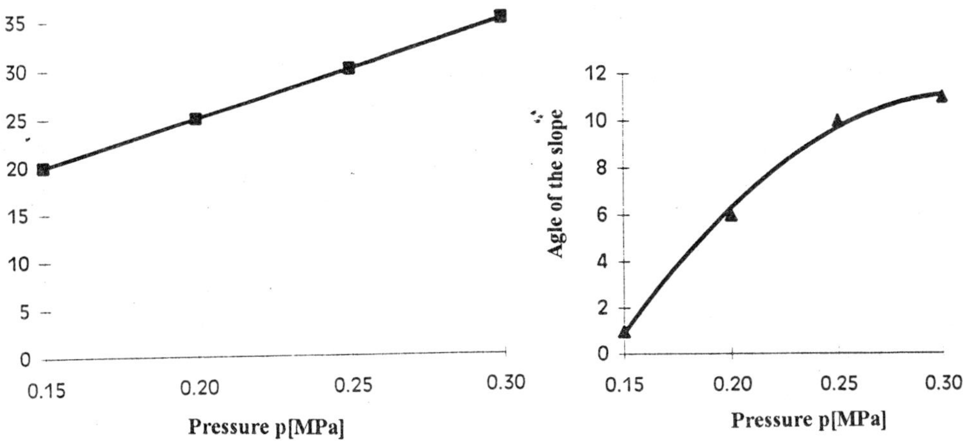


Fig.60. The results of the experiments
a) relationship between velocity and pressure on the flat ground
b) relationship between the angle of the slope and pressure

## 2.8.7 Possible applications and perspectives

The further development of MM depends on possible applications. The good examples of such applications were shown in the years 1991-93. To them belongs medical micromanipulators (endoscope), robots for inspection [26]. The list of possible models is rather long and includes motors, turbines, micro-actuator, walking machines. The development of MM in the future (mobile robots, actuators, mechanisms of micro motion, machine service, assembly etc.) deepens strongly on the investigations of living organisms on the mili, micro and nano level., The next century can be the century of micro and nano engineering based on the micro structure of organic world.

In medicine the future can bring microsize machines that investigate and repair damage in the cardiovascular, rendl and digestive systems. They can perform urgent operations on the inner ear, nose, cutting and suturing even on individual nerve fibres. In agriculture armies of crawling or flying insect - like micromechanisms may be used for pollination, planting seeds, targeting chemical spray, cell implants and past control in remote locomotion elements will appear like: micro motors, micro actuators, turbines, propellers, bearings, generators, sensors, micro optic devices. In JPL in California a new prototype of accelerometer was built, which measure the changes of acceleration smaller than $10^{-6}$g. It is expected that the industry of MM will appear. The new philosophy of MM design is expected.

## 3. REFERENCES


[1]  A. Morecki, J. Ekiel, K. Fidelus, Cybernetic Systems of Limb Moments in Man, Animals and Robots. PWN-Polish Scientific Publisher, Warsaw. Ellis Horwood Limited Publisher-Chichester, 1984, pp. 55-61, 167-174.

[2]  Footprints of Time, Time Australia, July 31,1995, p. 61.

[3]  Biomechanical Modelling of Human Walking. Proceed. of the Ninth World Congress on the Theory of Machines and Mechanisms. Vol. 3, , Milan, Italy, 1995, pp.2400 - 2404.

[4]  A. Morecki, K. Jaworek, J. Olszewski, S. Koozekanani, R. McGhee, R. Rahmani, Reduced Order Dynamic Model for Computer Analysis of Human Gait. Proceed. of the 4th Symposium on Theory and Practice of Robots and Manipulators. Eds. A. Morecki, G. Bianchi, K. Kędzior. PWN-Polish Scientific Publishers, Warsaw, 1981, pp.368-381.

[5]  J. Olszewski, An investigation of Human Motion Models in Dynamical Conditions. Ph.D.. Dissertation, Warsaw Technical Univ. 1977 (in Polish), under supervision of Prof.. A. Morecki.

[6]  K. Jaworek and A. Morecki, Method of verification of kinematic and Dynamic Properties of a Biped Locomotion Model. XIII Inter. Conference on Dynamics of Machines, Warsaw, April 6 - 10, 1981, pp. 212-217

[7]  A. Morecki, R. McGhee, S. H. Koozekanani, J. Olszewski, C. N. Burnett and K. Jaworek, Two Methods for Automatic Computer Analysis of Human Motion from Optical Images, Proceed. of the 7th Inter. Congress of Biomechanics, Sept.18-21, 1979, Warsaw, Poland, PWN-University Park Press Baltimore 1981, pp.133-140.

[8]  A. Morecki, Identification, Modelling and Rehabilitation Problems in Modern Biomechanics. Biomechanics of Motion (Ed. by A. Morecki), Springer-Verlag 1980, pp. 1-40.

[9]  K. Kędzior, A. Morecki, M. Wojtyra, T. Zagrajek and T. Zielińska, A. Goswami, M. Waldron, K. Waldron, Development of a Mechanical Simulation of Human Walking. Proceed. of Ro.Man.Sy'11th, Theory and Practice of Robots and Manipulators, Ed. by A. Morecki, G. Bianchi and C. Rzymkowski, Springer-Verlag, 1997 (in printing) pp.

[10] Polish-American Marie Sklodowska-Curie Fund. „Development of a Mechanical Simulation of Human Walking". Grant No MEN/NSF-94-159 between The Ohio State University and Warsaw University of Technology, 1994.

[11] K. Kędzior, M. Wojtyra, T. Zagrajek, Dynamic Model of Human Lover Extremity. Book of Abstracts, XVth Congress of the ISB, Jywaskyla, July 1955, pp. 58 - 59.

[12] A. Morecki, K. Waldron et. al, Development of a Mechanical Simulation of Human Walking. Second Polish-American Maria Sklodowska-Curie Foundation Grant, No MEN/NSF 9-159, Report Nov. 1955.

[13] R.D.Cop. „A Methodology for the Understanding of Time-Varying Leg-Muscle Forces During Human Walking. Doct. disser, the Ohio State University, 1986.

[14] Shin-Ming Song and K. J. Waldron, Machines that Walk: The Adaptive Suspension Vehicle, The MIT Press, Cambridge, Massachusetts 1989.

[15] P. T. Tschebyshev, Selected works (in Russian) Publisher AN CCCP, 1955, pp. 906-908.

[16] A.M orecki, Modelling, Mathematical Description, Measurements and Control of the Selected Animal and Human Body Manipulation and Locomotion Movements. Biomechanics of Engineering. Modelling, Simulation, Control. Ed. by A. Morecki, CISM Courses and Lectures No 291 Springer-Verlag 1987, pp. 1 - 83.

[17] T.Młynarski, Generalize Analytical Method for Kinematic Analysis of Planar Mechanisms Techn. University of Cracow, Monograph 165, Cracow; Position Analysis of planar linkages using the method of modification of kinematic units, MMT Journal, No. 6, pp. 831-838, 1996.

[18] T. Emura and A. Arakava, A study of walking robot controlled with of attitude sensor. Proceed. of the 4th Inter. Conf. of Adv. Robotics, Springer-Verlag 1989, pp. 640-651.

[19] K. Jaworek and W. Pogorzelski, Walking Machines (in Polish) in Basic Problems of Modern Technik, PWN, Vol. XXV, Robotics, Warsaw 1987, pp. 327-359.

[20] A. Morecki and T. Zielińska, Locomotion of a Machine of a Static Crawler type: Gait Modelling, Proceed. of the 4th Inter. Conf. of Adv. Robotics. Springer-Verlag, 1989, pp.664 - 675.

[21] A. Morecki and T. Zielińska, Quadruped Walking Machine-creation of the model of motion. Proceed. Robots and Biological Systems. Towards a New Bionics? Ed. by Dario P., Sandini G., Acbicher P., NATO ASI Series F, Vol. 102, 1993, pp. 206-222.

[22] J. A. Kizono, M. Iwasaki, T. Nemoto, A. Asakura, Development on Walking Robot for Underwater Inspection. K. J. Waldron (Ed.) Advanced Robotic 1989, Springer-Verlag, pp. 652-663

[23] John Bares, Lessons from Dante II, 93'ICAR

[24] IS Robotics, Exploring the Future: Twin City Office Centre 22, McGroth Highway, Somerville, MA 02143, USA.

[25] P. Szabelak, Parameters identification of walking machine, Hermes II, MSc Dissertation (in Polish), June 1996, Warsaw Univ. of Technology (supervisor T. Zielińska).

[26] T. Hayashi, On Micromechanisms and their Researchers and Developments. Proceed. „Ro.Man.sy'9", Springer-Verlag, London, 1993, pp.3-12.

[27] A. Morecki, Micromechanisms and Microwalking Robots. System Modelling Control Vol.1, 8, 1995 (Ed.E.Kącki) Published by Polish Society of Medical Informatics, Łódź 1995, pp. 37 - 40.

[28] H. Miura, Robot Intelligence and Microrobot, Procees. Ninth World Congress on the TMM, Vol. 1, 1995, pp. LXII-LXV.

[29] Suzumori, F. Kondo and H. Tanaka, Applications of a Flexible Microactuator to Microrobots. 1st Inter. MM Symp. Tokyo, June 1993, pp. 50-54.

[30] Niećko, The construction of the mobile micromechanism family driven by electromagnetic force (in polish). MSc dissertation, Dec.1994, Warsaw University of Technology, (Supervisor A. Morecki).

[31] Masuto Mizukami, Kunio Koyabu and Fumikozu Ohira, $ICM^3$ Miniaturised Mobile Machine Driven by Electromagnetic Force, 1st, IFToMM International Micromechanism Symposium. Proceed. Tokyo, 1-3 June 1993, pp. 41-45.

[32] H. Nabada, S. Sawada and A. Watabe, A 10-mm Cube Miniaturised Vehicle with Air-Driven Turbines. Proceed. 1st IFToMM International Micromechanism Symposium, June 1993, TIT, Japan, pp. 46-49.

[33] K. Baran, Micromobile vehicle driven by gas turbine (in Polish) MSc Dissertation, June 1996 . Warsaw Univ. of Technology, (Supervisor A. Morecki).

[34] D.A. Kugath, D.R. Wilt, Problems in selection of design parameters effecting manipulators performance, First CISM-IFToMM Symposium „Ro.Man.Sy'73", Vol. II, Udine 1974, Springer-Verlag, pp.169-189.

[35] R.B. McGhee and D.E. Orin, An Interactive Computer-Control System for a Quadruped Robot First CISM-IFToMM Symposium „RoMan.Sy'73", Vol. I, Udine 1974, Springer-Verlag, pp. 25-40.

[36] Plustech. Tempere. Finland. http://www.plutech.fi/.

[37] Dudziński, A. Soliński, A.Seyfried,; Computer Dyno Graphy - the characteristics of the system for measurements of reaction forces during locomotion, Postępy Rehabilitacji, 1996 (in printing).

[38] Ariel Performance Analysis System (APAS), User's Manual Diego California 1995.

[39] A.A. Grishin, A.M. Formalsky, A. Lensky, S.V.Zhitomirsky, Dynamic Walking of a Vehicle with Two Telescopics Legs Conltrolled by Two Drives; The International Journal of Robotics Research, Vol. 13, No 2, April 1994, pp. 137-147.

# CHARACTERISTICS OF HUMAN LOCOMOTION


**N. Berme, E. Oggero and G. Pagnacco**
**The Ohio State University, Columbus, OH, USA**



## ABSTRACT

The human locomotive apparatus is fascinating in its versatility, sophistication and performance. Its main characteristic is versatility. The locomotive apparatus appears to be optimized for an enormous variety of activities, not just for a few specific ones. While many animals can outperform humans in specific situations, none can perform as well in a multitude of conditions. This has very important repercussions in the study of human locomotion. Given the complexity and flexibility of the human locomotive apparatus the characterization of all the possible kinds of human locomotion is a daunting task. For this reason often only very specific situations are analyzed; the most common is certainly walking on a flat, prepared surface: the normal, level gait or simply gait.

## 1. INTRODUCTION

Since the antiquity there has been an interest in studying motion of humans and animals.  Plato, Aristotle, Leonardo da Vinci, Galileo Galilei, Borelli, and Marey, just to name a few, explored the field and prepared the bases for future investigation.  However, the quantitative characterization of movement has been possible only in the last century and a half, thanks to the enormous advances in instrumentation and imaging technology.  For the study of human locomotion the new era begun in 1836 with the work by the Weber brothers who introduced the scientific investigation of the mechanics of gait.  Since then, the advances in this field happened at an exponential rate, especially in the last thirty years [1].

Given the incredible complexity of the human locomotive system, a complete characterization of human locomotion is an enormous task.  Even after decades of study, much is still to be discovered, especially in the area of the neurological control behind all human movements.  For these reasons and for the obvious space constraints only some of the most important characteristics of human locomotion will be presented here.

### 1.1 Human locomotion

The term *locomotion* indicates the act of going from one place to another.  It derives from the combination of two Latin words, *loco* ablative of *locus* meaning to a location or place and *motus*, past participle of the verb *movere* meaning moved.  The meaning of the term is very broad, not indicating the specifics but just the act itself.  According to this definition, the expression *human locomotion* indicates the general act of moving from one location to another as performed by humans.  Under this definition the locomotion can be implemented in a very large number of possible ways; walking, running, jumping, swimming, skiing, and even driving a car or riding a bus are all forms of human locomotion.


## 2. PRINCIPAL CHARACTERISTICS OF THE HUMAN LOCOMOTIVE APPARATUS

The human locomotive apparatus is fascinating in its versatility, sophistication and performance.  Its main char-

acteristic can be found in its versatility.  Humans are able
to move on all kinds of terrain and surfaces: they can climb
mountains, trees and obstacles, walk or run on snow, sand,
gravel and other natural surfaces as well as on artificial
ones like asphalt and concrete.  It can be safely stated
that the only locomotive activity forbidden to a human
being, at least without an external aid, is flying.  This is
the result of millennia of evolution involving the whole
human body, from the skeleton, to the muscles, to the nervous system.

This versatility also manifests itself in the ability to
compensate for pathological conditions that might occur
almost anywhere in the locomotive system.  Even the inabil-
ity to use some muscles, or the loss of mobility of some
joints often does not prevent a person from successfully
moving from one place to another.

For locomotive purposes, humans normally employ an
upright bipedal gait.  This is one of the characteristics
that differentiate them from almost all the other animals,
and is one of the reasons of the locomotive versatility.  In
studying human locomotion we might be inclined to concentrate our attention to the lower limbs.  We have to remember, however, that a very important role is performed by the
other parts of the body, especially the upper limbs.  Apart
from some activities like swimming, where the upper limbs
provide most of the propulsive action, they are commonly
employed to improve both static and dynamic equilibrium and
to provide support in difficult situations.  Sometimes, like
for instance on a steep uneven surface, humans prefer to
actually move as quadrupeds in order to maximize equilibrium.

The inherent instability of the upright position
requires a sophisticated control of the position and movement of all body segments.  This is realized by a highly
complex nervous system, which is capable of finely regulating a large number of muscles.  Much of the functioning of
this system is still not very well understood.  A very
important fact about the nervous system is the presence of
considerable transmission and processing delays, often in
the range of tens of milliseconds and sometimes even several
hundreds of milliseconds.  This makes the control of movements much more complex that it might otherwise appear.

Versatility is also the result of the presence of a complex foot structure, which can adapt to the terrain and provide the nervous system with accurate information on the pressure distribution on the foot itself.

All considered, it appears that the human locomotive apparatus is optimized not for just a specific activity, but for an enormous variety of them. While many animals can outperform humans in specific situations, none can perform so well in a multitude of conditions. This has very important repercussions in the study of human locomotion.

One of the most profound consequences is that while some of the components of the locomotive apparatus or their characteristics might appear unimportant for a specific activity, they might be paramount for other activities. As anyone has probably experienced at one time or another, many of the muscles acting on the lower limbs are not used very much in most of the everyday activities, but sometimes when a new activity is performed, we feel the tension in muscles we did not even think existed.

Also, different motion patterns are used to better adapt to the requirements of the contingent situation. For instance, when walking on a flat surface, the feet usually start contacting the ground at the heel and break the contact at the toes. However, this is not the motion used by soldiers or expert mountaineers when walking on flat, but slippery or unstable surfaces like ice. In such situations, the feet make and break contact remaining parallel with the ground in order to increase the area of contact and therefore reducing the local pressure. Another example can be found in running: in long distance runs the heels make contact with the ground, while in sprints they do not.

All that has been said up to this point should help to clarify that it is impossible to define more detailed characteristics of the human locomotion without first focusing the attention to a specific locomotive action. It also points out the possible presence of different movement patterns and their consequential transitorial phases in the overall action of going from one place to another. Because of the inherent greater complexity involved with the study of transitorial conditions, the study of human locomotion is often focused on steady state walking.

## 3. CHARACTERISTICS OF GAIT

If specific movements are considered, the most common is
certainly walking on a flat, prepared surface: the normal,
level gait or simply gait.  This kind of locomotion is characterized by the fact that at least one foot is always in
contact with the ground.  For this reason two distinct
phases are present: the single support and the double support, respectively meaning one or both feet are in contact
with the ground.  From an energetic point of view, it is
characterized by the continuous transfer of energy from
potential to kinetic, so when one is maximum, the other is
minimum [2].

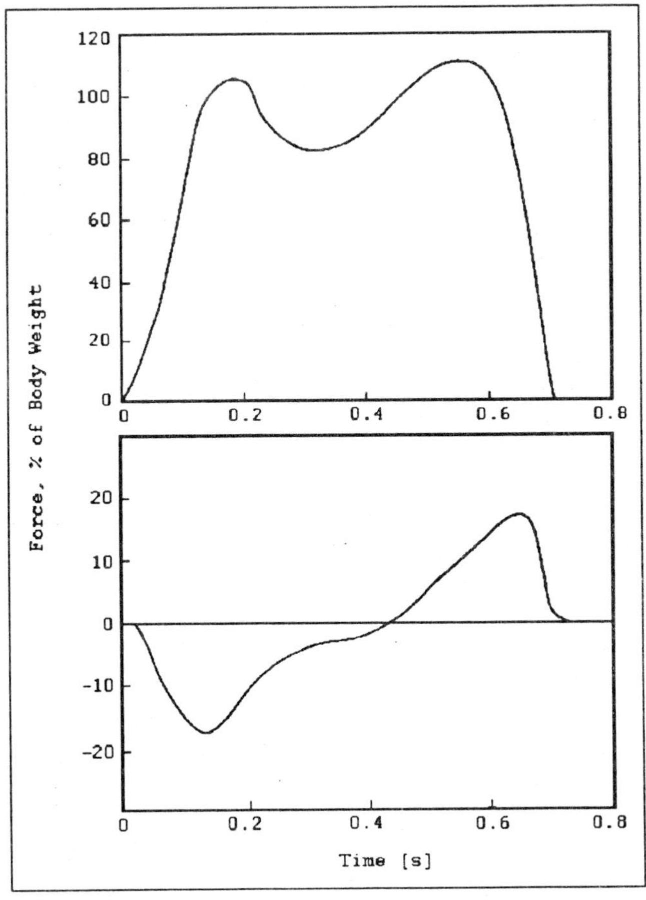


Figure 1: Typical ground reaction forces in gait

Another important characteristic of this locomotion is the movement of the feet.  Typically, they first contact the ground at the heels.  Then, the contact does a continuous motion from the heel to the toes.

From a quantitative point of view, the ground reactions generated during a physiological gait cycle have the characteristic shape shown in Figure 1.

Important characteristics of the human gait where discovered by Saunders and coworkers [3] by observing the motion of the pelvis, as representing the center of mass of the body.  They found that in the plane of progression the center of mass describes a smooth regular sinusoidal curve with two cycles for every gait cycle, i.e. the center of mass is displaced in the vertical direction twice during the gait cycle, from the heel strike of one foot to the subsequent heel strike of the same foot.  The summits of this fluctuation happens at the middle of the stance phase of the supporting limb.  They further found that in the horizontal plane the trajectory also takes a sinusoidal shape, where the center of mass is displaced to the right and to the left, in phase with the weight-bearing extremity.  Combining these two motions, in a single gait cycle from the right heel strike to the left toe off, the center of mass may be followed as it rises smoothly to a summit at about 25% of the cycle; but at the same time it deviates to the right. As the center begins to descent, it smoothly deviates toward the left to continue this side to side movement as it once more begins to rise to a second summit at about 75% of the cycle.  When the second summit is reached and the center of mass proceeds to fall, it begins to return gradually to the right and has reached the central axis of the forward motion as the cycle is completed.

Considering the energy expenditure, Saunders et al. suggested that the set of movements performed during a gait cycle is directed toward the overall optimization of the displacement of the center of mass.  The rational here is that the minimization of the energy loss is necessary because of the non efficient energy expenditure of the human muscles.

By comparing the human gait with a compass kind of movement, they were able to identify six determinants of gait. These are:

- Pelvic Rotation: in normal level walking, the pelvis
  rotates alternatively to the right and to the left relative to the line of progression.  This rotation, of
  about 8 degrees in magnitude, flattens the arc described
  by the center of mass in compass gait.

- Pelvic Tilt: it occurs while the body is passing over
  the vertical supporting member, and consists of a rotation of the pelvis of about 5 degrees towards the non
  supported side.  This motion again results in a flattening of the summit of the trajectory of the center of
  mass.

- Knee flexion in the stance phase: the supportive limb
  enters the stance phase at heel strike with the knee
  joint in near-full extension.  The knee joint is then
  flexed up to a maximum of about 15 degrees and then
  extended again before toe off.  This motion results once
  more in a flattening of the summit of the trajectory of
  the center of mass.

- Foot and Knee mechanisms (4th and 5th determinants): the
  flexion-extension movement of the knee combined with the
  rotation of the foot, first around the heel and then
  around the fore part of the foot itself, result in the
  obliteration of the abrupt inflections otherwise present
  at the intersections of the arcs described by the path
  of the center of mass.  The overall result is a smooth
  sinusoidal pathway for the center of mass in the plane
  of progression.

- Lateral displacement of the pelvis: excessive motion of
  the center of mass in the frontal plane is avoided by
  the presence of the tibiofemoral angle, which, together
  with relative adduction at the hip, reduces the lateral
  displacement to a little more than half of what would
  otherwise be needed in order to maintain balance.

In their study Saunders and coworkers did not consider
the upper body.  By doing so they were not able to identify
the important role that its motions have in minimizing the
energy expenditure.  These motions and their effects are:

- The oscillatory motion of the upper limbs: it generates
  a sinusoidal up and down motion of the center of mass.
  This motion is in phase opposition with the one produced

by the lower limbs, therefore reducing the actual vertical motion of the center of mass.

- Trunk rotation: induced by the movements of the upper limbs, it is in opposition with the pelvic rotation. This actually facilitates the pelvis rotation by introducing a torsional oscillation.

## 4. CONCLUSION

Given the complexity and flexibility of the human locomotive apparatus the characterization of all the possible kinds of human locomotion is a daunting task. For this reason often only very specific situations are analyzed. While this is generally a necessity and can provide very good insights, it is of the foremost importance to understand the boundaries that define the validity of the results of such analyses. General conclusions rarely can be obtained from considering all too limiting conditions. This is especially true in the case of the human locomotive system that appears not to be specialized for a specific movement but for a huge number of movements and situations, probably more so than any other animal.

## REFERENCES

1. Nigg, B.M. and Herzog, W., Biomechanics of the musculoskeletal system. John Wiley & Sons, 1995.
2. Cavagna, G. A., Aspects of efficiency and inefficiency of terrestrial locomotion. Biomechanics VI-A, Ed. Asmussen, E. and Jorgensen, K., University Park Press, Baltimore, 1978, 3-22.
3. Saunders, M., Inman, V.T. and Eberhart, H.D., The major determinants in normal and pathological gait. The Journal of Bone and Joint Surgery, 35-A (1953), 543-558.

# MODELING AND SIMULATION OF HUMAN LOCOMOTION


**N. Berme, E. Oggero and G. Pagnacco**
**The Ohio State University, Columbus, OH, USA**



ABSTRACT

The human locomotive system is probably the most sophisticated and complex locomotive apparatus that ever existed.
In order to understand how the models of such system are
built, it is useful to consider the meaning and implication
of modeling and simulation as an attempt to represent reality. The human locomotive apparatus can be considered as
constituted of three systems (i.e. skeletal, muscular, and
nervous systems) coupled together. Models can include a
representation of one, two, or all three systems. The purpose and possibilities of each system are very different,
and the accuracy of the results depends on the assumptions
and formulation of the model. The possibility to verify
such hypotheses relies on the state-of-the-art of measurement systems, currently available, for noninvasive assessment of human locomotion parameters.

## 1. INTRODUCTION

The human locomotive system is probably the most sophisticated and complex locomotive apparatus that ever existed.
The great number of its components as well as the variety of
its possible motion patterns make the modeling of such apparatus and the simulation of its movements a very challenging
task.  However, even the crude representation, currently
possible, of such a system can provide useful insight to its
workings.

Models and simulations of the human locomotion have many
purposes, but generally, they fall in one or more of the
following categories:

- to provide insight and increase the knowledge of how the
  human locomotion is achieved, in both normal as well as
  pathological conditions;

- to help diagnosing and to provide a way to improve
  pathological situations;

- to provide possible ways to optimize specific locomotion
  actions.

Before proceeding further, it is perhaps useful to consider the meaning and implications of the terms "human locomotion", "modeling" and "simulation".

### 1.1 Human Locomotion

The term *locomotion* indicates the act of going from one
place to another, irrespective of the method used for
achieving this goal.  In relation to modeling, however, "human locomotion" is generally used to indicate the act of
walking.  Probably, the primary reason for this is that the
science of modeling is still in its infancy, and most
research is concentrated on steady state walking on a level
surface.

### 1.2 Modeling

In general modeling, or creation of models, is an act
that is common to all human activities.  A model can be
defined as an attempt to represent reality, usually in a
simplified manner.  Models are used not only in the scientific and technical studies, but also in everyday life.  In
our minds reality is represented by models, and all mental

planning activities use them.  Even thinking what to do during the day is nothing more than a model of the day.

Models employed for scientific or technical purposes have one or both the following aims: (I) to increase knowledge and insight about reality, and (II) to estimate or predict variables of interest [1].  The first goal seems contradictory with the fact that knowledge and insight are obviously required to develop the model itself.  However, a model can be built according to hypotheses made about reality and then used to verify them.  Thus, increasing knowledge of reality.  This is how most models are used in scientific research.

While a model created for the first purpose, generally, can also be used for estimating or predicting variables of interest, the opposite is not necessarily true.  The fact that the results obtained from a model are very accurate, does not mean that the model itself is a correct representation of reality, and therefore, can be used for improving knowledge.  For instance, models created by using artificial neural networks are often able to predict the variables of interest with enough accuracy, but they do not provide much insight to the system they represent.

The construction of models relies on two types of information: knowledge of the system being modeled, and experimental data that constitute the inputs and/or outputs of such a system [1].  In the case of models used in biomechanics, the former comes from the disciplines of anatomy and physiology, while the latter are generally found in the literature, or can be determined experimentally.  These experiments may utilize electromyograms (EMG), force plates, accelerometers, goniometers, motion analysis systems, or others, as required by the specific situation.

Since a model is usually a simplified representation of reality, a very important aspect of modeling is to decide what should be included and what should be omitted.  It seems obvious that all important aspects should be included, and that all unimportant aspects may be neglected.  However, attempting to list rules and guidelines is not easy.  The general theory of modeling requires that all a priori information available on the structure and function of the system to be modeled are included [2].  Unfortunately, this might, and often does, lead to a model too complicated to be useful.  On the other hand, in general one may suggest that

simpler is better.  However there is always the danger that
a simple model may not agree with reality, since some
aspects have been left out.  It appears that the choice of
including or excluding certain aspects is more of an art
than a science.

   If a choice must be made, it must be driven by the goals
of the model.  A model can not provide information on what
has been left out during its development.  For instance, the
forces on the cruciate ligaments are not predictable if in
the model the knee is represented by a pin joint and not by
its actual geometry; the deformation of bones and tissues
can not be estimated if a lumped parameter formulation is
used instead of a distributed parameter one; the effects of
body segments not included in the model can not be considered.

   The two attributes determining the adequacy of a model
are its validity and its verifiability [3].  The validity of
the model refers to its ability to predict system responses
which agree, within predetermined limits of accuracy, with
the corresponding responses of the real system.  This
attribute is fundamental, since all models are judged by
their ability to provide results which are in agreement with
the observable reality.

   A model can be validated through the use of direct or
indirect measurements.  In the former case the variables of
interest are measured in a set of experiments and then compared with what is predicted by the model.  If the experimental and the estimated results agree, the model is validated.  However, the validity of a model is not general but
is related to the boundary or initial conditions for which a
comparison between predicted and experimental results has
been made.  A model valid for some conditions is not necessarily valid for others.  The fact that a model has been
validated for many conditions might improve one's confidence
in the model's ability to be successfully used in similar
but different conditions.  Still, only an experiment with
the real system can confirm that what a model predicts is
correct.

   When it is impossible to make experimental measurements
of internal variables, as is often the case when studying
the human body, direct validation cannot be performed.
Examples of this situation are the forces acting on joints
or the force in ligaments and muscles.  However, in some

cases, it may be possible to measure another variable, which
is conceptually related to the one of interest but not
needed in the model, and compare such variable with the
model prediction.  This is called an indirect measurement.
For instance, if a model is developed to predict the intersegmental forces, a direct measurement is generally not possible.  Nevertheless, if the model is able to predict correctly the ground reaction forces, one might feel comfortable about its potential to provide an estimate of the
intersegmental loads.  Examples of commonly used indirect
measurements include EMG measurements for the estimation of
muscle forces, and kinematics and ground reaction force
measurements for the estimation of inertial, gravitational
and intersegmental loads in general.

Generally, the use of indirect measurements is a weaker
method to validate a model than the use of direct measurements.  For example, several different models developed to
predict the same variables and indirectly validated, often
predict, under the same conditions, different values for the
same variable [4].  This generally happens because of the
different assumptions made in the development of the models.
Since in reality, in a specific situation, each and every
variable can assume only a single value, most, if not all
these models, provide an inaccurate estimation.  If a direct
validation of these models could be possible it would allow
an easy identification of which model, if any, is the correct one.  The indirect validation provides only the knowledge that a model might be correct, not that it actually is.
Indirect validation can not be considered therefore a true
validation but rather an often weak evaluation of the potential of a model to do the task for which it was created.

Even if a model is valid, it does not mean that its
structure represent, or is even similar, to the real system.
The attribute of verifiability is tied to the ability of a
model to represent adequately the underlying conceptual
reality.  This is strictly related to the choice of what and
how to model, and is especially important if the purpose is
to gain insight to the real system the model represents.
Sometimes the best models for estimating variables of interest are conceptually inaccurate, but the sensitivity of the
results to such inaccuracies is very small.  Other times,
models are created as "black boxes", like is often the case

with artificial neural networks, without even trying to represent the underlying reality.

## 1.3 Simulation

There are many possible definitions of simulation.  Two relevant ones as stated in the American Heritage Dictionary (1992) are: *1.  Imitation or representation as of a potential situation or in experimental testing; 2.  Representation of the operation or features of one process or system through the use of another.*  Another possible definition is: *predicting the behavior of a complex system by repeatedly applying simple principles* [5].

In the study of human movement, simulations generally do not use the system whose behavior they are trying to reproduce, but rather a mathematical model of it.  This is done for many reasons, but mostly because of the flexibility and the greater reproducibility granted by working on a model and the possibility of estimating internal variables experimentally not measurable.

The purposes of simulations of human locomotive movements are usually the same ones of models: to increase knowledge and insight about reality, and to estimate or predict variables of interest; the main difference lies in the fact that models represent a system while simulations represent a situation or a process.

## 2. SYSTEMS CONSTITUTING THE HUMAN LOCOMOTIVE APPARATUS AND THEIR MODELS

The human locomotive apparatus can be considered as constituted of three systems:

- the skeletal system, constituted of bones, joints and ligaments providing the frame;

- the muscular system, constituted of the muscles and tendons providing the force to actuate the movements;

- the nervous system, that provides the control for the muscles.

The muscular system is coupled with the skeletal one by the geometry of the insertion points.  The nervous system is in turn coupled with the muscular one by means of the motoneurons and the proprioceptors that provide, respectively,

the activation of the innervated muscles and part of the
feedback necessary to control the motion.

Models of the entire locomotive apparatus can include a
representation of one, two, or all the three systems.  Specifically, because of the mutual relationships between them,
only the skeletal system can be modeled alone.  If the muscular system is to be included, necessarily the skeletal one
must also be modeled since it provides the geometrical
information about the muscular insertion points as well as
representing the bodies on which the muscular action can be
exploited.  Similarly, to model the neural system, the muscular one must be considered since it represent both the
object controlled and the source of part of the feedback
information.  Because of these mutual dependencies, three
kinds of models can exist:

- skeletal models;

- musculo-skeletal models;

- neuro-musculo-skeletal models.

It is possible to create models that fall in one of
these three classes by appropriately combining together models of one or more of the three systems constituting the
human locomotive apparatus.  For this reason, it is appropriate to consider these systems separately.

2.1 Skeletal system

As previously said, the skeletal system is constituted
of the bones, joints and ligaments that provide the frame of
the human body.  Usually, it is modeled as a series of rigid
links interconnected by simple joints.  While the use of
rigid bodies is a good approximation for the long bones and
the pelvis, it is not as good a representation for complex
structures like the foot, unless, of course, multiple links
are used to account for its numerous degrees of freedom.
Articulations are usually modeled as simple pin or spherical
joints.  While the spherical joint is a good approximation
of reality when used for the hip, pin joints are a very
crude approximation of the complex articulations such as the
knee.  The knee, like most joints of the human body is
three-dimensional.  It is, in fact, constituted of complicated bone surfaces covered with cartilage, sliding or roll-
ing on each other with complex trajectories of their instantaneous centers of rotation.  The excursion of their move-

ments is constrained by ligaments, as well as the bone surfaces themselves. While there have been efforts to produce
more physiological models using both rigid bodies and finite
element techniques, they are so much more complicated and
computationally intensive that they are normally not used in
simulating the skeletal system as a whole.

2.2 Muscular system

The muscular system is constituted of a very large number of muscles and tendons, each with its own characteristics. Some of the muscles in the lower limbs span only one
joint, exerting their action only on two skeletal segments
at a time. Some span two joints, and therefore, apply force
to three skeletal segments simultaneously. In every movement, muscles can be grouped, according to their functional
role, in four categories: agonistic, antagonistic, fixator,
and synergistic. They represent respectively the muscles
that perform the movement, the muscles that oppose the movement, the ones that help in fixing the positions of body
parts not involved in the movement and the ones that facilitate the action of the agonistic muscles by stabilizing the
articular joints involved in the movement.

Many different muscle models have been developed. Most
of them are variations of the famous muscle model proposed
by Hill in 1938 [6]. This model expresses the force-
velocity relationship using the following equation:

$$v = b \frac{(F_0 - F)}{F + a} \tag{2-1}$$

where $v$ is the velocity of shortening, $F_0$ is the maximal
force at zero velocity and optimal muscle length, $F$ is the
instantaneous force and $a$ and $b$ are constants which are specific for a muscle.

Muscles affect the motion of the system by generating
moments around the joints. Since the muscles involved in
the locomotive movements usually generate very significant
forces with relatively small moment arms around the articular centers, the generated torques are very sensitive to
errors in the estimation of the geometrical configuration.

For the sake of simplicity, it is common to group many
muscles according to the motion they generate about the
joints (e.g. knee flexors and extensors) and their structure, or to consider only the larger and more active muscles

for a specific movement.  This helps to simplify the problem
by avoiding the complication of including a large number of
muscles whose characteristics are not always sufficiently
known.

Since muscles affect the motion of the system by generating a torque around the joints, it is also a common practice to model group of muscles as pure torque generators.
This greatly reduces the overall complication of the model
and prevents errors induced by the incorrect estimation of
the geometric variables.  However, it also excludes many
important characteristics of the muscular actions.  In particular, it makes it impossible to consider the nonlinearities introduced by the changing geometry as well as
contraction velocities.  Yet, this crude approximation is
useful, especially when the goal is to solve the inverse
dynamics problem.

2.2 Nervous system
The central and peripheral nervous systems are the controllers of the muscular actions, and therefore, of the
movements.  They are constituted of many different components dedicated to gather the information required to control the movements, to process such information, as well as
the conscious commands, and finally, to appropriately activate the muscles.

The knowledge about the movements and the surroundings
of the body is obtained by various muscle proprioceptors
that provide information on the length, contraction speed,
and force generated by every muscle; by a very large number
of other sensory cells providing information on external and
reaction forces acting on the body; and by the vestibular
and visual systems.  The processing of all this information
is performed by a very complex network of neurons, and ends
at the motoneurons that innervate the muscles and ultimately
provide their activation.

Even today, little is known about how movement patterns
are generated and controlled, and how balance is maintained.
Since this is the least known of the three systems constituting the locomotive apparatus, it is where nowadays most
of the research is concentrated.

Beside its complexities, what differentiates the nervous
system from most controls designed by humans is the presence
of significant delays in the transmission of information

across the neural system.  Such delays exist both at the synaptic level as well as in the transmission along the nerves.  The total time for the sensory information coming from the muscle proprioceptors to reach the central nervous system is in the order of hundreds of milliseconds.  Of analogous magnitude is the time taken by the commands issued by the central nervous system to reach the muscles.  This makes impossible the use of a control strategy based on feedback from the sensory elements to the central nervous system.  This is particularly true if, instead of locomotive movements, maintaining a balanced upright position is considered.

Many theories have been formulated on how balance and movements are controlled.  What is known is the presence of several reflexes at the spinal level, as well as the impossibility to perform any controlled movement in case of a spinal injury.  This suggests that motion patterns are generated at the cortical level, and that the spinal circuits, being close to the muscles, can provide some kind of relatively fast feedback type of control.  However, the ability of such spinal circuits to compensate for external perturbations appears to be limited.  If the discrepancy between the actual and desired movement exceed certain thresholds, the central nervous system has to respond to compensate. Because of the large transmission delays, this compensatory interventions of the central nervous system appears to be feasible only to correct major perturbations or to provide a correction during the next planned movement cycle.

Because of all these complexities, models of the entire locomotive apparatus almost never consider all the characteristics of the nervous system.  Most of the time the reflexes and the delays are neglected, and the muscle activations are given as open-loop and pre-planned.  Often, the information on when and how much to activate a muscle is obtained by analyzing the electromyograms (EMG) of the muscles.  A promising way of creating more realistic models comes from artificial neural networks.  Including the transmission delays, and what is known about the dynamics of the motor control of the nervous system in such models might lead to a better way of representing the complex neural interactions, which make control of movements and balance possible.

## 3. CLASSIFICATION AND CHARACTERISTICS OF THE MODELS OF THE HUMAN LOCOMOTIVE APPARATUS

As previously stated, there are three general classes of models of the human locomotive system. The simplest are the skeletal models, where only the skeletal apparatus is considered. Next come the musculo-skeletal models, where the muscles and their interactions with the skeletal system are also present. Finally, there are the neuro-musculo-skeletal models that consider also the control of the muscles performed by the nervous system. The purpose and possibilities of these three classes of models are very different.

### 3.1 Skeletal Models

Skeletal models can be used to investigate the kinematics of movement as well as to provide information about the intersegmental loads due to inertial, gravitational and external forces in various location of the skeletal system, mainly the joints. An example of such models is the one developed by Saunders and coworkers to identify the determinants of gait [7]. Since their interest was only in the kinematics, not even the inertial characteristics had to be included.

### 3.2 Musculo-skeletal Models

Musculo-skeletal models are characterized by the addition of some representation of the muscular system to what might otherwise be considered a skeletal model. However, since in this class of models the control system of the muscles (i.e. the nervous system) is not included, they can only be used to analyze human movement, and not for synthesis or simulation. These kind of models are mostly used to solve the inverse dynamic problem. This consists in solving the dynamic equations governing the motion of a system using the kinematics as well as the gravitational and external forces as known terms. The actuation forces and torques are the unknowns. Mathematically it can be expressed by the equation

$$\{F\} = [M]\{\ddot{q}\} - \{G\}\{B\} \qquad\qquad (3\text{-}1)$$

where $\{F\}$ represents the actuation forces and moments, $\{G\}$ the gravitational and external forces, and $\{B\}$ the elastic and damping forces. This category of problems are called inverse or indirect dynamic problems, because the logical process of obtaining motion from actuators is inverted.

The models used for this purpose generally consider muscles as pure torque generators. This is consistent with the fact that, the mathematical formulation of the problem allows only a single actuation force or moment to be estimated for each and every degree of freedom present in the model. If the skeletal system is represented as a linkage, the only degrees of freedom are the joint angles. Therefore, the only actuations that can be determined are the net intersegmental moments.

In order to investigate the forces developed by each muscle, it is necessary to create a model which includes a more physiological representation of the muscular system. However, such models contain larger number of muscles than the number of degrees of freedom. Therefore, the problem of estimating muscular forces is an underdetermined one, and is usually approached as an optimization problem. The procedure in such a case is to first determine the net intersegmental moments at a particular instant and then use static optimization procedures to distribute the forces necessary to create such moments among the various muscles [8][9]. Useful information to reduce the under-determination and help solving such optimization problems come from electromyograms, as well as from known muscle characteristics such as size and cross-sectional area.

In reality we do not know what functional, if any, is minimized in the human locomotive system under the specific conditions considered. Therefore, such optimization techniques can only offer estimations of possible muscle forces, and not actual values.

Nevertheless, even estimating the net intersegmental moments alone can be used effectively for clinical and research purposes.

3.3 Neuro-musculo-skeletal models

In this class of models both the actuators and their controls are present, and all kinetic models used for the synthesis of human movements fall in this category. Even models that consider purely ballistic motions can be regarded as neuro-musculo-skeletal models. It can, in fact, be argued that the absence of muscular actuation is a per-

fectly possible control strategy. Incidentally, it is also
the one that minimizes the metabolic energy consumption.

In these models the skeletal system is generally represented by relatively complicated linkages. Often, in order
to reduce the complexity of the model, not all the degrees
of freedom present in the human body are modeled. One common simplification is, for instance, not to consider the
ankle inversion-eversion. Also common is to neglect the
upper body motion, and model the upper body as a lumped
inertia. Skeletal articulations are often represented as
ideal frictionless spherical or cylindrical joints. However, sometimes separate articulation models have been used
to better estimate the resultant moments generated by muscular forces.

The muscular system is commonly represented in a simplified way by ideal torque generators or by grouping together
muscles with similar function and structure. In the latter
case, usually a weighted average is used to define the
equivalent origin and insertion points.

The goals of the simulation drive how the nervous system
is modeled. If the goal is optimization of a specific movement, muscle activations are found by using optimization
procedures. Here, an open loop type of control is assumed.
If the goal is to reproduce a locomotive activity and to
investigate specific control strategies however, different
solutions are implemented according to the hypothesized control strategy. Some models estimate muscle activation levels by trial and error starting from data obtained by electromyographic measurements. Others impose the trajectories
of some segments or points and find the activations necessary to perform such a movement.

Because of the complications involved in modeling a
feedback based control system, such models are typically
used when only a small part of the body, such a single limb,
is investigated. In models of the entire locomotive apparatus quite often an open loop control is implemented.
Because of the absence of feedback, these models have the
significant limitation of not being able to compensate for
errors, which are both numerical as well as due to the muscle activations considered. This makes cyclic movements,
like the ones used for locomotion, not perfectly repeatable
from cycle to cycle. For this reason most of the models
loose their balance after few motion cycles.

Important aspects of human motor control are the neural delays, as well as the fact that coordinated movements are performed. The expression coordinated movements refers to the simultaneous movement of all the body segments through their trajectories. To perform a coordinated movement is significantly different and much more difficult than sequentially moving multiple joints from their initial to final configurations, as it is commonly done in robotics or with upper extremity prostheses. The task of controlling such coordinated movements appears even more difficult when it is considered that the action of each muscle effects the entire system. This can be seen if the system of equations representing the direct dynamic problem is considered [10].

$$\{\ddot{q}\} = [M]^{-1}(\{F\} + \{G\} + \{B\})\qquad(3\text{-}2)$$

Focusing the attention only on the effects of the actuators

$$\{\ddot{q}\}_F = [M]^{-1}\{F\}\qquad(3\text{-}3)$$

Decomposing the actuation vector to show the contribution of each muscle

$$\{F\} = \sum_i \{F\}_i\qquad(3\text{-}4)$$

The accelerations of body segments produced by each muscle are therefore

$$\{\ddot{q}\}_{F_i} = [M]^{-1}\{F\}_i\qquad(3\text{-}5)$$

Even if the vector $\{F\}_i$ will have only two or three non zero terms corresponding to the segments on which the specific muscle applies a moment, the matrix $[M]^{-1}$ is generally a full matrix. it therefore produces a vector of segmental accelerations $\{\ddot{q}\}_{F_i}$ with mostly non zero terms.

All these complexities, added to the fact that the neurological motor control is still one of the less known aspects of the human body, make the creation of accurate representations of the human locomotive system very difficult. Notwithstanding all the necessary simplifications, the neuro-muscolo-skeletal models offer an invaluable way to simulate possible control strategies, the effects of pathological conditions, and eventual ways to correct them, and

can offer significant insights on the human system.  They
have been successfully used to quantify the influence of
individual gait determinants on the ground reaction forces
generated during normal, level walking; to investigate the
possibility of functional neuromuscolar stimulation; and to
optimize specific movements.

3.4 Example: a three dimensional simulation of single support
     In 1989, Pandy and Berme presented a three dimensional
model to simulate the entire single leg support of normal
level walking [11][12].

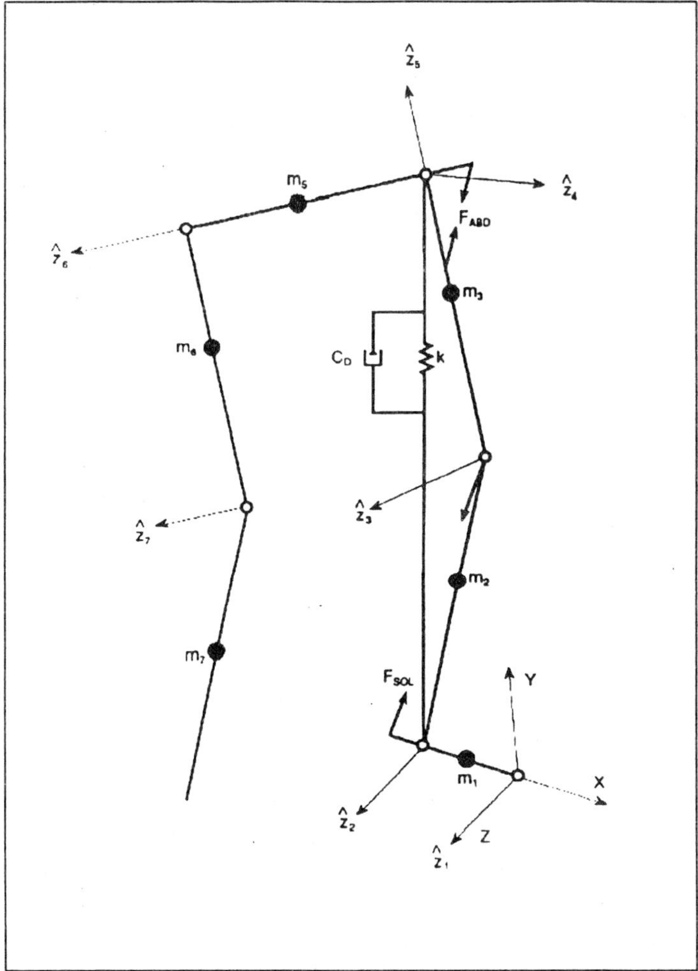


Figure 3-1: A 6-link, 7 DOF, 3D model for simulating the dynamics of the
     single-leg support phase of normal level walking [11][12].

In this model the skeletal system of the lower limbs is represented by a six-link, seven-degree-of-freedom, three-dimensional linkage, and the articulations are modeled by frictionless revolute joints (Figure 3-1). Since the ankle joint is represented by a single degree of freedom, this model possesses only five of the six determinants of gait. Here, it should be noted that in order to allow the lateral displacement of the pelvis, it is in fact necessary to include in the model the degree of freedom representing the ankle inversioneversion. The upper body is modeled by a lumped mass at the pelvic level with the assumption that its motion do not contribute significantly to the overall dynamic behavior of the system. The muscular system is modeled by ideal torque generators acting on every joint. Also present are two single-joint muscles modeled as ideal force actuators. One of these muscles represents a hip abductor, while the another provides the ankle plantarflexion action upon the stance limb by generating a force between a point below the knee and the heel.

Also present during the initial stance phase, from opposite toe-off to heel-off, is a linear massless, damped spring placed between the hip and the ankle. This element is introduced to reproduce the flexion-extension characteristic of the stance knee. After heel-off, this is substituted by a damped torsional spring at the knee joint.

The joint moments and the muscle forces to produce the motion are given as inputs of the simulation. The authors grossly designed them by trial and error to reproduce segmental motions and realistic ground reaction forces. This approach supposes an open loop control strategy of the movements.

The purposes of the simulations performed using this model were two: to show that it is possible to generate a gait cycle with very simple actuators and controls, and to quantify the influence of individual gait determinants on the ground reaction forces generated during normal, level walking. The influence of the gait determinants was studied by selectively reducing the degrees of freedom of the model to simulate pathological conditions, where one or more determinants of gait are missing.

The simulations performed using this model suggest that pelvic list is not as dominant a dynamic determinant as either stance knee flexionextension or foot and knee interaction.  Specifically, the first peak in the vertical reaction force appears to be primarily due to the stance knee flexionextension while the second peak is the result of the plantarflexor muscle activity.  Transverse pelvic rotation appears to make an important contribution by limiting the magnitude of the horizontal ground reaction prior to opposite heel strike.

This model is a very simplified representation of the human locomotive apparatus.  Not all the determinants on gait are included and the effects of the motion of the upper body is neglected.  While these are common simplifications made when modeling the human gait, they are nevertheless significant.  Moreover, in this model the complex muscular system is reduced to a series of ideal force and torque generators, without considering the complex dynamic behavior of muscles and tendons.  Yet, even in its simplicity this model proved to be very able to offer significant insight into the influence of body segmental motion during human walking.


## 4. FUTURE DEVELOPMENTS IN MODELING AND SIMULATION OF HUMAN LOCOMOTION

The modeling and simulation of human movement in general, and of locomotion in particular, still appear to be in their infancy.

Today's models are often a simplified representation of the human locomotive system.  Although this has various reasons, most importantly it is related to the lack of ability to effectively deal with complex models.  While a lot has yet to be discovered about the nervous system and how movements are controlled, there is a vast knowledge of the skeletal and muscular systems available to create more realistic models.  However, the inclusion of such knowledge brings with it a significant increase in the complexity of the models.

Since models and simulations are mostly implemented by using digital computers, their evolution as well as that of the programming and modeling software, will provide ever growing possibilities to effectively create more complex and realistic representations of the human body.

One significant practical limit of most of the current models is that they are not created in a modular way: it is very difficult to substitute one muscle or joint representation with another without a major time and coding effort. Software development technologies, like object oriented programming, or the use of more flexible simulation computer programs could help changing this, allowing models to grow in complexity without requiring to "reinvent the wheel" every time.

Significant improvements could also come from the evolution in measurement techniques. The ability to measure some of the now inaccessible variables of the human locomotive system would significantly improve the knowledge of how such apparatus works.

In the area of neurological motor control, the use of artificial neural networks appears to be very promising. While few studies have yet been made to adapt the classical forms of artificial neural networks to represent more realistically the dynamics of the human nervous system, they have the potential to offer a new approach to the difficult quest for a better understanding of motor control.


## REFERENCES


1. Nigg, B.M. (1994), "General comments about modelling", in *Biomechanics of the musculo-skeletal system*, ed. B.M. Nigg and W. Herzog, John Wiley & Sons.
2. Karplus, W.J. (1976), "The spectrum of mathematical modeling and systems simulation", in *Simulation of systems*, ed. L. Dekker, pp.5-13, Delft.
3. Hatze, H. (1990), "Synthesis of Human Motion", in *Biomechanics of Human Movement*, ed. N. Berme and A. Cappozzo, Bertec, Columbus, OH.
4. Herzog, W and Leonart, T.R (1991), "Validation of Optimization Models that Estimate the Forces Exerted by Synergistic Muscles", *Journal of Biomechanics*, 24(S1): pp. 31-39.
5. Nigg, B.M. and van den Bogert, A.J. (1994), "Simulation", in Biomechanics of the musculo-skeletal system, ed. B.M. Nigg and W. Herzog, John Wiley & Sons, 1995.
6. Hill, A.V. (1938), "The Heat of Shortening and the Dynamic Constants of Muscle", *Proceedings of the Royal Society*, 126(B): pp. 136-195.

7. Saunders, M., Inman, V.T. and Eberhart, H.D. (1953), The major determinants in normal and pathological gait, *The Journal of Bone and Joint Surgery*, 35-A: pp. 543-58.
8. Pedotti, A., Krishnan, V.V., and Starke, L. (1978), "Optimization of Muscle-force Sequencing in Human Locomotion", *Mathematical Bioscience,* 38: pp. 57-76.
9. Herzog, W. (1987), "Individual Muscle Force Estimation Using a nonlinear Optimal Design", *Journal of Neuroscience Methods*, 21, pp. 167-179.
10. Zajac, F.E. and Gordon, M.E. (1989), "Determining muscle's force and action in multi-articular movement", *Exercise and Sport Science Reviews*, ed. K Pandolf, Williams & Wilkins, Baltimore, MD, 17, pp. 187-230.
11. Pandy, M.G. and Berme, N. (1989a), "Quantitative assessment of gait determinants during single stance via a three-dimensional model - Part 1. Normal gait", *Journal of Biomechanics*, 22: pp. 717-24.
12. Pandy, M.G. and Berme, N. (1989b), "Quantitative assessment of gait determinants during single stance via a three-dimensional model - Part 2. Pathological gait", *Journal of Biomechanics*, 22: pp. 725-33.

# SOME THEORETICAL AND PRACTICAL ASPECTS
# OF MODELLING AND SIMULATION OF
# THE HUMAN MUSCULOSKELETAL SYSTEM


**M. Dietrich, K. Kedzior and C. Rzymkowski**

**Warsaw University of Technology, Warsaw, Poland**


## ABSTRACT


The aim of this revue is to set the information about the fundamental aspects of application of the mathematical modelling and computer simulation in biomechanics of human movement. The typical steps taken in this process are presented (Fig. 1). Computer assisted methods of formulation of the mathematical models of the human musculoskeletal system and computer aided methods of collecting and processing of the experimental data are discussed.


## 1. INTRODUCTION

Modelling has always been one of the fundamental methods applied to scientific investigations. Due to real object complexity (especially in living organisms), and a complex nature of their activity (e.g. locomotion), the necessity for experimental investigations of theoretical research into simplified substitutes (called models) of the real objects arises and this trend will probably remain unchanged.

Sometimes, the material model of real object is designed at the preliminary stage of experimental investigations. We can mention here some typical examples; e.g., manually operated biomechanical model of a gymnast on a high bar made of wood, rubber bands and strings investigated by Bauer [1], or epoxy resin models of vertebrae of the human lumbar spine used by Dietrich and Kurowski [6,7] for experimental verification of the hypothesis of mechanical causes of spondylolysis.

However, a basic research method employed nowadays in biomechanics of the human motion is abstract modelling, usually realised in terms of computer simulation. Transformation of a physical model into a mathematical one is therefore required, which can be easily converted then into a computer coded (analog or, more often, digital) simulation model.

Abstract modelling, i.e. the formulating of a model [38], may be considered an art, since not only knowledge and experience but also the researcher's intuition is here of crucial importance. Intuition is most important at the initial stage of modelling, when - having in mind the aim of research - the researcher makes decisions about a model type, structure, approximation level of the real object, etc., [18,19]. At that stage of modelling it is much more suitable to deal with a model, form of which is close to the real (material) one, i.e., the physical model. The physical model of real object is an abstract system composed of physical parameters (e.g., mass, stiffness, damping) chosen on the basis of a known or presumed structure and operation of the real system, considering also both internal and environmental interactions.

Nowadays, a majority of research works into biomechanics are carried out by means of computer simulation. This trend has been accelerated by a substantial improvement of performance, widespread availability as well as relatively low exploitation costs of computers, observed in the past decade, and the availability of universal software of straightforward utility (user-friendly), especially in the field of computer graphics [5]. Therefore, below we will discuss only this method of modelling.

Figure 1 shows typical steps taken in the process of abstract modelling. Formulating of a physical model (idealisation), as mentioned above, is one of the tasks, which must be performed by the researcher himself. Professional software packages (systems), available nowadays, assist the researcher when transforming the physical model to a mathematical one (formalisation) and then in conversion into a computer code (programming). However, the analysis of simulation results consisting in estimation of their predictive value and, what is of crucial importance, proving the modelling steps validity, has to be carried out by the researcher himself ("user" in Fig. 1). It seems that "idealisation", "prediction" and "validation" will remain duties of the scientists for good.


## 2. MODEL TYPES AND THEIR DESIGN

Two basic types of physical models can be distinguished: models of concentrated parameters (e.g., mass, stiffness, damping) and those of distributed parameters.

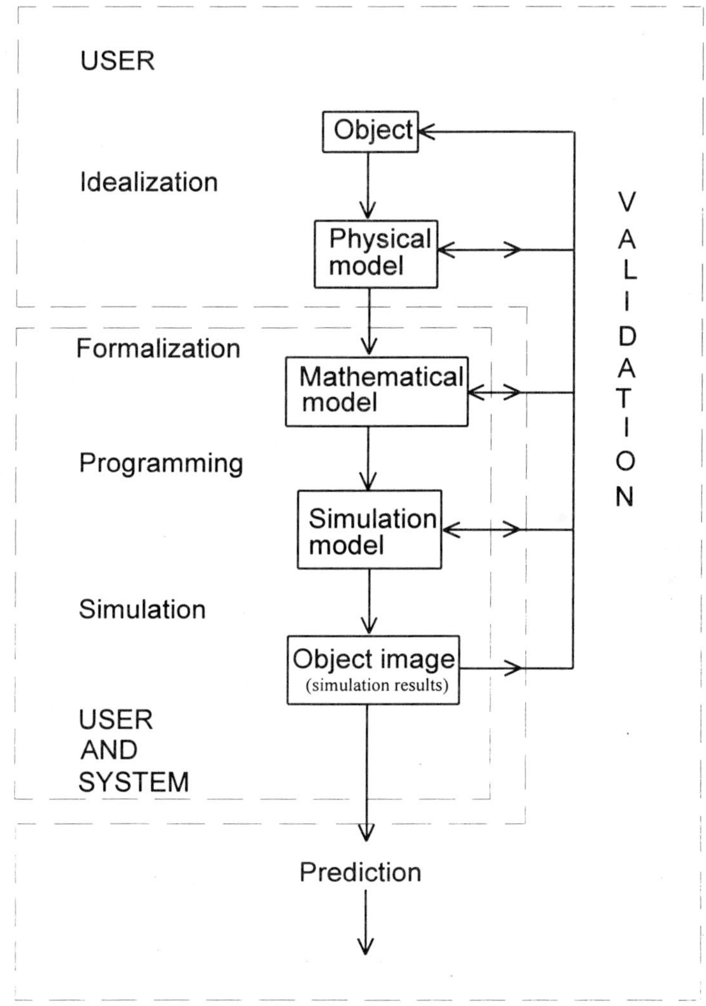


Fig. 1. Block diagram of abstract modelling and simulation

Models of the first type predominate in biomechanics of human body motion. Ordinary differential equations or combined differential and algebraic set of equations represent such models. The first case refers to the situation, where the physical model consists of one rigid element (concentrated mass, [4,20,21]) or several rigid elements connected by kinematic pairs into a simple [15,25] or branched [2,3,34] open kinematic chain. In the second case, when the physical model contains one or more closed kinematic chains [26] it is necessary to employ additional algebraic equations for the phenomenon to be accounted for.

A majority of the models used nowadays, except for the simplest cases when a biomechanical system is represented by one element only, have the form of the so-called multi-body systems. When formulating the equations of motion (i.e., designing the mathematical model) for such systems the principles of mechanics having the form of either differential (integral) variational principles or balance equations of inertial and active forces should be employed. Practical applications have proved that the latter one suits better to modelling of the multi-body systems. There are some balance equations used most often nowadays; i.e., Newton-Euler equations, Lagrange's equations, and becoming more and more applicable Kane's equations [31].

For systems with a small number of degrees of freedom (1÷3) the set of equations of motion can be formulated straightforward (e.g. writing on a sheet of paper). This approach has, however two main disadvantages, it is very toilsome and prone to the errors, being very difficult to avoid when transforming a large number of mathematical expressions. Therefore special computer programs are widely applied to formulation of the equations of motion.

The following two approaches should be mentioned here. The first one, called symbolic manipulation consists generally in direct imitation of real, manual operations by means of the appropriate computer programs, which generate automatically the analytic expressions, being fragments of the equations of motion. The user has only to enter the structure data (division of the modelled system into elements and their arrangements) and parameters of the system (geometry, mass, etc.). While formulating the symbolic equations computer introduces some simplifications at the same time (e.g. reduction of similar terms, etc.). Basic advantage of the symbolic method consists in the fact that for one physical model the equations have to be formulated only once and then can be applied many times to solving both direct and inverse problems of mechanics (see Section 3). The main disadvantage, in turn, is a huge RAM usage, which imposes a serious limitation on the method application, especially when dealing with systems with a large number of degrees of freedom and having microcomputers at one's disposal.

The second approach i.e. numerical formulation of the equations of motion consists in designing the algorithm, which calculates numerical values of the adequate terms, without storing their analytical form in a computer memory. Therefore, even when solving one problem, the process of equations formulation is repeated many times. However, since all operations are done on numbers the process is swift. A basic advantage of the method is the fact that it allows systems with larger number of degrees of freedom to be modelled, still having microcomputer of small RAM at one's disposal.

Thus, when it is necessary to formulate the equations of motion representing a biomechanical multi-body system one should consider the possibility of using an available package of computer programs for assistance in completing such a task. The package usually facilitates also both solving the equations and presentations of the results obtained, using modern computer graphics (diagrams, animation, etc. [5]). The world software market offers nowadays a rich variety of such packages, applicable both to big and fast computers (main-frame type) and microcomputers [36].

MACSYMA (a package suitable for generation of equations of motion in symbolic form) [32] and DADS (a numerical package) [13] are among those, which have been first to win renown. Most popular packages (including short operational description of each of them), as well as the list of most important items of the literature devoted to the analysis of multi-body systems are presented in paper [35] and monograph [36].

Specialised systems were developed for solving simulation tasks in case of impact loading conditions. MADYMO-3D [27] is a good example of such systems.

One of the advanced Polish packages is CAMIR [33]. It enables symbolic generation of the equations of motion in terms of Lagrange's equations for both open and closed kinematic chains.

The physical models of second type, i.e. those of distributed parameters can be either transformed into mathematical models having the form of partial differential equations or one of the equivalent numerical methods should be employed; i.e., the Finite Element Method (FEM) or the Boundary Element Method (BEM). Such models are used when describing motion of human body fluids, tensions and deformations in the human musculoskeletal system, tensions and deformations of lungs during the respiration process, etc. Particularly, the FEM has become lately more and more popular in modelling of the musculoskeletal system. The following, main advantages of the FEM should be mentioned:

- It is easy to represent spatial musculoskeletal system and model its spatial elements (bones, vertebrae, ribs, intervertebral disks, muscles, ligaments);
- It is possible to examine static, dynamical and stability problems appearing in the system under various everyday life and emergency conditions (norm, pathology, work, sport, etc.);
- It is possible to adopt different optimisation criteria when modelling the way of muscle tension control realised by the human nervous system (See Section 4);
- It is easy to change both geometrical and mechanical parameters of the model.

The FEM is widely applied in mechanical engineering [41]. However, when modelling the musculoskeletal system some adjustments reflecting some specific properties of the biological objects should be introduced. Primarily, it should be taken into consideration that:

- Materials of bones, ligaments and muscles are anisotropic, and therefore the main direction of stiffness (e.g. the direction of muscle fibbers), for which the experimental data are known best, changes its orientation;
- Values of stiffness parameters for bones, e.g., the Young's modulus ($10000 \div 15000$ MN/m$^2$) are much higher then the corresponding ones for intervertebral discs, muscles and ligaments ($0.4 \div 160$ MN/m$^2$), which results in wrong conditioning of the final system of equations representing the musculoskeletal system;
- Muscle tension is caused not only by the change in a distance between intersections (the so-called tension passive component) but also by the activation controlled by the nervous system (tension active component);
- Nuclei pulposi of intervertebral discs and the abdominal cavity are almost incompressible;
- Limb joints, intervertebral discs and rib cage joints impose constraints upon the relative movements of bones, vertebrae and ribs;
- Pressures in the nuclei pulposi of intervertebral discs, abdominal cavity and rib cage are of non-conservative character.

None of the FEM packages available in the market allows meeting of all the requirements mentioned above (e.g. [14]). We were therefore forced to create our own FEM package allowing all the requirements to be satisfied [8,9,10,11,12,23].

To complete our discussion, we should also mention another type of models used in the human muscle system modelling, i.e. "black box" models describing interaction between the activation reaching the muscle along the neural way (input signal) and the force exerted by the muscle (output signal), accounting at the same time for the length and velocity of the muscle contraction. These models are mainly applied to interpretation of the measurement results of dynamic biomechanical characteristics of main human muscle groups. A sample model is presented in papers [22,24].


## 3. TASKS OF MODELLING

The typical problems investigated within the framework of the human musculoskeletal system can be divided into two classes of tasks:
- investigation of big motions of the organism, in which considerable amplitudes of angles of rotation appear in joints (e.g. during locomotion, manipulations, physical work process, etc.);
- examination of small dislocations, deformations of body elements and their internal tension affected by the external loads and inertial forces.

Sometimes, both these tasks should be completed at the same time.

The problems of the first type are usually solved employing the multi-body system models, which however can be realised in two ways. The first one consists in formulating and solving the so-called direct problem of mechanics. Knowing the physical model of human body (or man-machine system) and the set of external and muscular loads acting upon it, we can formulate and then solve (analytically or numerically) equations representing the mathematical model. Trajectories of the body motion and/or its parts are obtained after solving the direct problem of mechanics.

Knowing from experiment the kinematic parameters of motion (see Section 5) we can formulate the so-called inverse problem of mechanics (i.e. the second one of the ways mentioned above), which aims at determination of the muscular forces (force moments). Thus, the question how the central nervous system controls the motion act considered can be answered indirectly. It is also possible to assume kinematic parameters of motion (trajectories, velocities and accelerations of the body elements), and then employ the method of inverse problem of mechanics and provide an answer to the question how the central nervous system should control the motion act considered, for the required kinematic parameters of the motion to be achieved.

The problems appearing in the second class of tasks (small dislocations and deformations) are usually solved using the FEM-type models, in which the direct problems predominate, i.e. dislocations and tensions caused by the action of known external forces should be determined. The inverse problem, i.e. determination of the forces affecting the analysed distribution of tensions and deformations in body elements, except for some very simple cases has no explicit solution. Therefore, additional information about forces (e.g. the specifying nature - concentrated, distributed or kind - inertial, real, etc.) is necessary.


## 4. OPTIMISATION

Sometimes, when solving both direct or inverse problem, it may be necessary to apply at the same time optimisation procedure to analysis of the human musculoskeletal system.

Optimisation in biomechanics consists in finding the best solution for a chosen criterion when completing a given physical task. Similarly as in the other fields, two approaches can be taken when dealing with optimisation problems in biomechanics; i.e., parametric optimisation and functional optimisation.

Numerical values of one or more parameters, e.g. the values of joint angles of the upper limb representing the position of hand in the working space, which ensures the lowest moments of muscular forces [25] are obtained in result of the parametric optimisation. On the other hand, time functions result from the functional optimisation, e.g. the histories (time courses) of angles describing the posture of a ski jumper during flight, which allows him to reach the maximal jump distance [15]. In most tasks carried out in biomechanics of the human motion the second approach should be taken, which, however, is very difficult to follow successfully.

Besides the mathematical model discussed above (see Sections 1 and 2), a formal (mathematical) description of each task has to comprise also a merit criterion (also called the objective function) of the process to be optimised (maximised or minimised). When optimisation is employed for improving the motion technique in sport, this criterion is usually established for maximisation of the result, e.g., minimal time of a certain distance run, maximal lifted weight, etc. In many cases, however maximisation of the sport results may be most important but not the only criterion of optimisation of a given motion. The following criteria are also often taken into consideration; e.g., minimisation of a competitor's work during a long-lasting motion (long distance run, cycling, rowing, etc.), minimisation of loads in joints and tendons (jumps, weight lifting, etc.). When several merit criteria have to be considered simultaneously we deal with the multi-criterial optimisation.

Solving optimisation problems is, except for some obvious cases, rather a difficult process to carry out. Usually, even when dealing with the parametric optimisation it is almost impossible to arrive at the analytical solution, some examples however do exist [28]. Therefore, most problems are solved numerically. Reviews of the applicable algorithms can be found in specialistic handbooks, there are also universal program packages available in the market (e.g. [17]).

In most optimisation tasks undertaken when analysing the human motion technique the functional optimisation approach should be followed. Moreover, since a large number of optimised constant or functional parameters (the so-called decisive variables) appear in these problems, the necessity for big and fast computers arises. Unilateral constraints i.e., those represented mathematically in terms of inequalities, pose serious obstacles to completing the optimisation tasks. Unfortunately, those constraints usually appear when solving optimisation problems in analysis of the human motion, e.g., the condition that a force (e.g. reaction between foot and base) or a moment (e.g. moment exerted by a group of flexor or extensor muscles) shall be of a certain sign (base cannot pull foot, muscles cannot push). When completing such an optimisation task application of the sequential gradient restoration algorithm (SGRA) [30] is recommended.

Another obstacle, often met when solving the optimisation problems in biomechanics is a large number of decisive variables, i.e. those affecting the value of optimised objective function (i.e. the function representing the optimality criterion). The objective function is then multi-dimensional, and often non-linear with respect to decisive variables. Its shape in multi-dimensional space reveals a large number of local extrema, which makes it difficult or sometimes even impossible to find a solution i.e., a set of decisive variables values, for which the objective function reaches its optimal value (minimal or maximal) by means of most popular nowadays gradient optimisation procedures. The stochastic procedure (Monte Carlo Method) appears to be most efficient in these cases, sample application is given in [25].

To complete our discussion the so-called inverse optimisation task, appearing also in biomechanics should be mentioned. When looking at some examples from the sport field the cases can be highlighted when it is assumed (having in mind, however, that this assumption might be false) that a sport champion's motion (registered e.g. on a film) has been executed optimally or at least perfectly (the so-called "master pattern"). For training purposes it could be helpful to have information on histories (time courses) of the resulting moments of muscular forces in joints of a champion, examining therefore his motion technique. In some cases such a formulation of task represents just the inverse problem of mechanics (i.e. known - kinematic motion parameters, searched - muscular force moments in joints). Sometimes, however, such problems cannot be explicitly solved since when executing the analysed motion the number of independent active muscle drives (groups) is greater than the number of driven degrees of freedom (according to the assumed model of competitor's body). In these cases the solution can sometimes be obtained after completing the kinematic data with time courses of some external forces in relation to parts of the champion's body (e.g. reactions between foot and base, foot and bicycle, gymnast's hand and bar, etc.). It enables some searched muscular forces (moments of forces) to be determined from additional equations. When such data are not available the task can be completed only by assuming a certain additional optimisation (merit) criterion, i.e. this "adopted" by the champion. The inverse problem of mechanics transforms then into an optimisation task.

Observations show, that the way of human muscles co-operation depends of various physiological factors and, if any, on pathological changes, which can be clearly seen when comparing the actions performed by a child and a grown up person. Training improves the co-operation of muscles when performing the practised action. Physiological factors may cause chronic tensions in whole muscle groups and thus affect mechanical properties of the respective area. Such protection is very often realised by muscles of the lumbar-sacral spine, in which tension called the protective contracture appears. It seems that the way of muscle control depends also on the conditions under which those actions are performed. For example, the action when the subject is frightened considerably increases the human motoric efficiency, manifesting itself in a speed and precision of the action, there arises also the possibility for developing muscle forces the magnitudes of which exceed considerably those appearing in every day motoric activity. Strong irritation affects increased muscle tension. State of health, fatigue, time of the day and season, as well as emotions evoked by the action performed are also important. The above considerations show that it is extremely difficult to give accurate description in terms of mathematical relationships of such a complex operation of the human muscle and practically even impossible without having more detailed information.

A literature survey shows that most often it is assumed that the nervous system controls muscles following a certain optimisation algorithm, i.e. the organism tries to minimise any unfavourable effects or maximise the favourable ones. Optimisation criteria (objective functions) are presented in details in monograph [37] and paper [9].


## 5. COMPUTER AIDED EXPERIMENTAL INVESTIGATIONS

Usually, the experiments should be carried out first, when the input data for a numerical simulation model of the human motion are to be obtained (e.g. for solving the inverse problem of mechanics - see Section 3). These investigations, however are labour- and time- consuming, especially at the stage of analysis and processing of the results obtained into a form applicable to a numerical model. The computer assistance is therefore necessary.

There are much more computer programs available, which have been designed to assist the researcher in biomechanical experimental investigations, than those applicable to modelling and simulation. The main reason for this lies in the same ranges of signal amplitudes and frequencies appearing both in biomechanics and engineering, and therefore typical software applicable to numerical results (the so-called time series) processing can be used.

Typical signals registered in biomechanics are: displacements (linear and angular), forces (force moments) and electromyograms, which in fact are continuous functions of time. Using an analog to digital converter (A/D) we obtain a digital form of these functions comprising the values (samples) at a given number of points of a time interval. The sampling frequency should be selected carefully: too high values of it demand for a big computer memory and require time-consuming calculations, while too low values enable some information represented in the signal to be lost. Most signals, after being registered, undergo the following processing: smoothing (filtration), differentiation once or two times (in the case of displacements for velocities and accelerations to be obtained), spectral analysis (especially of electromyograms), statistical analysis and presentation of results.

All the signal registered should be filtered for the noise signals to be attenuated, which result from both measurement errors and disturbances. The way of sampling may introduce high frequency noises into the signal registered (this also is the reason for choosing moderate sampling frequencies). When the signal should undergo differentiation, filtration shall be done first, since even small noises interfering with the original signal are being amplified substantially when differentiated.

One of the filtration method, however not applied very often is the Fourier Transform, which enables the signal components of given frequencies (being known from other sources as not contributing to the signal under investigation) to be separated (e.g. higher harmonics cut-off) with a reasonable accuracy.

There are, however, several more popular methods:

- Fitting calculus, relatively effective and fast tool, applicable on-line, especially when during measurement there arises the necessity for derivatives of the measured signal to be known, e.g. for control purposes;
- Approximation in terms of SPLINE functions, becoming more and more popular nowadays, very fast in the cases when the measured signal should be filtered and derivatives of the required order should be calculated. These methods are slower, however, in comparison to fitting calculus methods, on the other hand they enable proper control of the smoothing quality and precise assessment of the differentiation errors;
- Polynomial approximation, applied often in the cases when the researcher wants the investigated signal to be represented by one function only over the whole time interval.

The Fast Fourier Transform (FFT) algorithm, being a more efficient modification of the Fourier Transform method is most often applied to analysis of electromyograms. This method enables suitable grouping of arithmetical operations for their sequence to be changed, which reduces a number of floating point calculations many times and therefore the time of computation is considerably shorter, even for samples of huge sizes.

In practice, when applying one of the methods given above the researcher should only use one of the relevant computer packages being available, since writing a program for each case is very laborious task and the experience is also of crucial importance.

There are several universal packages available when dealing with such problems, e.g., MATLAB and DADiSP.

The first one is designed for analysis of automatic control systems, enabling at the same time data smoothing, calculating the FFT and statistical analysis. A good quality of the results presentation is also ensured (depending, of course, on the graphical display equipment).

The latter one (DADiSP) can be applied, first of all, to signal analysis, having great capabilities. It is a multi-window system, in which the signals processed can undergo many mathematical operations, and the information may be transmitted from one window to another. A very good graphical presentation quality is also ensured.

Many graphical packages, e.g., AXUM, GRAPHER and SURFER (the last two very popular), enable presentation of the processed data, as well as determination of the regression curves coefficients and statistical parameters of the analysed data set.

Some universal packages, e.g. the user-friendly DERIVE of simple hardware configuration requirements, or one of the biggest packages MATHEMATICA [39], enable straightforward realisation of the data processing, even those very complex. The MATHEMATICA system enables also formulation of very complex programs in terms of procedures included in the library supplied, using a special language. These programs can be designed for data processing and their graphical presentation, employing 3D effects and advanced graphical display hardware, including the PostScript printers.

Wide possibilities open up when employing the specialistic libraries of procedures realising the functions used in one's own program. The program can therefore, after some straightforward operations, meet satisfactorily the requirements imposed having capabilities comparable with those of known packages. The "Science and Engineering Tools" library proposed by Quin-Curtis (USA) seems to be very interesting. It is compatible with most popular both Microsoft (FORTRAN, C, Basic) and Borland (Turbo C, Turbo Pascal) compilers. This low-price library contains a large number of procedures for statistical analysis, data smoothing, Fourier analysis, matrix operations, numerical differentiation and integration. It has also great graphical capabilities (2D and 3D graphics, drivers for different graphical cards, printers and plotters, as well as optional HPGL and PostScript output formats).

Very useful libraries are available also at universities (usually with no charge for scientific purposes), e.g. the GCVSPL [40] is very popular among researchers in the field of biomechanics.


# 6. CONCLUSIONS

Basing on the presented review one can conclude that the methods for modelling and numerical simulation of the human musculoskeletal system applied nowadays limit the number of biological aspects accounted for. The models are usually worked out mainly (and sometimes solely) on the basis of principles of mechanics. Generally, they do not reflect or give only vague description of the processes typical for biological phenomena; e.g., physiological aspects of the decision process realised by the central nervous system, controlling of the motion of separated muscles or the whole body, fatigue of the living tissue, growth and remodelling of the living bone tissue ( a very interesting series of papers [29]), etc. Therefore one can predict that in future the development of the musculoskeletal system modelling will demand formulation of models of non-stationary phenomena in terms of random processes and fuzzy sets theories. Thus the prospects of future research are very interesting and vast.

## 7. ACKNOWLEDGEMENT

The study has been supported by the Polish State Research Committee, grant No 3 P 401 026 06.

## REFERENCES

1. Bauer W.L.: A manually operated biomechanical model of an internally energized self-oscillatory system, Winter D.A. et al. (eds.), Biomechanics IX-B, Human Kinetics Pub., Champaign, Illinois, 1985, 383-388.

2. Borowski S., Dietrich M., Kędzior K., Rzymkowski C., Zagrajek T.: Modelling of dynamic loads acting upon the human-operator musculoskeletal system, Proc. VIII World Congress on Theory of Machines and Mechanisms, Prague 1991, 3, 781-784.

3. Borowski S., Dietrich M., Kędzior K., Rzymkowski C.: Simulating model of man-operator in emergency situation, Lecture Notes of the ICB Seminar, International Center of Biocybernetics, Warsaw 1992, 10, 27-37.

4. Czyżkowski T.M., Kędzior K., Macukow B.: Biomechanical factors in design of bobsled and luge run, Jonsson B. (ed.), Biomechanics X-B, Human Kinetics Pub., Champaign, Illinois, 1987, 785-789.

5. Delp D., Delp S.: Understanding human movement with computer graphics, SOMA, Engineering for the Human Body, 1989, 3, 3, 17-25.

6. Dietrich M., Kurowski P.: The importance of mechanical factors in the etiology of spondylolysis; A model analysis of loads and stress in human lumbar spine, Spine, 1985, 10, 6, 532-542.

7.  Dietrich M., Kurowski P.: On the mechanical properties of lumbar spine, Bautista E. et al. (eds.), The Theory of Machines and Mechanisms, Pergamon Press, Oxford 1987, 3, 1861-1864.

8.  Dietrich M., Kędzior K., Zagrajek T.: Finite element method analysis of human spine segment, De Groot G. et al. (eds.) Biomechanics XI-A, Free University Press, Amsterdam 2988, 333-337.

9.  Dietrich M., Kędzior K., Zagrajek T.: Modelling of muscle action and stability of the human spine, Witners J.M., Woo S.L-Y. (eds.), Multiple Muscle Systems, Biomechanics and Movement Organization, Springer-Verlag, New York 1990, 451-460.

10. Dietrich M., Kędzior K., Zagrajek; T.: A. biomechanical model of the human spinal system, Proc. Intstn. Mech. Eng., Part H. Journal of Eng. in Medicine, 1991, 205, 19-26.

11. Dietrich M., Kędzior K., Miller K., Zagrajek T.: Computer simulation of discopathy treatment, U. Stanič, T. Bajd (eds.), Proc. 7th Int. Conf. Mechanics Med. Biol., Ljubljana-Pörtschach, 1991, 49-50.

12. Dietrich M., Kędzior K., Zagrajek T.: Biomechanical modelling of human spine system, Lecture Notes of the ICB Seminar, International Center of Biocybernetics, Warsaw 1992, 10, 38-59.

13. Haug E.J.: Computer Aided Kinematics of Mechanical Systems, Vol.1, Basic Methods, Allyn and Bacons, Boston, 1989.

14. Haug E.J.: Biomechanical models in vehicle accident simulation, PAM User Meeting, Nov.7, San Diego 1995.

15. Hubbard M., Komor A.: Optimal ski flight mechanics, 7th Biomechanical Engineering Symposium, Univ. of California, Davis, 1989, 12-13.

16. de Jalón Javier G., Bayo E.: Kinematic and Dynamic Simulation of Multibody Systems - The Real-Time Challenge, Springer-Verlag, New York, 1994.

17. Jennings L.S., Fisher E., Teo K.L., Goh C.J.: MISER3 Optimal Control Software; Theory and User Manual, EMCOSS Pty Ltd., 7 Topaz Place, Carine, WA 6020, Australia, 1990.

18. Kędzior K., Komor A., Maryniak J., Morawski J.: Methodological and cognitive aspects of modelling and computer simulation in biomechanics, Biology of Sport, 1988, 5, Suppl. 1, 5-27.

19. Kędzior K., Komor A., Maryniak J., Morawski J.: Modelling and computer simulation in biomechanics, Lecture Notes of the ICB Seminar, International Center of Biocybernetics; Warsaw, 1989, 5, 50-77.

20. Kędzior K., Macukow B., Ostrowski J.: Computer simulation of bobsled and luge downhill run, Biology of Sport, 1988, 5, Suppl. 1, 92-107.

21. Kędzior K., Macukow B., Ostrowski J.: Safety problems in bobsled and luge run design, De Groot G., et al. (eds.), Biomechanics XI-B, Free University Press, Amsterdam, 1988, 874-877.

22. Kędzior K., Lackowski J.: Simulation model of a skeletal muscle, Lectures Notes of the ICB Seminar, Intern. Center of Biocybernetics., Warsaw, 1992, 10, 97-107.

23. Kędzior K., Miller K., Zagrajek T.: Computer simulation of discopathy treatment (initial study), Lecture Notes of the ICB Seminar, Intern. Center of Biocybernetics, Warsaw, 1992, 10, 108-118.

24. Kędzior K., Niwiński W., Wit A.: Investigation and modelling of human muscle groups, Lecture Notes of the ICB Seminar, Intern. Center of Biocybernetics, Warsaw, 1992, 10, 119-126.

25. Kędzior K., Roman D., Rzymkowski C.: Modelling of upper extremity effort under static working conditions, Lecture Notes in Control and Information Sciences, Vol.187, Springer-Verlag, London 1993, 333-338.

26. Komor A., Kubań W., Parfianowicz L.: An improved model and computer simulation of cycling motion technique, Bergman G. et al., Biomechanics - Basic and Applied Research, Martinus Nijhoff Pub., Dordrecht 1987, 653-658.

27. MADYMO User's Manual 3D, TNO Road-Vehicles Research Institute, Delft, The Netherlands, 1992.

28. Maroński R.: An optimal running downhill on skis, J. Biomechanics, 1990, 23, 5, 435-439.

29. Mattheck C., Huber-Betzer H.: CAO - computer simulation of adaptive growth in bones and trees, K.H. Held et al. (eds.), Computers in Medicine, Computational Mechanics Publications, Southampton, Boston, 1991, 243-252.

30. Miele A.: Gradient algorithms for the optimization of dynamic systems; Leondes C.T. (ed.), Control and Dynamic Systems, Advances in Theory and Application, Academic Press, New York, 1980, 16, 1-32.

31. Nielan P.E., Kane T.R.: Symbolic generation of efficient simulation / Control routines for multi-body systems, Bianchi G., Schiehlen W. (eds.). Dynamics of Multibody Systems, Springer-Verlag, Berlin, Heidelberg. 1986, 153-164.

32. Rand R.H.: Computer Algebra in Applied Mathematics: An Introduction to MACSYMA, Pitman Publishing Inc., Boston, 1984.

33. Rzymkowski C.: A package of computer programs for equations of motion - biomechanics applications, Biology of Sport, 1988, 5, Suppl. 1, 188-192.

34. Rzymkowski C., Kędzior K.: Modelling and simulation of walking machine jump over obstacle, Proc. VIII CISM-IFToMM Symp. on Theory and Practice of Robots and Manipulators Ro.Man.Sy'90, Cracow, June 1990, 359-366.

35. Schwertassek R., Robertson R.E.: A perspective on computer oriented multibody dynamical formalism and their implementations, Bianchi G., Schiehlen W. (eds.), Dynamics of Multibody Systems, Springer-Verlag, Berlin, Heidelberg, 1986, 261-274.

36. Schiehlen W.: Multibody Systems Handbook, Springer-Verlag, Berlin, 1990.

37. Seireg A., Arvikar R.: Biomechanical Analysis of the Musculoskeletal Structure for Medicine and Sport, Hemisphere Publishing Co., New York, 1989.

38. Shtoff W.: Modelling and Philosophy, Izd. Nauka, Moscow-Leningrad, 1968 (in Russian).

39. Wolfram S.: Mathematica - A System for Doing Mathematics by Computer (2nd ed.). Addison Wesley Pub. Co., Redwood City, California 1991.

40. Woltring H.J.: A FORTRAN package for generalized, cross-validatory spline smoothing and differentiation. Advanced Engineering Software, 8, 2, Computational Mechanics Publications 1986, 104-113.

41. Zienkiewicz O.C., Taylor R.L.: The Finite Element Method, McGraw-Hill (fourth edition), London, 1991.

# A BIOMECHANICAL MODEL OF
# THE HUMAN MUSCULOSKELETAL SYSTEM


**K. Kedzior and T. Zagrajek**

**Warsaw University of Technology, Warsaw, Poland**



## ABSTRACT

The three-dimensional model of human musculoskeletal system consists of 45 rigid bodies (Fig. 1) connected by means of the spring-damper elements representing joints. The model is considered as a kinematic chain having about 270 degrees of freedom driven by 250 muscle actuators. The force-length-velocity characteristic of muscles as well as force-time characteristic (the rate of muscle force change due to the change of activation) are introduced into the model. The software package acts according to the block diagram shown in Fig. 8. It enables the muscle forces and reactive forces in joints to be determined from the registered (or assumed) kinematic data of human motion.


## 1. INTRODUCTION

The epidemiological data prove that a large number of people engaged in different types of physical activities suffer from various musculoskeletal system illnesses. That number includes not only labourers, i.e. those doing manual works, but also; e.g., nurses looking after bedridden people, surgeons, dentists, sportsmen and housewives. The computer operators should be noted here, being more the white- then the blue-collar workers, since their health is also affected by musculoskeletal diseases. Therefore the necessity arises for the research into biomechanics of motion to be pursued, focusing on the problem of loads to which the elements of human body (bones, muscles, tendons, intervertebral discs, etc.) are subject when performing various motion acts. This is the reason why a good model simulating the human musculoskeletal system is needed. Such a model should enable determination of the loads, under both static and dynamic conditions, to which all the elements of musculoskeletal system are subject, in order to predict all damages to human health likely to appear due to those loads.

The attempts at designing such models have been undertaken for many years, most of them, however, failed and no model satisfying all the requirements imposed has been designed yet. There are many biomechanical simulation models available in the software market nowadays, the majority of them, however, represent the human body as a system of rigid or flexible bodies connected by means of kinematic pairs (multi-body type of models). They are applied mainly to determination of the reactive forces and moments acting upon main human joints under the static [2,24] or dynamic [22,23] conditions, respectively. When applying those models, it is usually impossible to determine the forces developed by particular muscles, magnitudes of which should be known if the distribution of loads in all elements of the human body is to be assessed exactly. There is, however, the package [24] with the aid of which one can assess, under static conditions, the forces exerted by some muscles of the human trunk as well as the forces compressing certain intervertebral discs. There are also the software packages available, in which the Finite Element Method (FEM) [21] has been employed in designing a model of the human body [8]. They can be successfully applied when the stress distributions in some human tissues (e.g. bones, skin, eyes) are to be determined under huge dynamic loads (appearing e.g. in result of the car crash), i.e., in the cases when the body element loads due to muscle forces are negligible in comparison with the external and inertial forces. Therefore, these packages cannot be used when solving typical problems of biomechanics of work, in which the forces exerted by muscles determine the load distribution within the musculo-tendino-skeletal system.

On the other hand, some substantial limitations can be recognised also in the simulation models known from literature, i.e. those models, which may appear in a near future in the software market. The highest degree of development reveals the multi-body type model (skeleton represented in terms of rigid bodies driven by muscles) proposed by Seireg and Arvikar [14]. Using this model one can determine the forces in all human skeletal muscles under kineto-static conditions, i.e., the inertial forces cannot be determined by means of the procedures the model is supplied with; they can, however, be accounted for if their magnitudes are known, e.g. from experiment. Some simplifications, being of crucial importance to the results, have been assumed when designing this model. First, the problem of muscle co-operation has been solved (i.e. the forces exerted by particular muscles have been found) employing the linear programming (i.e. linear merit criteria). Furthermore, the force - length - velocity characteristics of muscles have not been introduced into the model. The linear programming approach affects considerably the simulation results, i.e. the solving algorithm is rather simply and the time of computing is much shorter, but on the other hand, the magnitudes of forces obtained are much too far from the reality. When adopting the linear optimisation criterion, the solution is arrived at, in which the forces exerted by many muscles are equal to zero; the only working muscles are those, which in the considered position of human body can exert in joints the moments of greatest magnitudes. This solution, however, is in contradiction to the experience (e.g. results of EMG measurements) and this is the reason why some researchers employ non-linear merit criteria (e.g. energetic [4] or soft saturation criterion [15]).

A sample application of another multi-body type model of the human upper extremity to ergonomic optimisation (under static conditions, non-linear merit criterion) of the work-space was presented in the paper [10]. An advanced multi-body type model of the human elbow joint complex (two-degree-of freedom system driven by eight muscle actuators) was presented in the paper [7]. The model can be applied both under static and dynamic conditions.

The FEM type model of the human trunk proposed by Dietrich et al. [3,4,5] enables the forces exerted by muscles of the human spinal system to be determined as well as the stress distributions in muscles and intervertebral discs. A non-linear merit criterion has been applied to solving the problem of muscle co-operation, which enabled more realistic results to be obtained. This model can be used, however, only when solving static [3,4,5] or kineto-static problems [1] or some selected issues of dynamics, e.g., man under vibration [6].

A new, original model of the human musculoskeletal system not suffering from the limitations mentioned above is presented below, being the result of developing the models presented before [11,12].

A physical model of the human musculoskeletal system consists of 45 rigid (non-deforming) bodies (Fig. 1) connected by means of the "spring - damper" elements representing joints. Therefore, this model can be considered as a biokinematic chain of the tree type with branches and closed loops having about 270 degrees of freedom, depending on the option of the feet-base or hands-base contact (e.g. if both feet are in contact with base, the closed loop appears in the model).

Rigid bodies represent the elements of human body being (e.g. bones) or those assumed as (spinal segments, feet, hands, etc.) much more stiff than the remaining ones (i.e., muscles, tendons, intervertebral discs, etc.). Unfortunately, the infinite stiffness being assumed does not allow the stress distribution inside the element to be determined.

Each rigid body is characterised in terms of its mass (sample data are shown in Table I) and inertial moments relative to the principal co-ordinate system. This system (its origin lies at the centre of mass, products of inertia vanish) will be called hereinafter the local system of a given body. It should be noted, however, that the assumption of products of inertia vanishing should be considered as a quite reasonable "practical" approximation. The local systems for particular rigid bodies were assumed in the way ensuring a straightforward mathematical description of the system, e.g. for long bones the $x$-axis always coincided with the long axis of the bone (see Fig. 1).

TABLE I

Inertial data of the rigid bodies representing chosen parts of the human body.

| Rigid element | Mass [kg] | $J_x$ [kgm$^2$] | $J_y$ [kgm$^2$] | $J_z$ [kgm$^2$] |
|---|---|---|---|---|
| Humerus | 1.90 | $1.19 \cdot 10^{-2}$ | $1.35 \cdot 10^{-3}$ | $1.35 \cdot 10^{-3}$ |
| Ulna | 0.65 | $3.97 \cdot 10^{-3}$ | $3.25 \cdot 10^{-4}$ | $3.25 \cdot 10^{-4}$ |
| Radius | 0.65 | $3.97 \cdot 10^{-3}$ | $3.25 \cdot 10^{-4}$ | $3.25 \cdot 10^{-4}$ |
| Wrist | $0.50 \cdot 10^{-2}$ | $1.00 \cdot 10^{-5}$ | $2.00 \cdot 10^{-6}$ | $2.00 \cdot 10^{-6}$ |
| Hand | 0.50 | $1.00 \cdot 10^{-3}$ | $2.00 \cdot 10^{-4}$ | $2.00 \cdot 10^{-4}$ |

## 2. PHYSICAL MODEL

Each rigid body has been assumed as having 6 degrees of freedom. Displacement of a given rigid body, i.e. all its points or those fixed on it - e.g. a marker introduced for the body motion registration purposes, can be expressed by three linear displacements of the body centre of mass within the local frame of reference and three angles of revolution about the local system axes. But this method can be applied only when describing the motion of a body or a point connected with it within a short time interval $\Delta t$. When considering the motion of a given point in longer time intervals a trajectory determined in the global system should be introduced. The trajectory is composed of short segments, each one of which is determined in the local system in the aforementioned way.

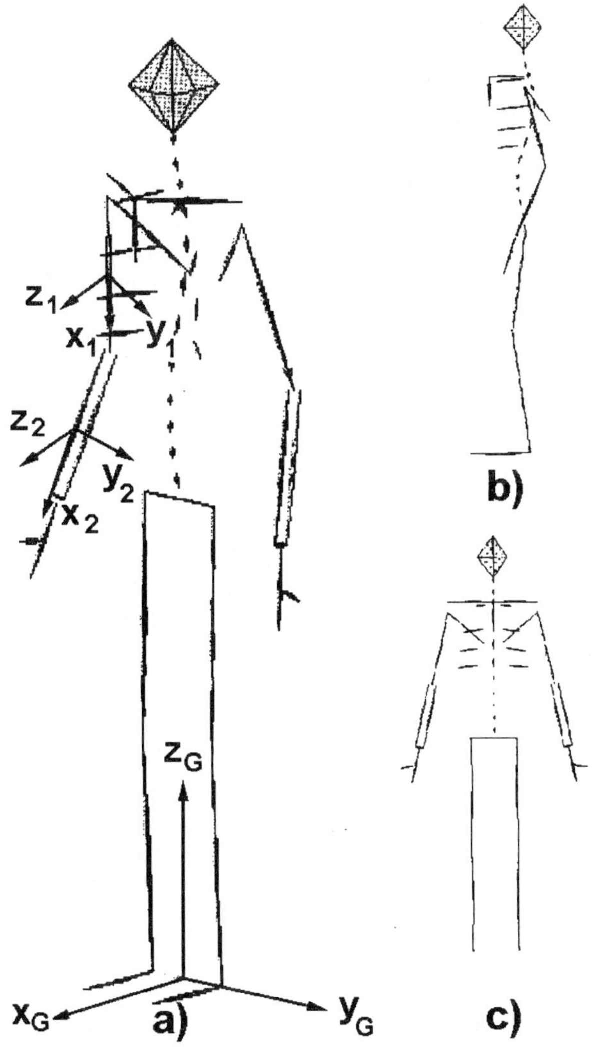



Fig. 1. Physical model of the human rigid bodies system: a) oblique, b) side and c) front views, respectively; the global ($x_G$, $y_G$, $z_G$) and a sample local ($x_1$, $y_1$, $z_1$ and $x_2$, $y_2$, $z_3$) co-ordinate systems marked out.

Each elastic and damping element ("spring-damper") representing a joint has the form of spring or beam.

Each element of the "spring - 6D" type connects two points of the two rigid bodies, co-ordinates of which in the global system are the same (it is assumed that the adjacent rigid bodies, when weightless and subject to neither external nor inertial forces have one point of contact only). The element is composed of the six "spring-damper" "sub-elements": three linear ones working in three perpendicular directions and three torsional (angular) ones. By assuming appropriate stiffness values for the springs forming a given element, different kinds of joints can be modelled; e.g., stiff junction fixing (6 springs of high stiffness), one degree-of-freedom hinge (5 springs very stiff and one angular of low stiffness), ball-and-socket joint (3 linear, very stiff springs and 3 angular of low stiffness), etc. Assuming appropriate length - force (or angle - torque) characteristics of the springs, both non-linear stiffness of the articular capsule and anatomic constraints of the motion in the joint can be taken into account. This approach enables the reactions in joints to be determined straightforward. The assumed values of damping coefficient of the "spring-damper" elements are very low and the only effect on simulation results they exert is smoothing the simulated motion act trajectory.

Simplified elements of the "spring - 3D" type (composed of the linear springs of high stiffness only) were employed when modelling the rigid body - marker fixing. The marker, as mentioned above enables registration of the human body motion. The approach simplifies the experimental data introduction to the simulation model. The motion of a given rigid body is explicitly determined by the trajectories (in the global or local system) of three markers, not collinear however, fixed on it.

Intervertebral discs, being flexible joints of rigid vertebrae (or rigid spinal segments) as well as the cartilages creating flexible joints of ribs and the sternum were represented in the model by elements of the "beam - 3D" type, being classical, often applied to engineering structures modelling 3D finite elements [20]. Each "beam - 3D" element has a given initial length and two nodes, each of them belongs both to this element and one of two adjacent rigid bodies being joined by it. Each node of the element has six degrees of freedom (3 linear and 3 angular displacements). Each element of the "beam - 3D" type can carry loads exerted by: compressive and tensile forces, bending moments acting in two perpendicular planes, torsional moments and shearing forces. The following parameters describe therefore mechanical properties of the element: tensile stiffness, bending stiffness (two different values assumed ·in two perpendicular planes), compressive and shearing stiffnesses, respectively. A mass per unit length and a damping coefficient, the value of which depends on a current mass and stiffness have been also assumed for each element.

Elements of the type "spar - 3D", being widely applied to modelling of engineering structures, were used when modelling ligaments and tendons (with long muscle tendons included). Each element has two nodes, belonging both to it and the adjacent rigid bodies being joined by this element. Each node has 3 degrees of freedom (linear displacements only). The "spar - 3D" element carries only tensile or compressive loads acting along the straight line connecting nodes. The following parameters describe the element: initial length l, mass per unit length, cross-sectional area A, tensile (compressive) stiffness (Young's modulus), and damping coefficient depending on mass and stiffness. The Young's modulus may be assumed constant or variable, depending on the sign and magnitudes of deformations; the element can therefore represent precisely e.g. non-linear characteristic of the tendon, tensile stiffness of which is significantly larger than the compressive one.

Rigid bodies connected by means of springs and beams form the structure (biomechanism) driven by muscles. A special modification of the "spar - 3D" element, called here the "active spar - 3D" element, being worked out, was applied to modelling of muscles. This element reveals all properties of the "spar - 3D" element but is additionally supplied with a generator of the tensile force acting upon it. The force appears due to activation modelling the stimulation from the nervous system. Therefore, the force exerted along a straight line connecting nodes (representing the insertions of a given muscle to the rigid body) can be treated as an algebraic sum of the following two components: passive component $F_p$ appearing due to changes in the muscle length (i.e. changes in the distance between insertions) and the active one $F_a$ appearing due to muscle activation.

The component $F_p$ represents passive deformation of the muscle tissue, the magnitude of which depends on the Young's modulus value being assumed for a given active "spar - 3D" element. As mentioned above, the Young's modulus may be considered as a non-linear function of the element elongation.

The magnitude of $F_a$ component at the instant t depends on: instantaneous muscle length l (i.e. the distance between insertions), instantaneous muscle contraction or elongation rate v and instantaneous value of activation u(t). The activation of given muscle u is considered as a current value of active component ratio to the maximal active component possible to exert by a given muscle at a given length and contraction or elongation rate, respectively. The activation $u$ is therefore a non-dimensional quantity taking values from the range $0 \leq u \leq 1$. The value of $u$ can be therefore considered as a ratio of the active (activated) muscle fibres number to the total number of fibres of a given muscle. From the skeletal muscles biomechanics it follows that the force - length characteristics (i.e. relations $F_a(l)$ at $v=const$ and $u=const$) as well as the force - velocity characteristics (i.e. relations $F_a(v)$ at $l=const$ and $u=const$) can be represented by algebraic functions, while the relation between $F_a$ and $u$ can be represented by a differential equation; ordinary differential equations of the first or second order are usually applied [9,18].

It has been assumed, after Kędzior and Lackowski [9] that the relation $F_a=F_a(l,v)$ at $u=const$ can be factorised. Additionally, to simplify the numerical calculations algorithm is has been assumed that the relation between $F_a$ and $u$ can be also represented by algebraic items, putting therefore aside the differential equation. The active component can be therefore written as

$$F_a(l,v,u) = F_a(l_0,0,1) \cdot f_1(l) \cdot f_2(v) \cdot u(t) \cdot f_3(t) \qquad (1)$$

where:

$l_0$ -         length, at which the muscle is capable of exerting the maximum active component in situ (i.e. in the body); it is the length of muscle attained at an angle $\cdot$ of revolution being approximately half of the physiologically permissible one in a given joint; this length is independent of $u$ and $v$;

$F_a(l_0,0,1)$ - maximal value of the muscle force active component, being exerted isometrically, during the full tetanic contraction at $l=l_0$, $v=0$ and $u=1$;

$f_{1,2,3}$ -    some functions of one argument, described below.

In the present model the forms of functions $f_{1,2}$ appearing in Eq. (1) have been assumed after Pierrynowski and Morrison [13]. The function $f_1$ has the form

$$f_1(l) = 0.32 + 0.71 \exp[-1.112(l/l_0 - 1.00)] \cdot \sin[3.722 (l/l_0 - 0.656)] \qquad (2)$$

and represents the force - length characteristic within the range from $0.58 l_0$ to $1.81 l_0$ (see Fig. 2).

The branch of $f_2$ function (see Fig. 3) for positive contraction rates (concentric work) satisfies Hill's equation and is smoothly joined with the negative contraction rates branch (eccentric work), in which there has been accounted for that the maximum active force exerted during eccentric work was $k$ times greater than the maximum isometric force.

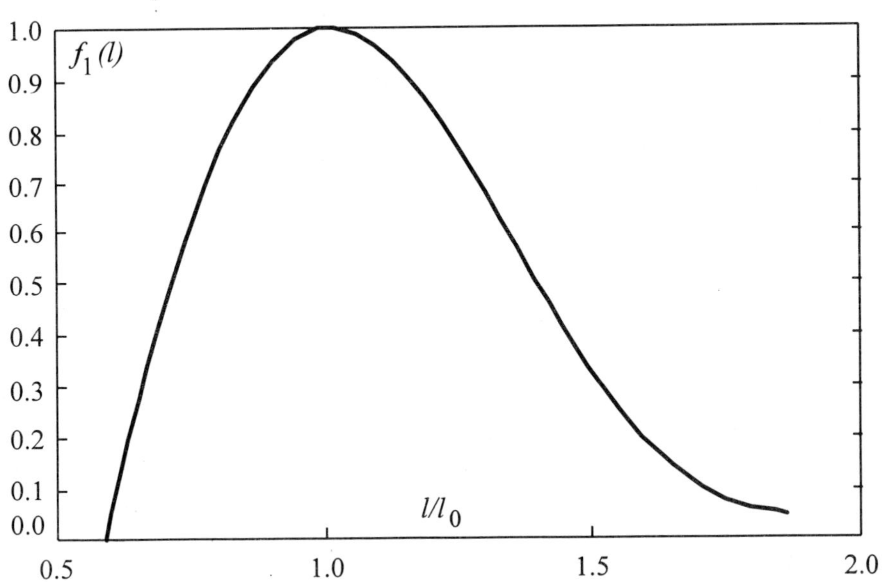



Fig. 2. Diagram of the dimensionless function $f_1(l)$.

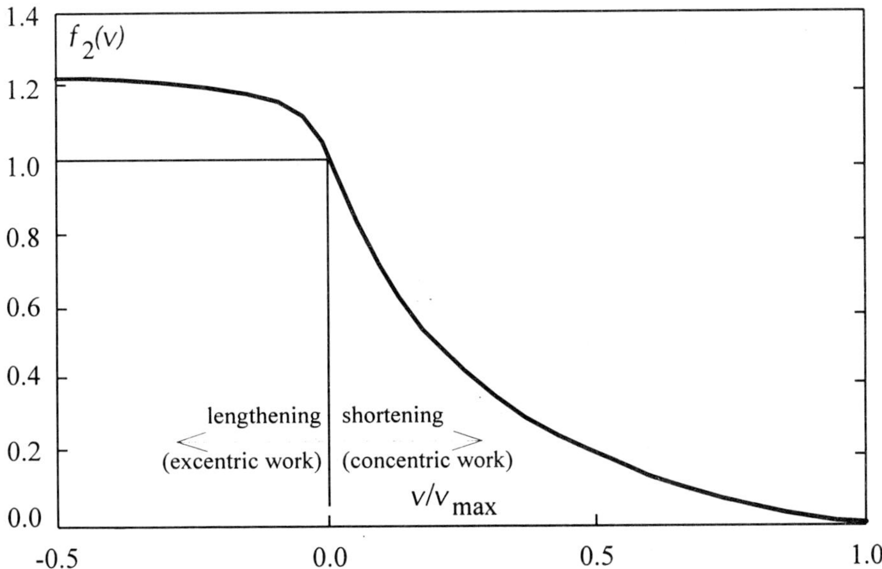



Fig. 3. Diagram of the dimensionless function $f_2(v)$.

$$f_2(v) = \begin{cases} 0.35[3.86 / (1 + 2.86v / v_{max}) - 1], & v \geq 0 \\ k - (k-1)^2 / (k - 1 - 3.86v / v_{max}), & v < 0 \end{cases} \qquad (3)$$

where $k$ takes the value 1.25 [13] and $v_{max}$ stands for the maximum velocity of active shortening of the muscle, taking the value [13]

$$v_{max}\,[m/s] = 6.43s^{-1}\,l_{fib}\,[m] \qquad (4)$$

where $l_{fib}$ denotes the length of contracting element of a given muscle, i.e., the distance between given muscle insertions measured along the muscle line of action minus the tendon lengths.

It should be noted that the relations (1), (2), (3) proposed in the paper [13] were obtained for the skeletal muscles of legs. Not having better results attainable the authors decided to apply them to description of all the muscles introduced into the present model.

The force exerted by a given muscle does not change immediately as the activation changes, which is reflected by the function $f_3(t)$ appearing in Eq. (1). The rate of muscle force change due to the change of activation is limited. Fig. 4 shows a sample course of $f_3$ function, which proves that the active muscle force (full tetanus, u=const, l=const) can increase its magnitude from zero to the maximal value in 0.2 s, while the regress to zero magnitude takes 0.18 s. The times 0.2 s and 0.18 s, respectively, were taken after Wittek [18]. Due to the lack of relevant data, we were forced to introduce this considerable simplification, having however in mind, that these values are different for different muscles. In the simulation program the function $f_3$ is realised in terms of constraints imposed on the rate of increase or decrease of the active component of muscle force.

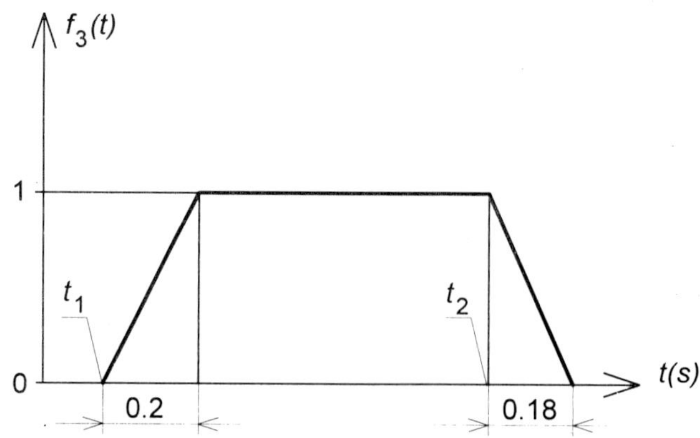


Fig. 4. Sample time course of the non-dimensional function $f_3(t)$; from the instant $t_1$ to the instant $t_2$ the muscle is stimulated by a constant activation u.

In the presents model it is additionally assumed that the magnitude of total force exerted by a given muscle $F = F_p + F_a$ must be lower than the permissible force $F_{max}$, having the form

$$F_{max} = A[m^2] \cdot 10^6 \, [N/m^2] \qquad (5)$$

where:
A -averaged physiological cross-section of a given muscle, i.e. the muscle volume divided by the value of $l_{fib}$, (see Eq. (4)).

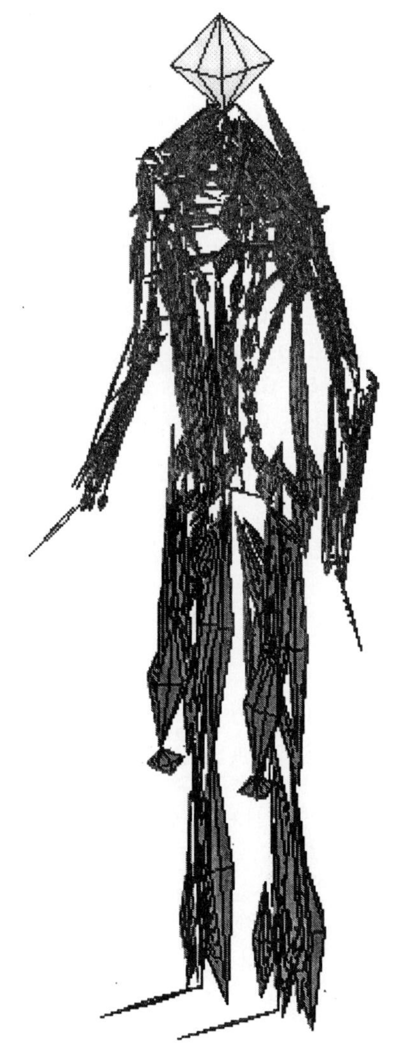

Fig. 5. General view of the scheme of the human musculoskeletal system physical model.

Two hundred fifty muscles, chosen arbitrarily from about 440 skeletal muscles of the human body, have been introduced into the model. Particular muscles, depending on their shape, number of insertions, division into particular actuators (e.g., caput breve and caput longum in the case of biceps) and possible wrapping around the axis of revolution in joint, etc., have been modelled in terms of one or several active spar- 3D elements. For example, the muscles wrapping around the joint are represented by the elements connected in series, with the obvious condition that the forces in elements shall be the same imposed. Finally, after taking the aforementioned division into account, the model comprises 290 muscle actuators acting separately; this number does not include, however the division into "in series" actuators, since in a given muscle they are acting together. The geometrical data, as well as masses were either taken from literature, e.g. from the monograph [14] and the work [20] or assessed on the base of anatomical atlases e.g.[16,17]. The radii of "muscle wrapping around the joint" were taken from the literature as well.

The scheme of the physical model of the human musculoskeletal system is shown in Fig. 5. It should be noted, that like in Fig. 1, due to its schematic character, particular elements presented in the pictures do not reveal the real anatomic shapes of the body elements (bones and muscles) being modelled, since it is not necessary. Bones and muscle are marked on the scheme by means of two cones of common base. In the case of muscle the area of a cone base is proportional to the averaged physiological cross-section of a given muscle. The elements of types "spring - 6D", "spring - 3D" and "beam - 3D", respectively, are not shown in the figures since having the form of numerical simulation data they are stored in a computer memory.

For better understanding of the modelling idea the scheme of skeletal system is presented in Fig. 6, while Fig. 7 and Fig. 8 show the schemes of musculoskeletal system of the right upper extremity and shoulder girdle. Insertion co-ordinates of some muscles of the upper extremity are given in Table II. The division of some muscles into acting separately "parallel" actuators (see e.g. muscle trapezius) and "in series" actuators (see e.g. muscle anconeus) winding round the joint and acting together (the same force exerted by each actuator modelling the muscle) can be easily seen from Fig. 7 and Fig. 8.

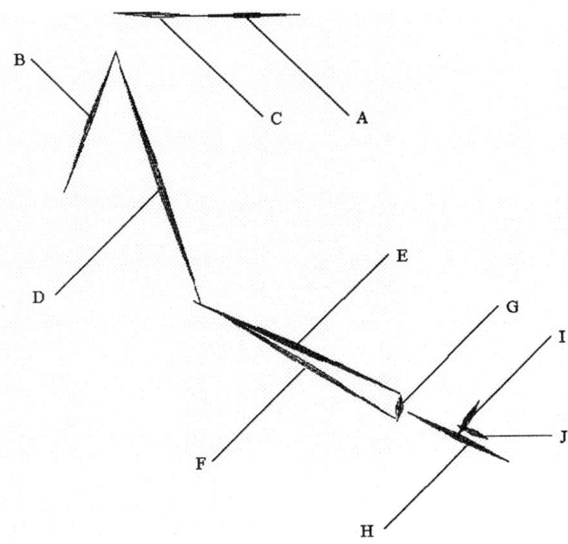

Fig. 6. Model of the rigid elements of right upper extremity
and shoulder girdle; side view, anatomical position:
A - torso, B - scapula, C - clavicle, D - humerus, E - radius,
F - ulna, G - wrist, H - hand, I - thumb, J - load.

TABLE II
Co-ordinates of the insertions of some upper extremity muscles.

| Muscle (number according to Fig. 7) | Proximal insertion located on humerus | | | Distal insertion located on radius | | |
|---|---|---|---|---|---|---|
| | $x_1[m]$ | $y_1[m]$ | $z_1[m]$ | $x_2[m]$ | $y_2[m]$ | $z_2[m]$ |
| Brachioradialis (18) | 0.135 | -0.025 | 0.005 | 0.125 | -0.010 | 0.005 |
| Supinator (24) | 0.165 | -0.028 | -0.013 | -0.055 | -0.006 | 0.006 |
| Pronator teres (25) | 0.155 | 0.035 | 0.005 | 0.015 | -0.010 | 0.005 |
| Biceps brachii caput longum (17) | -0.145 | -0.015 | 0.005 | -0.060 | 0.008 | 0.008 |
| Extensor capri radialis longus (26) | 0.140 | -0.028 | -0.015 | -0.135 | -0.015 | -0.015 |
| Extensor capri radialis brevis (27) | 0.140 | -0.023 | -0.015 | -0.135 | -0.007 | -0.015 |

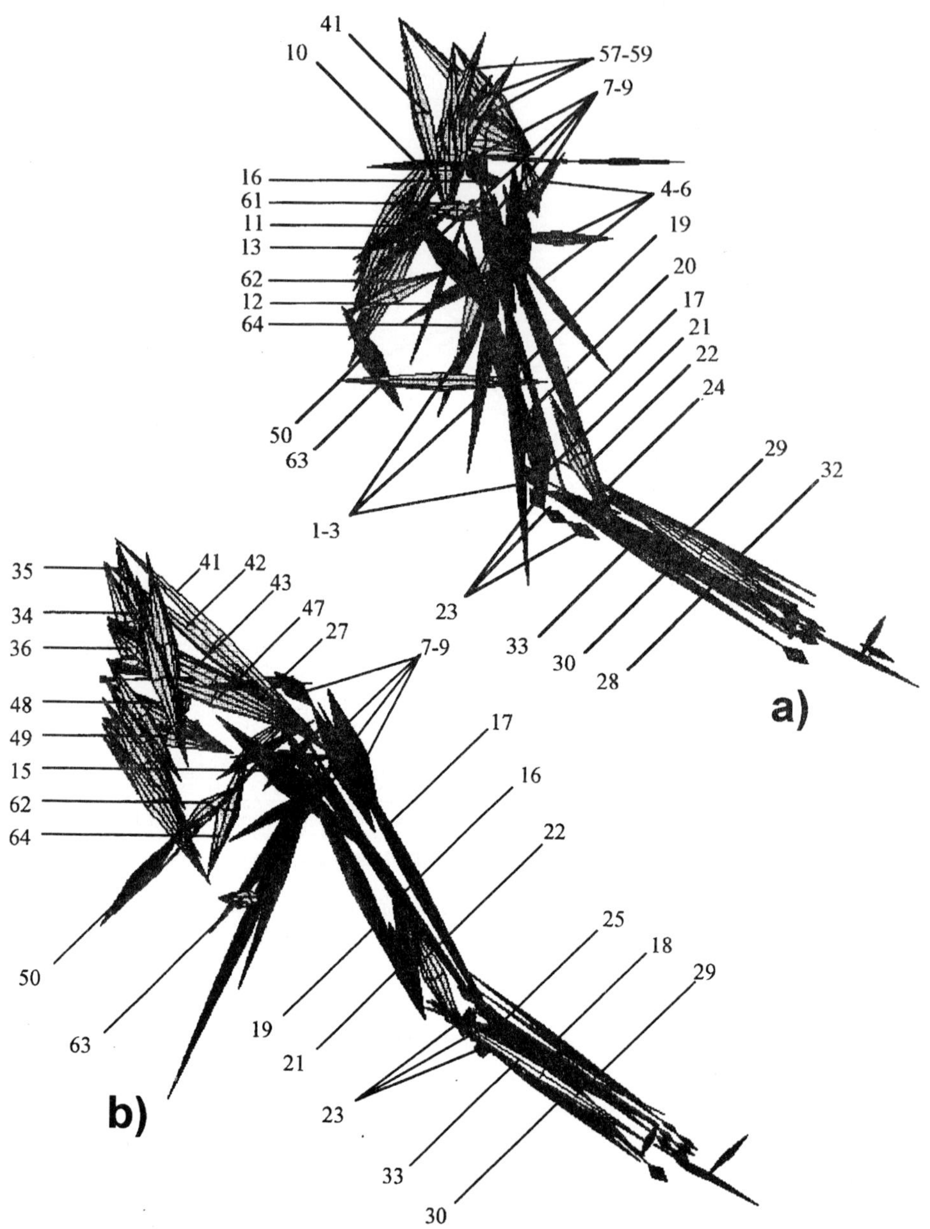



Fig. 7. Model of the right upper extremity and shoulder girdle, anatomical position: a) side view, b) rear view; for muscle numbers see the next page.

| | | | |
|---|---|---|---|
| 1. | latissimus dorsi "1" | 33. | flexor digit sublimis |
| 2. | latissimus dorsi "2" | 34. | trapezius "1" |
| 3. | latissimus dorsi "3" | 35. | trapezius "2" |
| 4. | pectorialis major "1" | 36. | trapezius "3" |
| 5. | pectorialis major "2" | *37. | trapezius "4" |
| 6. | pectorialis major "3" | *38. | trapezius "5" |
| 7. | deltoideus "1" | *39. | trapezius "6" |
| 8. | deltoideus "2" | *40. | trapezius "7" |
| 9. | deltoideus "3" | 41. | trapezius "8" |
| 10. | supraspinatus | 42. | trapezius "9" |
| 11. | infraspinatus | 43. | trapezius "10" |
| 12. | teres major | *44. | trapezius "11" |
| 13. | teres minor | *45. | trapezius "12" |
| *14. | subskapularis | *46. | trapezius "13" |
| 15. | coracobrachialis | 47. | trapezius "14" |
| 16. | biceps brachi caput breve | 48. | trapezius "15" |
| 17. | biceps brachi caput longum | 49. | trapezius "16" |
| 18. | brachioradialis | 50. | trapezius "17" |
| 19. | triceps brachi caput longum | *51. | trapezius "18" |
| 20. | triceps brachi caput mediale | *52. | rhomboid "1" |
| 21. | triceps brachi caput laterale | *53. | rhomboid "2" |
| 22. | brachialis | *54. | rhomboid "3" |
| 23. | anconeus | *55. | rhomboid "4" |
| 24. | supinator | *56. | rhomboid "5" |
| 25. | pronator teres | 57. | levator scapulae "1" |
| *26. | extensor carpi radialis longus | 58. | levator scapulae "2" |
| 27. | extensor carpi radialis brevis | 59. | levator scapulae "3"clavius |
| 28. | extensor digitorum communis | *60. | subclawius |
| 29. | extensor capri ulnaris | 61. | serratius anterior "1" |
| 30. | flexor capri ulnaris | 62. | serratius anterior "2" |
| *31. | flexor capri radialis | 63. | serratius anterior "3" |
| 32. | flexor pollicis longus | 64. | pectorialis minor |

Fig. 7 (cont.). Model of the right upper extremity and shoulder girdle, the list of muscles; "* " - muscle not marked in Fig. 7.


## 3. MATHEMATICAL MODEL

Since the physical model of the musculoskeletal system described in Section 2 has been built of rigid and elastic finite elements, it can be treated as the FEM type one. Following the procedure commonly used in the FEM [21], one obtains a matrix - vector set of ordinary differential equations describing the system motion. Due to large displacements of the rigid bodies as well as large deformations of the elastic bodies of non-linear mechanical properties these equations are non-linear.

This set, however, can be linearized at a given instant $t_0$, yielding a matrix - vector set of difference equations approximating the system motion within the time interval $\Delta t$ from $t_0$ to $t_1 = t_0 + \Delta t$ relative to local or global (in case of markers) systems of co-ordinates. The set can be written as

$$\mathbf{M}_0\ddot{\mathbf{q}}_1 + \mathbf{C}_0\dot{\mathbf{q}}_1 + \mathbf{R}_{E0} + \mathbf{K}_0(\mathbf{q}_1 - \mathbf{q}_0) = \mathbf{P}_{E0} + \Delta\mathbf{P}_E + \mathbf{P}_{M0} + \Delta\mathbf{P}_M \qquad (6)$$

where:

$\mathbf{q}_1$    - vector $\mathbf{q}$ of linear and angular generalised displacements of rigid bodies in local coordinate systems or generalised linear displacements of chosen points of the system, (markers) in global coordinate system at the instant $t_1$.

$\mathbf{q}_0$    - vector $\mathbf{q}$ of generalised displacements at the instant $t_0$.

$\dot{\mathbf{q}}_1$    - vector $\dot{\mathbf{q}}$ of generalised velocities at the instant $t_1$.

$\ddot{\mathbf{q}}_1$    - vector $\ddot{\mathbf{q}}$ of generalised accelerations at the instant $t_1$.

$\mathbf{M}_0$    - mass matrix $\mathbf{M}$ at the instant $t_0$.

$\mathbf{C}_0$    - damping matrix $\mathbf{C}$ at the instant $t_0$.

$\mathbf{K}_0$    - tangent stiffness matrix at the instant $t_0$.

$\mathbf{R}_{E0}$    - vector of internal generalised elastic forces (forces and moments) $\mathbf{R}_E$ at the instant $t_0$.

$\mathbf{P}_{E0}$    - vector of external generalised forces (forces and moments applied) $\mathbf{P}_E$ at the instant $t_0$.

$\Delta\mathbf{P}_E$    - increment of the vector $\mathbf{P}_E$ in the time interval $\Delta t = t_1 - t_0$.

$\mathbf{P}_{M0}$    - vector of generalised muscle forces $\mathbf{P}_M$ at the instant $t_0$.

$\Delta\mathbf{P}_M$    - increment (positive or negative) of the vector of generalised muscle forces in the time interval $\Delta t$.

Equation (6) is solved using the step-by-step method with the matrices $\mathbf{M}_0$, $\mathbf{C}_0$ and $\mathbf{K}_0$ being changed at successive time steps $\Delta t$ due to variable configuration of the physical model which represents at successive time steps a corresponding, variable position of the body. The mass matrix, for example is recalculated at each step. Masses of the elements representing muscles ("active spar - 3D"), tendons, discs and ligaments ("spar - 3D", "beam - 3D"), respectively, are reduced to the centres of mass of the corresponding rigid bodies, applying the principle that the system energy remains unchanged after the reduction. This approach enables the changes of the human body mass distribution due to motion (i.e. muscles dislocations relative to bones) to be reasonably approximated. The stiffness and damping are reduced in a similar way.

The vector $\Delta\mathbf{P_M}$ of muscle forces increments (and therefore also the vectors $\mathbf{P_M}$ and $\mathbf{P_{M0}}$) is related to the vector of total forces (active plus passive components) increments $\Delta\mathbf{F}$ exerted by muscles by the following equation

$$\Delta\mathbf{P_M} = \Delta\mathbf{F} \cdot \mathbf{D} \qquad (7)$$

It is a pure geometrical relation, in which the values of transformation matrix $\mathbf{D}$ entries are determined by a configuration of the physical model at a given instant $t$. The matrix $\mathbf{D}$ changes therefore at each time step $\Delta t$.

For each configuration of a given musculoskeletal system (or being more precise, for its physical model) the matrices $\mathbf{M_0}$, $\mathbf{C_0}$, and $\mathbf{R_{E0}}$ and $\mathbf{K_0}$ are known. The following two types of problems can be solved using Eq. (6), having in mind Eq. (7):

- The direct problem of mechanics applied to a biomechanical system, i.e. having known the time courses of $\Delta\mathbf{P_E}$ (external forces vector) and $\Delta\mathbf{P_M}$ (muscle forces vector) as well as the initial conditions, the time course of vector $\mathbf{q}$ (and its derivatives $\dot{\mathbf{q}}$ and $\ddot{\mathbf{q}}$) can be determined;
- The inverse problem of mechanics applied to biomechanical system, i.e. having known the time course of the vector $\mathbf{q}$ and its derivatives (e.g. from experiments consisting in registration of the motion of markers on film) together with the time course of $\Delta\mathbf{P_E}$ (external forces vector) and the initial conditions, the time course of muscle forces vector $\Delta\mathbf{P_M}$ (i.e. $\Delta\mathbf{F}$), which caused the motion considered can be found.

In biomechanics we deal with almost nothing but the latter problems. In this case an additional difficulty arises: the number of muscle forces in the human body is higher then the number of generalised displacements (it appears also in the present model), the problem, therefore becomes statically indeterminate. To overcome this obstacle in biomechanics, an additional "merit criterion" is introduced into the mathematical model. It is assumed that muscles in the human body follow a certain rational algorithm, e.g. minimise either the energy spent by the organism [4] or other factors (e.g. the sum of muscle forces or the sum of reactive forces in joints, etc.) [14] or satisfy the so-called "soft saturation" criterion [15]. The solution to Eq. (6), which satisfies also the adopted (but not necessary true) criterion is soughtafter. In the present model it has been assumed that muscles satisfy the so-called energetic criterion of the form

$$\frac{1}{2}\sum_{i=1}^{m}\frac{l_i F_i^2}{E_i A_i} = \min \qquad (8)$$

where:

$i = 1, ..., m$ -  index denoting a number of muscle actuator,

$F_i$ -  total force (active plus passive components) exerted by the i-th muscle actuator,

$A_i$ -  averaged physiological cross-section of the i-th muscle,

$E_i$ -  Young's modulus of the i-th "spar - 3D" element representing the i-th muscle actuator (passive component only).

It should be noted that the quantities appearing in Eq. (8) depend on each other. The force $F_i$ is a function of $l_i$, its derivative with respect to time - $v_i$ and the activation $u_i$ (see Eq. (1)). In the course of optimisation these dependencies should be introduced into the calculation algorithm.

Equation (6), which in fact is a set of equations written in a matrix form, cannot be numerically integrated directly, putting an additional obstacle before the researcher solving it. Big differences between the entries appearing in the matrix **K** (in the model there are elements of both very small (e.g. $10^{-1}$ N/m) and very large (e.g. $10^8$ N/m) stiffness) demand a very short integration step $\Delta t$ making direct integration a time-consuming procedure. Therefore the integration procedure proposed in the monograph [21] was applied, i.e. the modal superposition method. In this method, the considered motion of the system is represented in terms of linear combination of eigenvectors enabling Eq. (7) to be transformed to an unconjugate form, each equation of which can be integrated separately. Another advantage of the modal superposition method consists in the possibility that very high eigenfrequencies can be eliminated from the solution, what considerably raises stability, reducing at the same time numerical sensitivity of the problem, not affecting practically the results obtained.

Taking the above considerations into account, it can be stated that when solving the inverse problem of mechanics one deals with a typical optimisation task comprising the following items:

- The mathematical model of the task, i.e. Eqs (6) and (7);
- Constraints expressed by equation (1) (supplied additionally with Eqs (2), (3), (4)) and (5); the force exerted by a given muscle actuator must not exceed the magnitude calculated from Eq. (1) for the maximal activation u=1 at a given length and contraction rate; it should be noted that the final limitations come also from the forms of $f_3$ function and Eq. (5), respectively;
- The objective function (in biomechanics often called the "merit criterion") defined by Eq. (8).

From Eqs (1) - (8) it follows that the soughtafter variable being calculated at each time step $\Delta t$ is the vector of activation $\mathbf{u}$, components of which are activations of particular muscle actuators $u_i$.

It should be emphasised that the solution procedure described above is not a classical dynamic optimisation algorithm. In our case it consists in the optimisation of a dynamic process, being realised by means of a series of successive static optimisations performed at corresponding successive time steps. On the other hand, the way of muscle work control (if any) realised by the central nervous system is unknown. However, in some cases, e.g. single motion acts, it can be assumed that the optimisation procedure of the forces distribution over the muscles is realised in the way described above. While the genuine dynamic optimisation procedure is realised by the central nervous system by means of repeating a given motion many times (training). It can be therefore assumed that the optimisation method presented above works satisfactorily in the case when a single, untrained motion act is to be simulated.

## 4. SIMULATION MODEL

Equations (1) - (8) have been transformed into a numerical simulation model, the idea of which is shown schematically in Fig. 8. The scheme has a form typical for the multidimensional feedback control system, with the input - $\mathbf{q}_r(t)$ vector, being the required trajectory, i.e. the set of known, registered in experiment, trajectories in time of chosen points of the system rigid bodies (or markers fixed on them) to be followed; while the output - $\mathbf{q}(t)$ vector, being the calculated trajectory results from the simulation program. At the successive time steps $\Delta t$ the vector $\Delta \mathbf{q}$ is determined (called the control error), which corresponds to the vector $(\mathbf{q}_1 - \mathbf{q}_0)$ (in Eq. (6). The control system (the simulation program in fact) shall choose the muscle activation vector, $\mathbf{u}(t)$ for which the calculated trajectory $\mathbf{q}(t)$ is as close to the required trajectory $\mathbf{q}_r(t)$ as possible.

After the primary numerical simulation it has been found that unsatisfactory results came from the calculation algorithm based on the vector $\Delta \mathbf{q}(t)$ only, i.e. poor required trajectory reproduction has been obtained. Therefore the method, being well-known in the control theory and practice, has been employed, consisting in the subroutine simulating the proportional plus integral plus derivative controller action (PID controller, see Fig. 8) being built in. Using the trial-and-error method is has been found that best results could be obtained for the following function realised by the regulator

$$z(t) = k_1 \cdot \Delta\dot{q}(t) + k_2 \cdot \Delta q(t) + k_3 \cdot \Delta\ddot{q}(t) \qquad (9)$$

where:

$\Delta q(t) = q_1 - q_0$ (see Eq. (6))

$z(t)$ - new input vector to the simulation model, being substituted for the vector $\Delta q(t)$ from Eq. (6),

$k_1, k_2, k_3$ - constants, the values of which result from experiments.

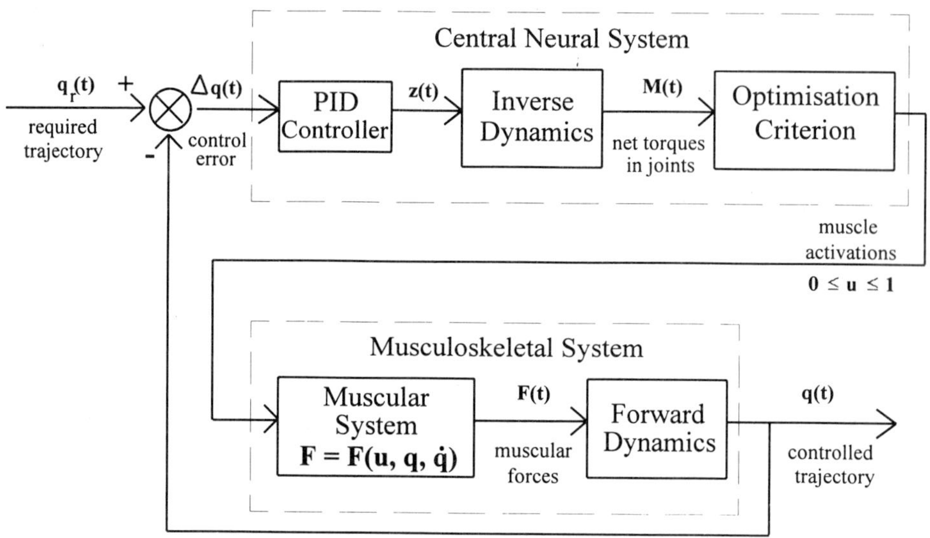


Fig. 8. Block diagram of the multidimensional control system of the human motion: $q_r(t)$, $q(t)$ - vectors of generalised co-ordinates, $F(t)$ - vector of muscular forces.

The new vector $z(t)$ carries the information about the displacements, velocities and accelerations of the system, respectively, and the PID controller imitates the control process realised by the central nervous system.

The number of co-ordinates of chosen points of the human body (in fact, it concerns the markers fixed on it) is always smaller that the number of generalised co-ordinates describing the physical model motion (i.e. the number of components the vector $q(t)$ is composed of - see Eq.(6)). However, since the solving algorithm of the inverse problem of mechanics is supplied with the optimisation procedure the solution, i.e. the activation vector $u(t)$ can be found in all cases.

When using the simulation program it has appeared that the simulation model is very sensitive to motion registration errors introduced by the input data. Careful data processing was therefore demanded, in which the package CCVSPL designed by Woltring [19] occurred to be very useful.

The simulation model is installed on the workstation SUN SPARC-20. The computation time varies, depending on the case considered, e.g. the simulation of a motion performed by one extremity (e.g. an arm) takes approximately 15 minutes, while the simulation of the whole body motion takes more then 2 hours. In each case about 80% of computation time is consumed by the optimisation procedure.

## 5. EXAMPLE

The following example demonstrates capabilities of the simulation model described above.

The manual handling task is considered. Fig. 9 shows several chosen positions of the body during the motion act. The modelled subject is loaded with 10 kg held in hands; the motion is symmetric in respect to the sagittal plane. Time courses of all muscular forces and reactions in joints have been obtained. Sample simulation results are presented in Fig. 10 ÷ Fig. 16.

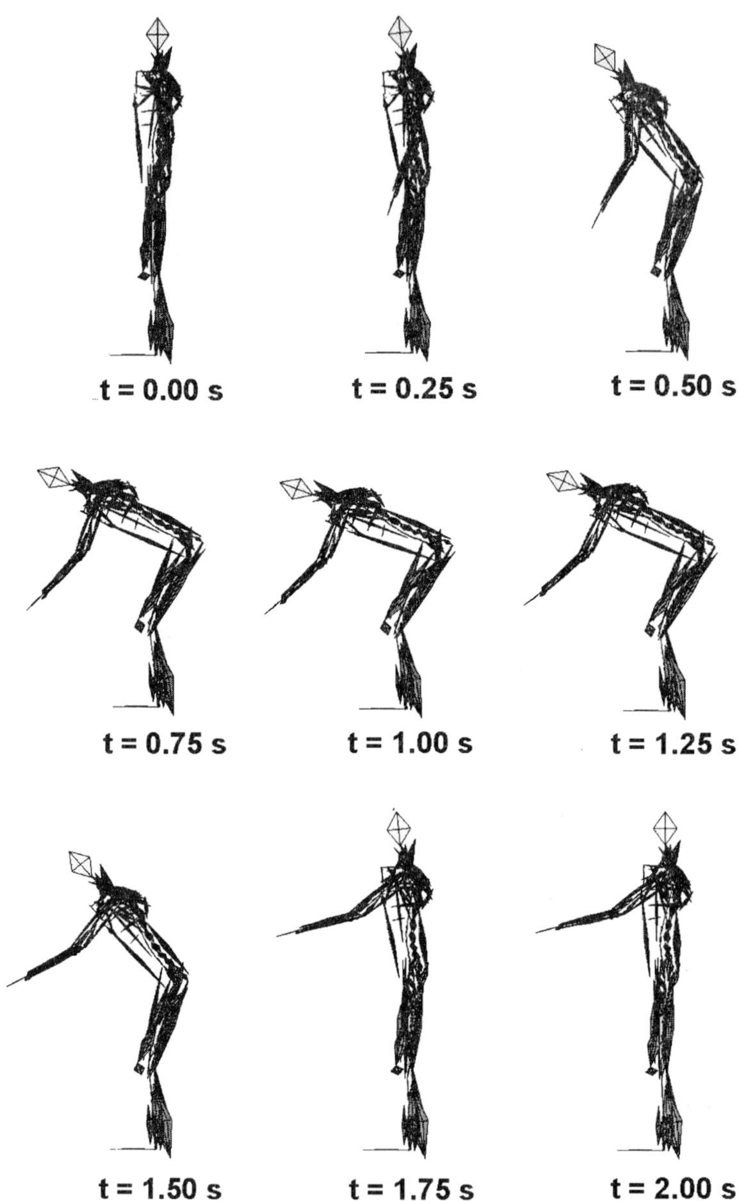

t = 0.00 s     t = 0.25 s     t = 0.50 s

t = 0.75 s     t = 1.00 s     t = 1.25 s

t = 1.50 s     t = 1.75 s     t = 2.00 s

Fig. 9. Configuration of the human body at successive instants (side view).

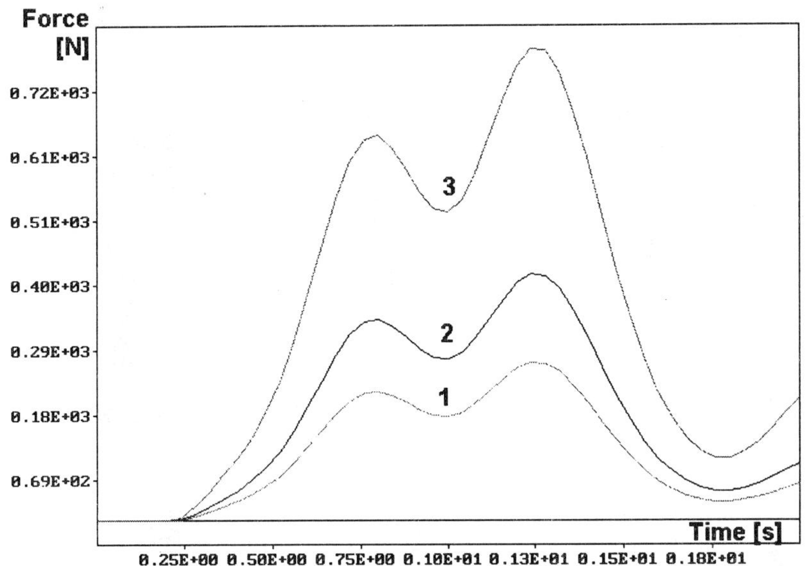



Fig. 10. Time courses of the forces exerted by chosen trunk muscles:
1) m. intertransversali, 2) m. interspinales, 3) iliocostalis.

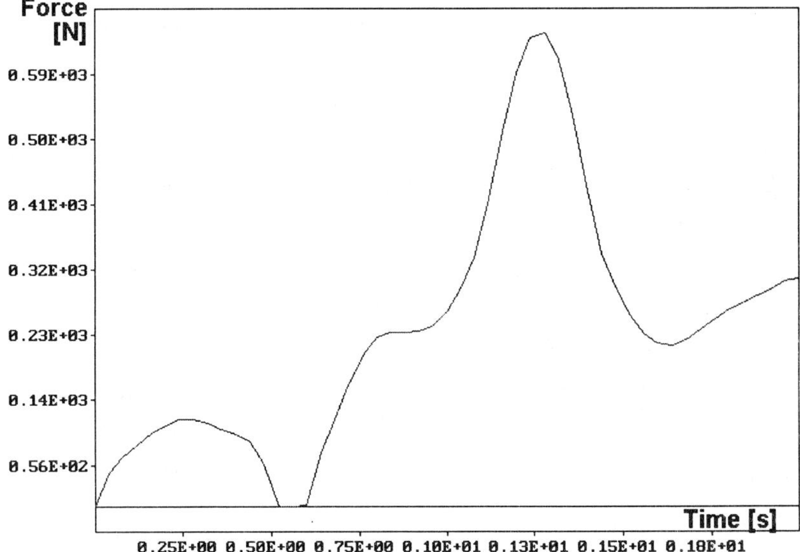



Fig. 11. Time courses of the force exerted by upper limb muscle biceps
brachii caput breve.

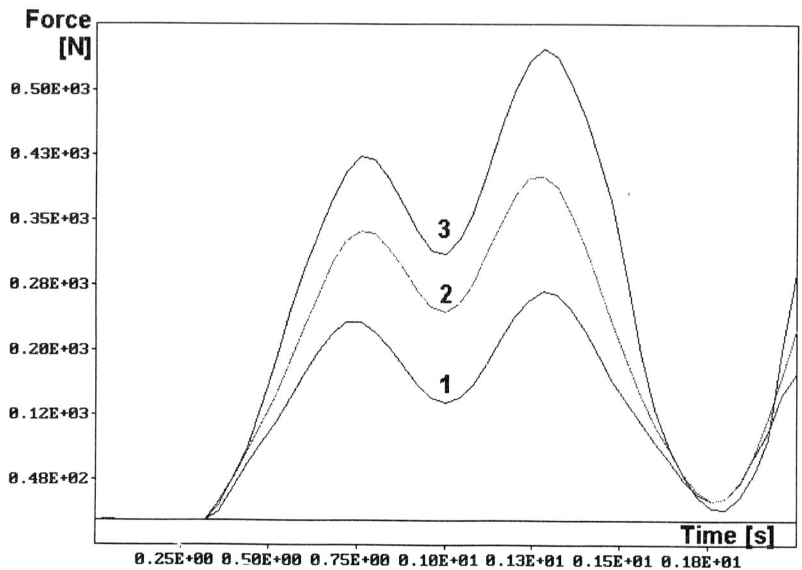

Fig. 12. Time courses of the forces exerted by chosen lower limb muscles:
1) m. semitendinosus, 2) semimembranosus, 3) biceps femoris.

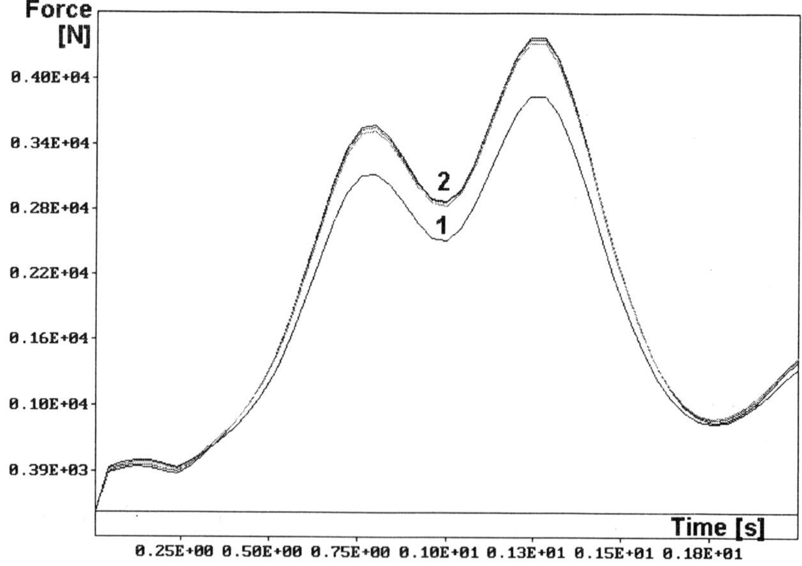

Fig. 13. Time courses of compressive forces acting on the intervertebral
discs: 1) L5/S1, 2) L1/L2, L2/L3, L3/L4, L4/L5.

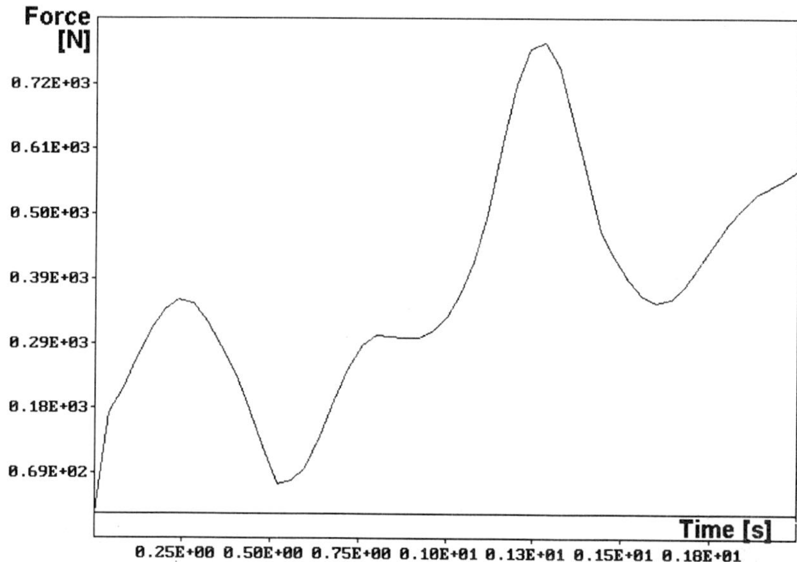



Fig. 14. Time course of the radius - humerus reactive force, the component acting along ulna.

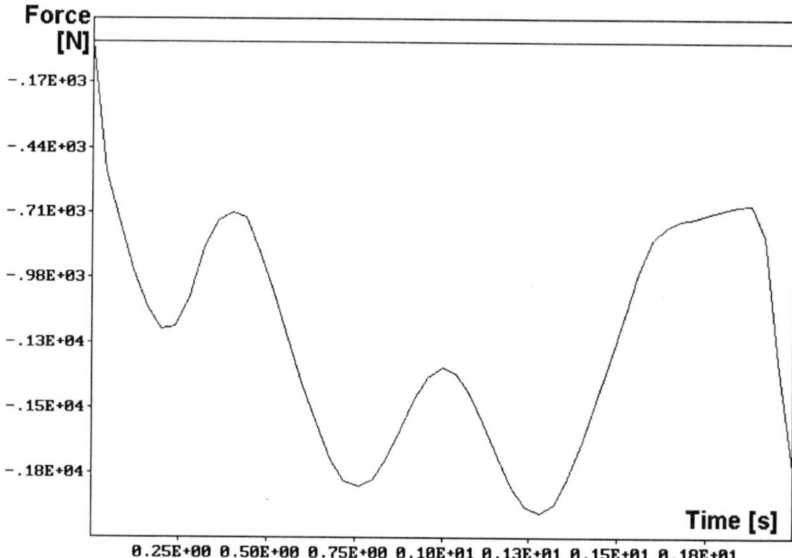



Fig. 15. Time course of the reactive force in the knee joint, the component acting along femur.

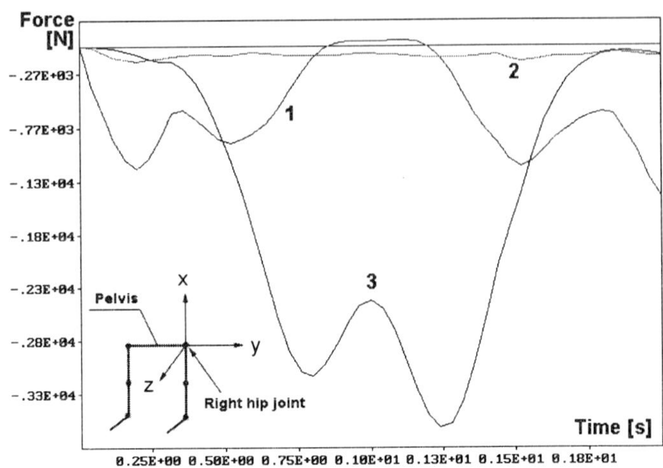


Fig. 16. Time courses of the reactive forces in the right hip joint:
1), 2), 3) - components along axis x, y, z according to the local
"pelvis" system of co-ordinates.


## 6. CONCLUSIONS

The model presented above has been tested on several examples. Basing on these tests it can be stated that:

- It enables the muscle forces and reactive forces in joints to be determined from the registered kinematic data of the human motion;
- Basic features making the present model different from other known ones are: capability of simulation of dynamic motion acts; possibility for the force-length-velocity characteristics of the muscle to be introduced into the model of muscle activity, as well as the so-called internal dynamics of muscle (function $f_3(t)$); non-linear, and therefore more realistic merit criterion, being applied to solving the problem of muscles co-operation;
- The model, like the other ones, needs validation. We are working on it.


## ACKNOWLEDGEMENTS

The assistance of Ms. Joanna Żabiuk, Mr. Marek Wojtyra, M.Sc., Ms. Beata Golmento-Enfer, M.Sc. and Mr. Jean-Stanisław Enfer, M.Sc., is gratefully acknowledged.

The study was supported by the Polish State Research Committee, under grant No 3 P 401 026 06.

## REFERENCES

1. Borowski S., Dietrich M., Kędzior K., Rzymkowski C., Zagrajek T.: Modelling of dynamic loads acting upon the human-operator musculoskeletal system. Proc. VIII World Congress on Theory of Machines and Mechanisms, Prague 1991, Vol.3, 781-784.

2. Chaffin D.B., Andersson G.B.J.: Occupational Biomechanics (2nd ed.). John Willey and Sons, New York 1991.

3. Dietrich M., Kędzior K., Miller K., Zagrajek T.: Statics and stability of human spine under working conditions. W.S. Marras et al. (eds.), The Ergonomics of Manual Work, Taylor and Francis, London - Washington D.C., 1993, 147-150.

4. Dietrich M., Kędzior K., Zagrajek T.: Modelling of muscle action and stability of the human spine. Winters J.M., Woo S.L-Y. (eds.), Multiple Muscle Systems, Biomechanics and Movement Organization, Springer-Verlag, New York 1990, 451-460.

5. Dietrich M., Kędzior K., Zagrajek T.: A biomechanical model of the human spinal system. Proc. Instn. Mech. Engrs., Vol. 205, (1991), Part H, Journal of Engineering in Medicine, 19-26.

6. Dietrich M., Kędzior K., Zagrajek T.: Three-dimensional FEM model of man-operator under vibration. Proc. of the Ninth World Congress on the Theory of Machines and Mechanisms, Politecnico di Milano, 1995, Vol.3, 2187-2190.

7. Gonzalez R.U., Hutchins E.L., Barr R.E., Abraham L.D.: Development and evaluation of a musculoskeletal model of the elbow joint complex. Transactions of the ASME, Journal of Biomechanical Engineering, Vol.118, Feb. 1996, 32-40.

8. Haug E.J.: Biomechanical models in vehicle accident simulation. PAM User Meeting, Nov.7, San Diego 1995.

9. Kędzior K., Lackowski J.: Simulation model of a skeletal muscle. Lectures Notes of the ICB Seminar, Intern. Centre of Biocybernetics., Warsaw, 1992, Vol.10, 97-107.

10. Kędzior K., Roman D., Rzymkowski C.: Modelling of upper extremity effort under static working conditions. Lecture Notes in Control and Information Sciences, Vol.187,Springer-Verlag, London 1993, 333-338.

11. Kędzior K., Wojtyra M., Zagrajek T.: Dynamic model of human lower extremity. Vth Int. Symposium on Computer Simulation in Biomechanics, University of Jyväskylä,June 1995, 58-59.

12. Kędzior K., Wojtyra M., Zagrajek T.: 3D dynamic model of human upper extremity. XVth Congress of International Society of Biomechanics, University of Jyväskylä, July 1995, 464-465.

13. Pierrynowski M.R., Morrison J.B.: A physiological model of muscular forces in human locomotion - theoretical aspects. Mathematical Biosciences, 75, 1985, 69-101.

14. Seireg A., Arvikar R.: Biomechanical Analysis of the Musculoskeletal Structure for Medicine and Sport. Hemisphere Publishing Co., New York 1989.

15. Siemieński A.: Soft saturation, an idea for load sharing between muscles − application to the study of human locomotion. A. Cappozzo, M. Marchetti, V. Tosi (eds.), Biolocomotion, a Century of Research Using Moving Pictures. Promograph, Rome 1992, 293-304.

16. Sinielnikov R.D.: An Atlas of Human Anatomy. State Medical Publ., Moscow 1963 (in Russian).

17. Thompson C.W., Floyd R.T.: Manual of Structural Kinesiology (12th ed.). Mosby - Year Book Inc., St. Louis 1994.

18. Wittek A.: Mathematical Models of Muscle for Analysis of the Human Musculoskeletal System Response to Transient Loads. Chalmers University of Technology, Dept. of Injury Prevention, Report RO32, Göteborg 1996.

19. Woltring H.J.: A FORTRAN package for generalized, cross-validatory spline smoothing and differentiation. Advances in Engineering Software, 8(2), Computational Mechanics Publications 1986, 104-113.

20. Yamaguchi G.T., Saw A.G.U., Moran D.W., Fessler M.J., Winters J.M.: A survey of human musculotendon actuator parameters. J.M. Winters, S.L-Y. Woo (eds.), Multiple Muscle Systems, Biomechanics and Movement Organization, Springer-Verlag, New York 1990, 717-773.

21. Zienkiewicz O.C., Taylor R.L.: The Finite Element Method, McGraw-Hill (fourth edition), London 1991.

22. ADAMS/Android, Mechanical Dynamics Inc., Ann Arbor, Michigan.

23. MADYMO 3D User's Manual, V. 5.1, TNO Road-Vehicles Research Institute, Delft, The Netherlands, May 1994.

24. 3D Static Strength Prediction Program™, User's Manual, Version 3.0. The University of Michigan, Center for Ergonomics.

# DYNAMIC MODELS, CONTROL SYNTHESIS AND STABILITY OF BIPED ROBOTS GAIT


**M. Vukobratovic**

**Mihajlo Pupin Institute, Belgrade, Yugoslavia**



## ABSTRACT

In this chapter modeling of artificial biped gait, control synthesis and stability analysis are presented. Beside that, in a separate section control of biped gait is considered, partly based on application of fuzzy logic theory.

Modeling of biped gait is based on introduction of the ZMP notion, representing point in which total reaction of the support surface onto the foot, belonging to the supporting leg, is acting. The leg trajectories are prescribed and the compensating movements of the trunk are calculated in such a way, that system stays in dynamic equilibrium.

In order to enable gait control of the biped system at the level of perturbed regimes, control was synthesized in two steps. First, in each joint of the system control with constrained accelerations is applied and then, on the global level, to some of the joints the stabilization task is assigned of the whole, where the basic task lies in ensuring the gait and preventing the overturning the system. For the system analysis the aggregation-decomposition method was applied, using vector functions in bounded regions of state space. In order to include in the stability analysis the unpowered degrees of freedom, too, models of the composite subsystems were formed, incorporating one powered and one unpowered degree of freedom. In that way it was enabled to apply the mentioned method for stability analysis, developed for the systems, in which all the degrees of freedom are powered.

In the last chapter, simulation experiments of biped control with a hybrid approach that combines the traditional model-based and fuzzy logic-based control techniques. The combined model is developed by extending a model-based decentralized control scheme by fuzzy logic-based tuners for modifying parameters of joint servo controllers. The simulation experiments performed on simplified two-legged mechanism demonstrate the suitability of fuzzy logoc-based methods for improving the performance of the robot control system.

## 1. INTRODUCTION

Twenty one years ago, the "Mihajlo Pupin" Institute published in English a comprehensive research monograph by M. Vukobratovic under the title LEGGED LOCOMOTION ROBOTS AND ANTHROPOMORPHIC MECHANISMS. In this monograph were presented results of seven-year work of a small research group in the Biocybernetics Department of the Institute "Mihajlo Pupin" , as well as results of researches from several other centres in the world. In 1976, the monograph was published in Japanese and Russian, and in 1983 in the Chinese language.

The period of vigorous research in the domain of mathematical modelling and motion synthesis of the legged locomotion mechanisms and machines was primarily concerned with the applications in the rehabilitation of disabled people and with the problems of specific (legged) transport.

Legged locomotion systems in general are mechanisms of variable kinematic structure. In fact, during the gait (walk) the legged locomotion system is supporting on different number of legs, depending on the adopted walking pattern and of the actual phase of the gait. For example, the anthropomorphic system is alternatively supported on one and both legs. Consequently, in one case, the legs and trunk form an open, and in the other case a closed kinematic chain. However, in single-support phase, the walking mechanism can change its structure, as illustrated in Fig. 1.1. During the gait process the foot can rotate

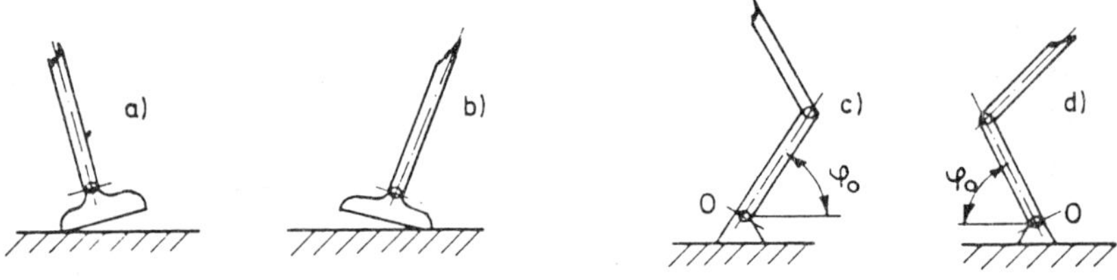


Fig. 1.1. Structural change of the legged mechanism

around its edges, as shown in Fig. 1.1. a) and b). The corresponding kinematic schemes are shown on Fig. 1.1. c) and Fig. 1.1. d) As it can be recognized when the foot relies upon one or the other edge, the position of the joint O changes stepwise.

Another characteristics of the walking vehicles is that some degrees of freedom are uncontrollable. All joints of the mechanism can be powered by appropriate drives, while the hinge O (Fig. 1.1. c) and d) ) cannot possess such a drive even if its position changes continually. Accordingly, the degree of freedom $\varphi_0$ cannot be controlled directly. Oh the other hand, change of $\varphi_0$ is very important, since at the greater $\varphi_0$ system can overturn. Thus, we face very specific situation: the motion of the mechanism should be controlled for some (passive) degree of freedom by means of acting upon the remaining (powered) degrees of freedom.

Next, the mechanism is connected to a fixed support only through the friction forces. Sketches on Fig. 1.1. c) and d) represent an idealization, and the friction force is sufficient to prevent the sliding of the leg.

The relevant references are given at the end of this Chapter.

## 2. MODELING OF BIPED DYNAMICS

Prescribed synergy method, in general, requires that to one part of the system dynamics is prescribed, whereas from the rest of the system such "compensating" dynamics is required to bring the system to equilibrium with respect to the task specifications and corresponding conditions of dynamic connections. In case of biped locomotion mechanisms, it is reasonable to impose prescribed motion to the legs (to ensure desired gait pattern) while motion of the upper part of the body have to be determined to ensure system's dynamic stability. Additionally, in this way dimensionality of the system is reduced without system's simplification or linearization.

### 2.1 Single-support phase

Let us suppose the system is in single-support phase and the contact with the ground is realized by the full foot. Then, it is possible to replace all vertical elementary reaction forces by the resultant $R_V$. If we reduce it to the center of the supporting area, the reaction force N and moment M will be obtained. Point where total reaction force is passing through the foot surface is named Zero Moment Point (ZMP). Obviously, the ZMP in single-support phase can not be out of the supporting area (area covered by one foot).

The basic idea used in artificial synergy synthesis is that the law of the change of total reaction force under foot is known in advance, or prescribed. The prescribed part of dynamic characteristics which, in a dynamic sense, additionally restricts the system , is named "dynamic connections". Thus, if a certain point represents the ZMP, and if the ground reaction forces $\vec{R}_V$ are reduced to it, then the moment $\vec{M}$ should be equal to zero. The vector $\vec{M}$ has always a horizontal direction and, hence, two dynamic conditions have to be satisfied: The projection of the moment on two mutually orthogonal axes X and Y in the horizontal plane should be equal to zero.

$$M_X = 0 \qquad M_Y = 0 \qquad\qquad (2.1)$$

As for the friction forces, it can be stated that their moment with respect to vertical axis V is equal to zero:

$$M_V = 0 \qquad\qquad (2.2)$$

The axis V can be chosen to be in any place, but if it passes through the ZMP, then axes X, Y and V constitute an orthogonal coordinate frame, and V will be denoted by Z. The external forces acting on the locomotion system are the gravity, friction, and ground reaction forces. Let reduce the inertial forces and moments of inertial forces of all links to the ZMP and denote them by $\vec{F}$ and $\vec{M}_F$, respectively. The system equilibrium conditions can be derived using D'Alembert's principle and conditions (2.1) can be rewritten as

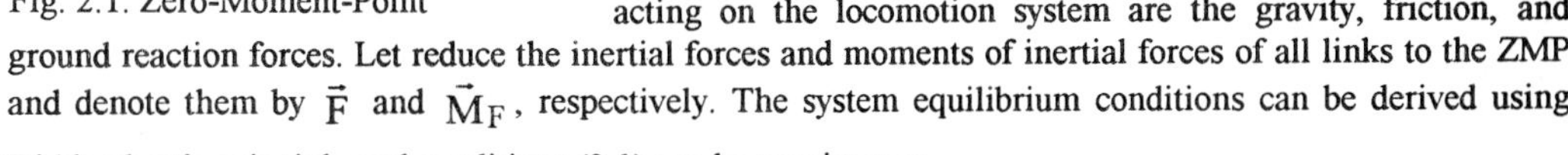

Fig. 2.1. Zero-Moment-Point

$$(\vec{M}_G + \vec{M}_F) \cdot \vec{e}_X = 0, \qquad (\vec{M}_G + \vec{M}_F) \cdot \vec{e}_Y = 0 \qquad\qquad (2.3)$$

Where $\vec{M}_G$ is the total moment of gravity forces with respect to ZMP, while $\vec{e}_X$ and $\vec{e}_Y$ are unit vectors of X and Y axes of the absolute coordinate frame. The third equation of dynamic connections (2.2) becomes:

$$(\vec{M}_F + \vec{\rho} \cdot \vec{F}) \cdot \vec{e}_V = 0 \qquad\qquad (2.4)$$

$\vec{\rho}$ is a vector from ZMP to the piercing point of the axis V trough the ground surface; $\vec{e}_V$ is axis V unit vector.

Let us adopt the relative angles between two links to be generalized coordinates and denote them by $q^i$. Let, additionally, suppose that the mechanism foot rests completely on the ground, so angle between them is zero, $q_0 \equiv 0$. Inertial force $\vec{F}$ and moment $\vec{M}_F$, in general case, can be represented in linear form of the generalized accelerations, in quadratic form of generalized velocities:

$$F^k = \sum_{i=1}^{n} a_i^k \cdot \ddot{q}^i + \sum_{i=1}^{n} \sum_{i=1}^{n} b_{ij}^k \cdot \dot{q}^i \dot{q}^i \ , \qquad\qquad k = 1, 2, 3$$

$$M_F^k = \sum_{i=1}^{n} c_i^k \cdot \ddot{q}^i + \sum_{i=1}^{n} \sum_{i=1}^{n} d_{ij}^k \cdot \dot{q}^i \dot{q}^i \ , \qquad\qquad k = 1, 2, 3 \qquad\qquad (2.5)$$

where coefficients $a_i^k, b_{ij}^k, c_i^k, d_{ij}^k$ ($k = 1, 2, 3$; and $= 1, ..., n$; $j = 1, ...n$) are the functions of the generalized coordinates , and $F^k$ and $M_F^k$ ($k = 1, 2, 3$) denotes projections of vectors $\vec{F}$ and $\vec{M}_F$. By introducing these expressions into (2.3) and (2.4) one obtains:

$$\vec{M}_G \cdot \vec{e}_X + \sum_{i=1}^{n} c_i^1 \cdot \ddot{q}^i + \sum_{i=1}^{n} \sum_{i=1}^{n} d_{ij}^1 \cdot \dot{q}^i \dot{q}^i = 0,$$

$$\vec{M}_G \cdot \vec{e}_Y + \sum_{i=1}^{n} c_i^2 \cdot \ddot{q}^i + \sum_{i=1}^{n} \sum_{i=1}^{n} d_{ij}^2 \cdot \dot{q}^i \dot{q}^i = 0$$

$$\sum_{i=1}^{n} c_i^3 \cdot \ddot{q}^i + \sum_{i=1}^{n} \sum_{i=1}^{n} d_{ij}^3 \cdot \dot{q}^i \dot{q}^i + \rho^X \left( \sum_{i=1}^{n} a_i^2 \cdot \ddot{q}^i + \sum_{i=1}^{n} \sum_{i=1}^{n} b_{ij}^2 \cdot \dot{q}^i \dot{q}^i \right) - \qquad\qquad (2.6)$$

$$- \rho^Y \left( \sum_{i=1}^{n} a_i^1 \cdot \ddot{q}^i + \sum_{i=1}^{n} \sum_{i=1}^{n} b_{ij}^1 \cdot \dot{q}^i \dot{q}^i \right) = 0$$

where superscripts X and Y denote the components in direction of the corresponding axis.

If the locomotion system has only three d.o.f., the trajectories for all angles $q^i$ can be computed from (2.6). If system has more than three d.o.f. (what, in fact, happen) the trajectories for the rest (n-3) coordinates should be prescribed in such a way to ensure the desired legs' trajectories (for example, measured from the human walk).

Now, set of coordinates can be divided in two subsets: the first one containing all coordinates whose motion is prescribed, denoted as $q^{0i}$, and the second subset comprising all coordinates whose motion is to be defined using the prescribed synergy method, denoted as $q^{Xi}$. Accordingly, condition (2.6) becomes:

$$\sum_{i=1}^{n} c_i^k \cdot \ddot{q}^{Xi} + \sum_{i=1}^{n} \sum_{i=1}^{n} d_{ij}^k \cdot \dot{q}^{Xi} \dot{q}^{Xi} + g^k = 0, \qquad\qquad k = 1, 2, 3 \qquad\qquad (2.7)$$

where $c_i^k$ and $d_{ij}^k$, ($k = 1, 2, 3$) are the vector coefficients dependent on $q^0$ and $q^X$, whereas vector $g^k$, ($k = 1, 2, 3$) is a function of $q^0$, $\dot{q}^0$, $\ddot{q}^0$ and $q^X$. Since the gait is symmetric, the repeatability conditions can be written in the form:

$$q^i(0) = \pm q^i\left(\frac{T}{2}\right), \quad \dot{q}^i(0) = \pm \dot{q}^i\left(\frac{T}{2}\right)$$

where sign depends on the physical nature of the appropriate coordinates and their derivatives; $\left(\dfrac{T}{2}\right)$ is the duration of the one half-step period. As the motion of the prescribed part of the mechanism has been already defined (repeatability conditions are implicitly satisfied), only for the rest of the mechanism whose motion has to be determined, repeatability conditions

$$q^{xi}(0)=\pm q^{xi}\left(\frac{T}{2}\right), \quad \dot{q}^{xi}(0)=\pm \dot{q}^{xi}\left(\frac{T}{2}\right) \tag{2.8}$$

are to be added to the original set of equations describing the mechanism motion.

System (2.7), together with conditions (2.8) enables one to obtain the necessary trajectories of the coordinates $q^{xi}$, i.e. to carry out the compensation synergy synthesis. Accordingly, the synergy synthesis for $q^{xi}$ coordinates is reduced to the solving of system (2.7), with conditions (2.8). Various iterative methods for solving the boundary value problem can be applied.

## 2.2 Double-support phase

In double-support phase both mechanism's feet are simultaneously in the contact with the ground. Then, kinematic chain playing the role of legs is closed, i.e. the unknown reaction forces to be determined act on its both ends.

The procedure for the synergy synthesis is in the most part analogous to that for single support phase. let the position of the axis V be selected within the dashed area in Fig. 2.2. Then, by writing the equilibrium equations with respect to three orthogonal axes passing through ZMP, and by setting the sum of all moments of external forces to zero, the compensating movements for the corresponding part of the body can be computed.

The next problem is how to choose the position of the axis V with respect to the ZMP. The information on ZMP and axis V is insufficient for computation of the driving torques. For this reason, it is necessary to provide some additional relations concerning the ground reaction force. The total teaction force under one foot can be expressed as a sum of three reaction forces and moment components in the direction of coordinate axes. The components $M_X$ and $M_Y$ can be equal to zero since the diagram of the vertical forces os of the same sign. The third component $M_V$ should also be equal to zero, according to following considerations. Generally speaking, the friction forces can produce moments, but in the synergy synthesis the moment $M_V$ should also be equal to zero. As a consequence, if moments of friction forces are generated, they should be of opposite sign under each foot. However, in such a case these moments do not affect the system motion but only load additionally the legs drives and joints. because of this, it is reasonable to synthesize the gait in such a way to reduce each of these moments to zero. Thus, it can be assumed that total moments of reaction forces under each foot are equal to zero,

$$\vec{M}_a=\vec{M}_b=0 \tag{2.9}$$

where the superscripts a and b denote the left and right foot, respectivelly. Characteristics of the friction bertween the foot and the ground can be represented by a friction cone (Fig. 2.3.). If the total ground raeaction force $\vec{R}$ is within the cone of angle $2\gamma$ its

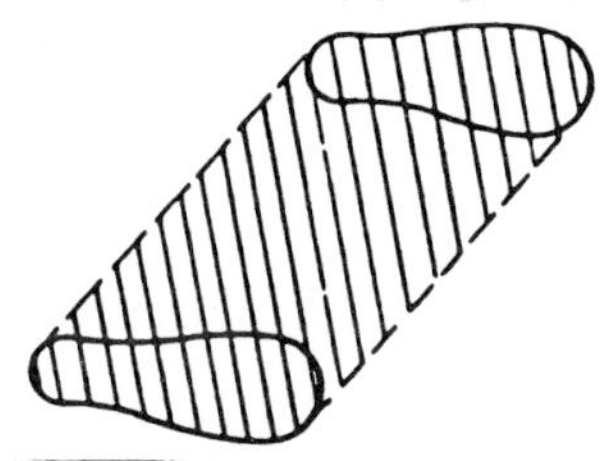

Fig. 2.2. Double support phase

horizontal component (i.e. friction force) will be of sufficient intensity to prevent an unwanted horizontal motion of the supporting foot over the ground surface. This can be expressed as:

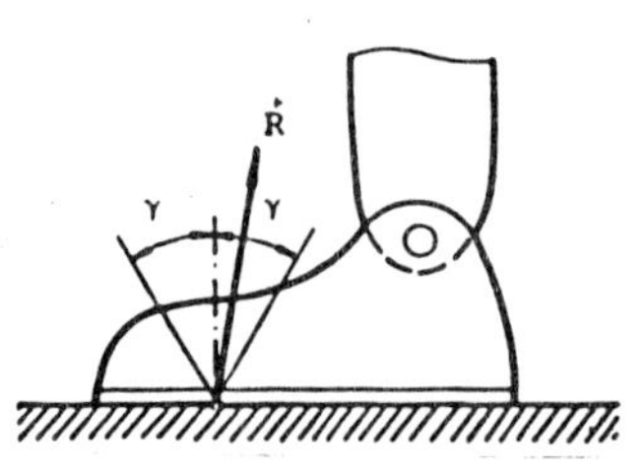

Fig. 2.3. Friction cone

$$\frac{\left|\vec{R}_X + \vec{R}_Y\right|}{\left|\vec{R}_V\right|} \le \text{tg}\gamma = \mu \tag{2.10}$$

where $\mu$ is the friction coefficient if the surfaces in contact. Thus, it is reasonable to distribute the horizontal components of ground reaction forces per foot proportionally to the normal pressure. the vertical components are inversely proportional to the distances between the ZMP and corresponding foot. So,

$$\frac{\left|\vec{R}_{Va}\right|}{\left|\vec{R}_{Vb}\right|} = \frac{\ell_b}{\ell_a} \tag{2.11}$$

Then, from (2.10):

$$\frac{\left|\vec{T}_a\right|}{\left|\vec{T}_b\right|} = \frac{\ell_b}{\ell_a} \tag{2.12}$$

Fig. 2.4. Friction force

holds for horizontal components, where $\vec{T}_a$ and $\vec{T}_a$ are the friction forces under corresponding foot (Fig. 2.4.). On the basis of similarity of the triangles $\triangle$ OAD and $\triangle$ OBC, it can be concluded that relation (2.12) does not depend on the direction of the force $\vec{T}$ (i.e. distances $\ell'_a$ and $\ell'_b$ ) but only on the distances between the feet, $\ell_a$ and $\ell_b$.

Thus, in order to have friction forces divided in proportion to the vertical pressures, a necessary and sufficient condition is that the axis $\ell'_a$ and $\ell'_b$ passes through the ZMP. Then, for the synergy synthesis in double support phase, the following vector equation holds

$$\sum_{i=1}^{n} \left(\vec{r}_i \times \left(\vec{G}_i + \vec{F}_i\right) + \vec{M}_i\right) = 0 \tag{2.13}$$

where $\vec{r}_i$ is a radius vector from the ZMP to the gravity centre of the i-th link, $\vec{F}_i$ and $\vec{M}_i$ are inertial force and corresponding moment of the i-th link reduced to its centre of gravity.

When synthesis of the compensating laws of motion is completed, it is possible to determine total horizontal and vertical reactions

$$R_Z = \sum_{i=1}^{n} \left(\vec{F}_{iz} + \vec{G}_i\right), \quad \vec{T} = \sum_{i=1}^{n} \left(\vec{F}_{iX} \cdot \vec{e}_X + \vec{F}_{iY} \cdot \vec{e}_Y\right) \tag{2.14}$$

where $\vec{F}_{iz}$ is the projection of $\vec{F}_i$ to the vertical axis and $\vec{F}_{iX}$ and $\vec{F}_{iY}$ to axes X and Y, respectively. Her, axis Z corresponds to vertical axis (previously denoted by V) which passes through ZMP. The axes X, Y and Z constitute the absolute orthogonal coordinate frame. Furthermore, the relations $\vec{T} = \vec{T}_a + \vec{T}_b$ and

$\vec{R} = \vec{R}_a + \vec{R}_b$ are obvious, and they, together with the relations

$$\vec{\ell}_a \times \vec{T}_a + \vec{\ell}_a \times \vec{T}_b = 0, \qquad \vec{\ell}_a \times \vec{R}_a + \vec{\ell}_a \times \vec{R}_b = 0 \qquad\qquad (2.15)$$

extend the posibility of defining the vertical reactions $\vec{R}_a$ and $\vec{R}_b$ , as well as the friction forces $\vec{T}_a$ and $\vec{T}_b$. $\vec{l}_a$ and $\vec{l}_a$ are vectors from the ZMP (denoted by 0) to the centres of the corresponding supporting aurfaces A and B, respectivelly.

## 2.3 Synthesis of nominal dynamics

The active spatial mechanism for realization of the artificial anthropomorphic gait belongs to the class of complex kinematic chains as shown in Fig. 2.5. During walking, chain representing legs change its

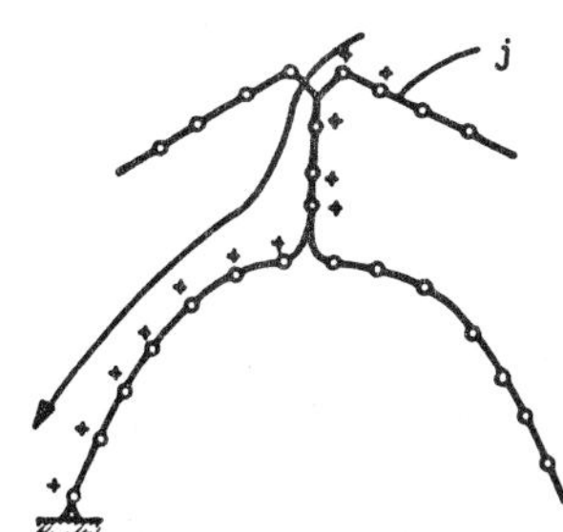

configuration from open to clesed kinematic chain, in single and double-support phase, respectivelly. For each phase there is a different procedure for forming dynamic equations, but it is based on well-known procedure for dynamic modeling of sinmple open kinematic chains for robotic manipulators. This procedure enables us to obtain following expression:

$$P = H(q,\theta)\cdot\ddot{q} + h(q,\dot{q},\theta) \qquad\qquad (2.16)$$

where: $P = [P_1, \ldots , P_n]$ is a vector of driving moments, $q = [q_1, \ldots , q_n]$ is a vector of joint coordinates, $\theta = [\theta_1, \ldots , \theta_n]$ is a geometric and dynamic parameters vector.

Fig. 2.5. Complex kinematic chain

In case of complex kinematic chains system have at least one link belonging to more then two kinematic chains, termed branching link. Calculation of the elements of matrix H and vector h of complex kinematic chains can be carried out by introducing the corresponding number of series of '+' joints. A series of '+' joints is formed in such a way that, when the chain is ruptured at a certain '+' joint, the j-th link should remain in the external part (not connected to the support) of the mechanism. Then, in the procedure of of forming differential equations, inertial force and moment of the j-th mechanism link is reduced only to its "own" '+' joint. Consequently, the following procedure is possible: the quantities $\vec{F}_j^{\,u}$ and $\vec{M}_j^{\,u}$ (total external force and moment) corresponding to the j-th link are succesivelly reduced to all '+' joints going from the j-th link towards the support. Then, after projecting the $\vec{F}_j^{\,u}$ and $\vec{M}_j^{\,u}$ onto the axis of the i-th joint, the resulting quantities denoted by $\Delta H_{ik}^{j}$ and $\Delta h_i^{j}$ van be caculated in the following way:

$$\Delta H_{ik}^{j} = -\vec{e}_i\left(\vec{b}_{jk} + \vec{r}_{ji} \times \vec{a}_{jk}\right), \qquad \Delta h_i^{j} = -\vec{e}_i\left(\vec{r}_{ji} \times \left(\vec{a}_j^{\,0} + \vec{G}_j\right) + \vec{b}_{jk}\right) \qquad\qquad (2.17)$$

Now, the components of matrix H and vector h are obtained by summing up the corresponding values from (2.17) with respect to all series of '+' joints

$$H_{ik}^{j} = \sum_{(j)} \Delta H_{ik}^{j} , \qquad h_i^{j} = \sum_{(j)} \Delta h_i^{j} \qquad\qquad (2.18)$$

Fig.2.6. illustrates a branching link having three kinematic pairs and which is the constituent of two series of '+' joints. In such a case the topological structure of the complex chain can be represented by the matrix MS. Each row of this matrix contains ordinal numbers of the corresponding series of '+' joints. The element MS(i,j) is the j-th joint in the i-th series of '+' joints. In addition, for each series of '+' joints, the ordinal number of the initial joint is also defined. The initial joint of the i-th series of '+' joints is the first joint of the i-th series differing from joints of the (i-1)-th series of '+' joints. The initial joint of the first series of '+'

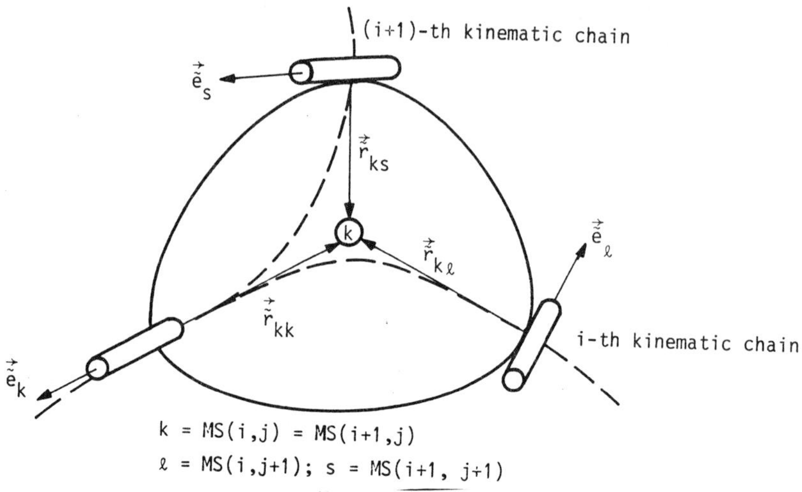


Fig. 2.6. Branching link

joints is MS(1,1). For the first link appearing in the first series of '+' joints, the matrix $Q_o^o$ ( $Q_i^o$ is a transformation matrix of the i-th link coordinate frame into reference frame) should be known. If a fixed support serves as a basis, the matrix $Q_o^o$ is a unit matrix. If we proceed to another chain, then the matrices $Q_i^o$ should be either stored or formed on the basis of procedure for forming dynamic equations of motion for open kinematic chain. The transformation matrix of the branching link serves to calculate the vectors $\vec{r}$ and $\bar{e}$. Besides, for branching links the information is beeded on their velocities ( $\bar{v}$ ) and accelerations ( $\bar{w}$ ) and the vectors coefficients $\vec{\alpha}$ , $\vec{\beta}$ , $\vec{\alpha}^o$ and $\vec{\beta}^o$ . It should be noted that all support vectors are equal to zero. These quantities for the mobile branching link should be stored when the preceding chain is analysed.


## 2.4 Example

For the following locomotion mechanism nominal dynamics has been synthesized. Mechanism (Figs. 2.7. and 2.8. ) consists of 14 links and 14 revolute joints. Links 5 and 10 are branching links. During motion mechanism hands are fixed on the chest. This structure can be split into three kinematic chains containing the joints 1-8, 9-12 and 13-14, in the first, second and third chain, respectivelly. The topological structure of the complex kinematic chain can be represented by a series of '+' joints in a matrix form:

$$MS = \begin{bmatrix} 1 & 2 & 3 & 4 & 5 & 6 & 7 & 8 & 0 \\ 1 & 2 & 3 & 4 & 5 & 9 & 10 & 11 & 12 \\ 1 & 2 & 3 & 4 & 5 & 9 & 10 & 13 & 14 \end{bmatrix}$$

Table 2.2. contains numerical values for the mechanical part of the mechanism. The prescribed part of the dynamics is adopted for the pairs 1-8, i.e. for the first chain. This part of the synergy (prescribed synergy) is defined based on measurements of the human gait as shown in Fig. 2.9. A set of prescribed ZMP trajectories for the single support gait phase is given in Fig. 2.10. Compensation has been synthesized for $q^9$ and $q^{10}$

to ensure the mechanism stability during motion, both in the sagittal and frontal plane (Fig. 2.12.). Some examples of results of compensating synergy are given in Fig. 2.12.

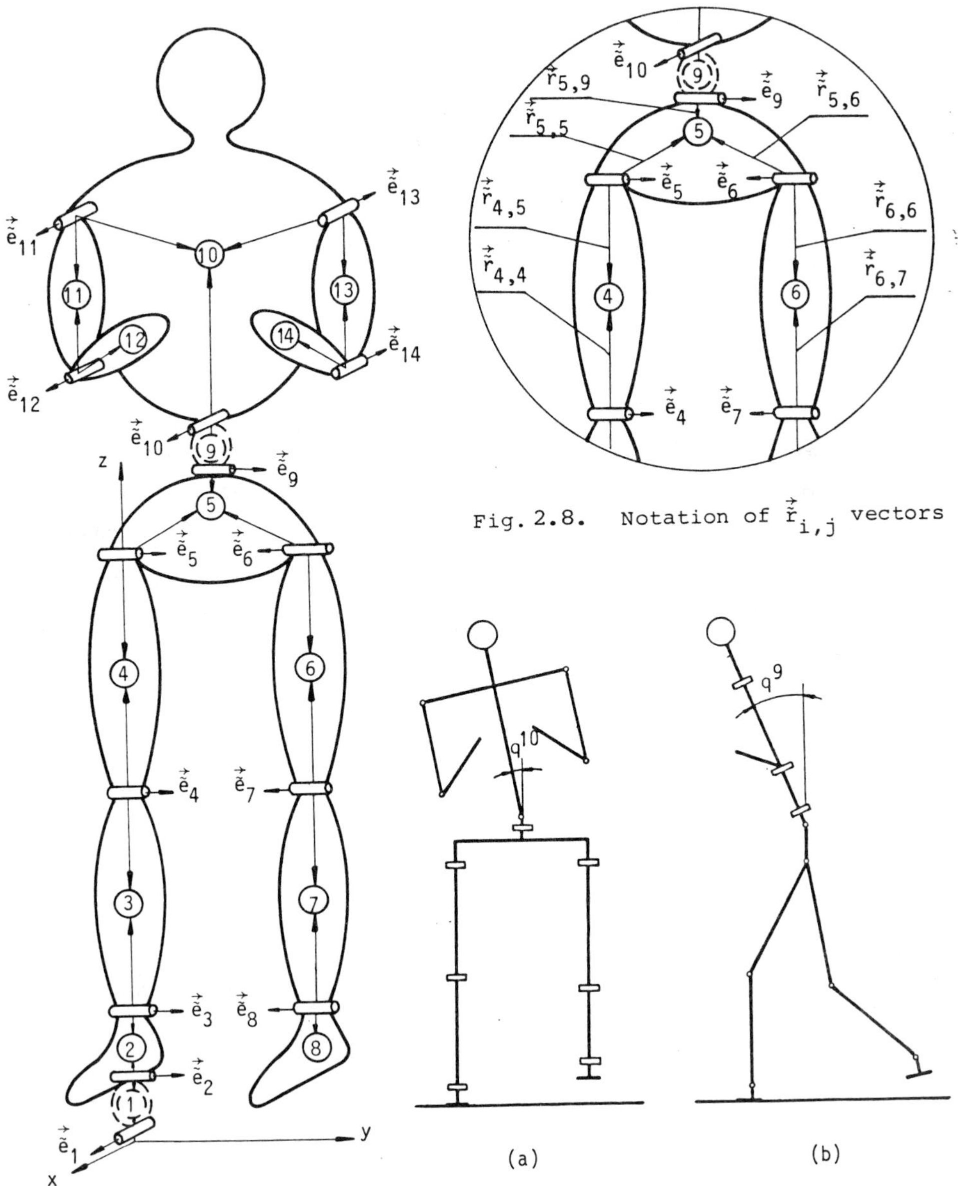

Fig. 2.8.  Notation of $\vec{\tilde{r}}_{i,j}$ vectors

Fig. 2.7.  Mechanical scheme of the anthropomorphic mechanism with fixed arms

Fig. 2.11.  Compensating d.o.f. in the frontal (a) and sagittal (b) plane

## Table 2.1. Kinematic and dynamic parameters of the mechanism

| Link | Mass [kg] | Moment of inertia [$kgm^2$] | | | Distance of the axes centres of joints from the link centre [m] | Joint unit axes |
|---|---|---|---|---|---|---|
| | | $J_x$ | $J_y$ | $J_z$ | | |
| 1 | 0.0 | 0.0 | 0.0 | 0.0 | $\vec{r}_{1,1} = (0, 0, 0.0001)^T$;   $\vec{r}_{1,2} = (0, 0, -0.0001)^T$ | $\vec{e}_1 = (1, 0, 0)^T$ |
| 2 | 1.53 | 0.00006 | 0.00055 | 0.00045 | $\vec{r}_{2,2} = (0, 0, 0.030)^T$;   $\vec{r}_{2,3} = (0, 0, -0.070)^T$ | $\vec{e}_2 = (0, 1, 0)^T$ |
| 3 | 3.21 | 0.00393 | 0.00393 | 0.00038 | $\vec{r}_{3,3} = (0, 0, 0.210)^T$;   $\vec{r}_{3,4} = (0, 0, -0.210)^T$ | $\vec{e}_3 = (0, 1, 0)^T$ |
| 4 | 8.41 | 0.01120 | 0.01200 | 0.00300 | $\vec{r}_{4,4} = (0, 0, 0.220)^T$;   $\vec{r}_{4,5} = (0, 0, -0.220)^T$ | $\vec{e}_4 = (0, 1, 0)^T$ |
| 5 | 6.96 | 0.00700 | 0.00565 | 0.00627 | $\vec{r}_{5,5} = (0, 0.135, 0.1)^T$;   $\vec{r}_{5,6} = (0, -0.135, 0.1)^T$;<br>$\vec{r}_{5,9} = (0, 0, -0.05)^T$ | $\vec{e}_5 = (0, 1, 0)^T$ |
| 6 | 8.41 | 0.01120 | 0.01200 | 0.00300 | $\vec{r}_{6,6} = (0, 0, -0.220)^T$;   $\vec{r}_{6,7} = (0, 0, 0.220)^T$ | $\vec{e}_6 = (0, -1, 0)^T$ |
| 7 | 3.21 | 0.00393 | 0.00393 | 0.00038 | $\vec{r}_{7,7} = (0, 0, -0.210)^T$;   $\vec{r}_{7,8} = (0, 0, 0.210)^T$ | $\vec{e}_7 = (0, -1, 0)^T$ |
| 8 | 1.53 | 0.00006 | 0.00055 | 0.00045 | $\vec{r}_{8,8} = (0, 0, -0.070)^T$ | $\vec{e}_8 = (0, -1, 0)^T$ |
| 9 | 0.0 | 0.0 | 0.0 | 0.0 | $\vec{r}_{9,9} = (0, 0, 0.0001)^T$;   $\vec{r}_{9,10} = (0, 0, -0.0001)^T$ | $\vec{e}_9 = (0, 1, 0)^T$ |
| 10 | 30.85 | 0.15140 | 0.13700 | 0.02830 | $\vec{r}_{10,10} = (0, 0, 0.34)^T$;   $\vec{r}_{10,11} = (0, 0.2, -0.06)^T$;<br>$\vec{r}_{10,13} = (0, -0.2, -0.06)^T$ | $\vec{e}_{10} = (1, 0, 0)^T$ |
| 11 | 2.07 | 0.00200 | 0.00200 | 0.00022 | $\vec{r}_{11,11} = (0, 0, -0.154)^T$;   $\vec{r}_{11,12} = (0, 0, 0.154)^T$ | $\vec{e}_{11} = (1, 0, 0)^T$ |
| 12 | 1.14 | 0.00250 | 0.00425 | 0.00014 | $\vec{r}_{12,12} = (0, 0, -0.132)^T$ | $\vec{e}_{12} = (1, 0, 0)^T$ |
| 13 | 2.07 | 0.00200 | 0.00200 | 0.00022 | $\vec{r}_{13,13} = (0, 0, -0.154)^T$;   $\vec{r}_{13,14} = (0, 0, 0.154)^T$ | $\vec{e}_{13} = (-1, 0, 0)^T$ |
| 14 | 1.14 | 0.00250 | 0.00425 | 0.00014 | $\vec{r}_{14,14} = (0, 0, -0.132)^T$ | $\vec{e}_{14} = (-1, 0, 0)^T$ |

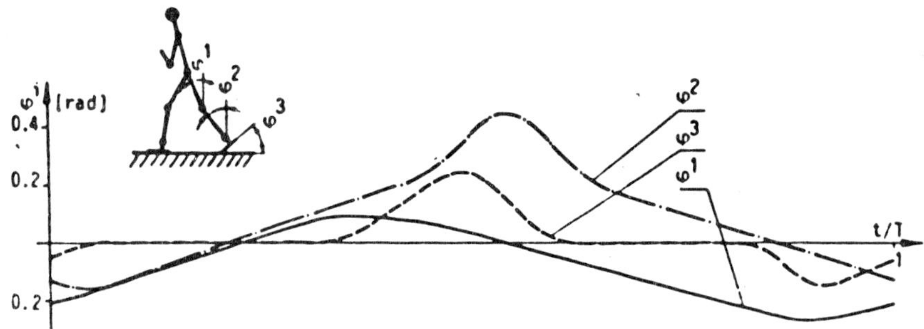


Fig.2.9. Synergy for walking upon level ground

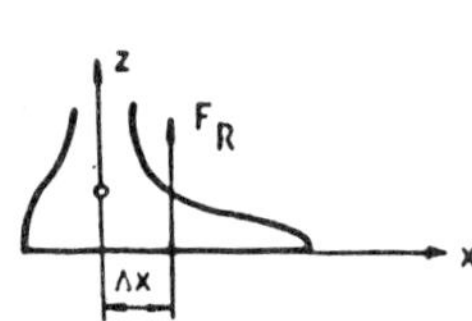


ZMP displacement

Fig.2.10. Set of ZMP trajectories for single-support gait phase

| CASE | t(sec) | $\Delta x$(m) |
|---|---|---|
| I | 0 ÷ T/2 | 0.0 |
| II | 0 ÷ 0.3<br>0.3 ÷ T/2 | 0.0<br>0.035 |
| III | 0 ÷ 0.5<br>0.5 ÷ T/2 | 0.0<br>0.035 |
| IV | 0 ÷ 0.2<br>0.2 ÷ 1.0<br>1.0 ÷ T/2 | -0.02<br>0.0<br>0.0 |
| V | 0 ÷ 0.2<br>0.2 ÷ 0.6<br>0.6 ÷ T/2 | -0.02<br>0.0<br>0.035 |

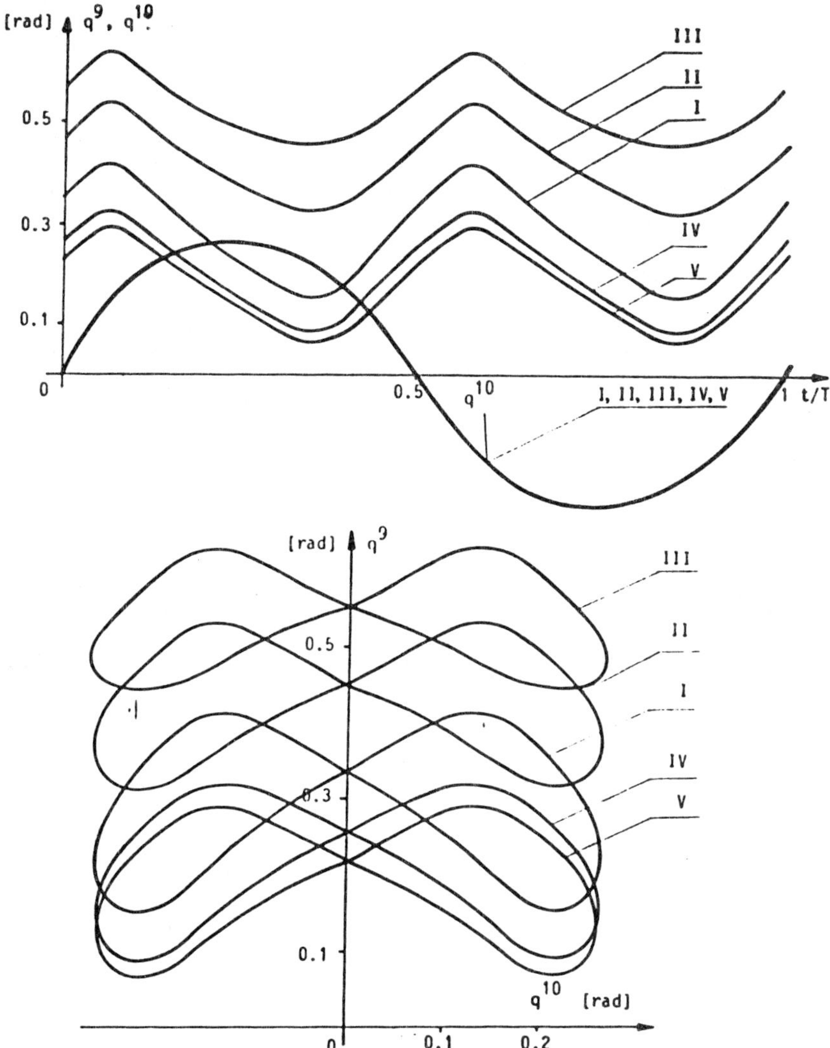


Fig.2.12. Compensating movements for the single-support gait upon level ground for T=1.5, S=0.6 and ZMP laws from Fig.1.9.

## 3. CONTROL SYNTHESIS OF BIPED GAIT

Hierarchy is a basic principle on which control of large systems, in general, is based. This also holds for robots. The hierarchical organization of the control system is most often vertical, so that each control level deals with some wider aspects of the overall system behavior than the lower level. A higher control level always refers to the lower ones, and it controls those system parameters that vary more slowly. A higher level communicates with a lower level, giving it instructions and receiving from it relevant information required for the decision-making. After obtaining the information from a lower level, each level makes decision taking into account general decisions obtained from higher level and forwards them to the lower level for execution.

## 3.1 Synthesis of Control with Limited Accelerations

Control synthesis has been done in two steps: a) level (stage) of nominal regimes, and b) level (stage) of perturbed regimes. At the level of nominal regimes, the control is computed on the basis of the complete (nonlinear) model with the permanent requirement for satisfying dynamic equilibrium conditions for the overall mechanism. This control should enable the system (in the absence if disturbance ) to follow the nominal trajectories. At the stage of perturbed regimes, control should force the actual state vector to its nominal value, i.e. to the nominal programmed trajectory. It is intuitively clear that the action should be "smooth", with no significant change in link acceleration, in order to keep its influence on unpowered degrees of freedom within an acceptable range.

Let us consider the overall system model defined as:

$$S: \quad \dot{x} = \hat{A}(x) + \hat{B}(x) \cdot N(u)$$

Let it be assumed that part of the system corresponding to powered d.o.f. can be rearranged as a set of subsystems $S_a^i$ which are coupled through the term $\left(f_c^i \cdot P_c^i\right)$. So

$$S_a^i: \quad \dot{x}_c^i = A_c^i x_c^i + b_c^i N(u^i) + f_c^i P_c^i, \qquad \forall i \in I_1$$

Let the nominal trajectory $x_c^o$, $x_c^o = \left(x_c^{o1^T}, x_c^{o2^T}, ..., x_c^{om^T}\right)^T$ and the nominal control $u^o$,

$u^o = \left(u^{o1}, u^{o2}, ..., u^{om}\right)^T$ be introduced in such a way to satisfy

$$S_a^i: \quad \dot{x}_c^{oi} = A_c^i x_c^{oi} + b_c^i N(u^{oi}) + f_c^i P_c^{oi}, \qquad \forall i \in I_1 \tag{3.1}$$

Then, the model of subsystem deviation from the nominal is considered in the form:

$$\Delta \dot{x}_c^i = A_c^i \Delta x_c^i + b_c^i N(\Delta u^i) + f_c^i \Delta P_c^i, \qquad \forall i \in I_1 \tag{3.2}$$

The purpose of the synthesis of disturbance compensating control $\left(\Delta u\right)$ is to force system deviation $\Delta x_c^i$, (i = 1, 2, ..., m) to zero to maintain the overall system stability.

We shall synthesize the local controller for the i-th actuator, i.e. for the $S_a^i$ subsystem whose model of state deviation around the nominal trajectory is given by (3.2). We want to define the controller for this subsystem which will reduce the state deviation $\Delta x_c^i(t)$ to zero, but in doing this we want to prevent the appearance of the too high accelerations. Therefore, we shall synthesize a controller which will ensure the acceleration of the corresponding joint $\Delta \ddot{q}^i$ is limited. To do this, we start from the simple problem of the second order linear system with limited accelerations.

Let us consider the classical time-minimum problem. Let the system be described by

$$\Delta \dot{q}_1^i(t) = \Delta q_2^i(t)$$

$$\Delta \dot{q}_2^i(t) = u_i^*(t) \qquad \left|u_i^*(t)\right| \leq \Omega^i \tag{3.3}$$

with initial conditions $\Delta q_1^i(0) = \alpha^i$ and $\Delta q_2^i(0) = \beta^i$ where $\Omega^i \in R^1$, $\Delta q_1^i \in R^1$ and $\Delta q_2^i \in R^1$. The value $u_i^*(t)$ should be computed in such a way to ensure that system (3.3) returns from the $\left(\alpha^i, \beta^i\right)$ to point (0, 0) in a minimal time interval.

Therefore, such a solution of (3.3) should be obtained that the functional

$$J = \int_{0}^{T^{*}} dt$$

is in minimum, where $T^{*} \in R^{1}$ defines unspecified time interval. Such type of problem is well known, and

for this particular case ($\Omega^{i} \neq 1$), its solution is given by the expression

$$u_{i}^{*} = \begin{cases} +\Omega^{i} & \text{if} \quad \Delta q_{1}^{i} < \dfrac{\Delta q_{2}^{i}|\Delta q_{2}^{i}|}{2\Omega^{i}} \quad \text{or} \quad \Delta q_{1}^{i} = \dfrac{\left(\Delta q_{2}^{i}\right)^{2}}{2\Omega^{i}} \cap \Delta q_{2}^{i} \leq 0 \\[4mm] -\Omega^{i} & \text{if} \quad \Delta q_{1}^{i} > \dfrac{-\Delta q_{2}^{i}|\Delta q_{2}^{i}|}{2\Omega^{i}} \quad \text{or} \quad \Delta q_{1}^{i} = \dfrac{-\left(\Delta q_{2}^{i}\right)^{2}}{2\Omega^{i}} \cap \Delta q_{2}^{i} \geq 0 \end{cases} \qquad (3.4)$$

We shall apply this solution to control one single actuator, i.e. the subsystems $S_{a}^{i}$ associated to the i-th joint.

Let us suppose the mechanism is powered by the DC motors whose models are given in the form (the state vector $\Delta x_{c}^{i} = (\Delta q^{i}, \Delta \dot{q}^{i}, \Delta i_{R}^{i})^{T}$:

$$\begin{bmatrix} \Delta \dot{q}^{i} \\ \Delta \ddot{q}^{i} \\ \Delta \dot{i}_{R}^{i} \end{bmatrix} = \begin{bmatrix} 0 & 1 & 0 \\ 0 & a_{22}^{i} & a_{23}^{i} \\ 0 & a_{32}^{i} & a_{33}^{i} \end{bmatrix} \begin{bmatrix} \Delta q^{i} \\ \Delta \dot{q}^{i} \\ \Delta i_{R}^{i} \end{bmatrix} + \begin{bmatrix} 0 \\ \bar{f}_{c}^{i} \\ 0 \end{bmatrix} \Delta P_{c}^{i*} + \begin{bmatrix} 0 \\ 0 \\ \bar{b}_{c}^{i} \end{bmatrix} \Delta u^{i} \qquad (3.5)$$

From the second equation of (3.5) we can write

$$\Delta i_{R}^{i*} = (u^{i*} - a_{22}^{i}\,\Delta \dot{q}^{i} - \bar{f}_{c}^{i}\,\Delta P_{c}^{i})/a_{23}^{i} \qquad (3.6)$$

where $\Delta \ddot{q}^{i}$ is replaced by the value of allowed link acceleration $u^{i*}$ from (3.4). Then, $\Delta i_{R}^{i*}$ in (3.6) is the

corresponding rotor current, and its derivative can be computed from the following expression:

$$\Delta \dot{i}_{R}^{i} = \left(\Delta i_{R}^{i*} - \Delta i_{R}^{i}\right)/\Delta t \qquad (3.7)$$

where $\Delta t \in R^{1}$ is the control sampling period. Now, we can determine the control for (3.5).

Let us assume that we want to limit acceleration of the actuator (joint) to be within limits $\Omega_{min}^{i}$ and

$\Omega_{max}^{i}$. Starting from the time-minimum control (3.4) we can adopt the following control.

From third equation of (3.5) the compensation control signal for i-th actuator is

$$\Delta u^{i} = k_{i1}^{L}\Delta q^{i} + k_{i2}^{L}\Delta \dot{q}^{i} + k_{i3}^{L}\Delta i_{R}^{i} + k_{i4}^{G}\Delta P_{c}^{i*} + k_{i5}^{G} \qquad (3.8)$$

where the constant feedback gains are: $k_{i1}^{L} = 0$, $\quad k_{i2}^{L} = \left(-a_{22}^{i} - a_{23}^{i} \cdot a_{32}^{i} \cdot \Delta t\right)/d$

$$k_{i3}^{L} = -a_{23}^{i}\left(1 + a_{33}^{i} \cdot \Delta t\right)/d \qquad k_{i4}^{G} = \bar{f}_{c}^{i}/d, \qquad k_{i5}^{G} = k_{i5}/d \qquad (3.9)$$

$$k_i^5 = \begin{cases} \Omega_{max}^i & if \quad \Delta q^i \lhd \dfrac{-0.5\Delta \dot{q}^i \left| \Delta \dot{q}^i \right|}{\Omega^i} \quad or \quad \Delta q^i = \dfrac{0.5\left(\Delta \dot{q}^i\right)^2}{\Omega^i} \cap \Delta \dot{q}^i \leq 0 \\[4ex] \Omega_{min}^i & if \quad \Delta q^i \rhd \dfrac{-0.5\Delta \dot{q}^i \left| \Delta \dot{q}^i \right|}{\Omega^i} \quad or \quad \Delta q^i = \dfrac{-0.5\left(\Delta \dot{q}^i\right)^2}{\Omega^i} \cap \Delta \dot{q}^i \geq 0 \end{cases}$$

where $d = a_{23}^i \bar{b}_c^i \Delta t$, $a_{jk}^i$, $\bar{b}_c^i$, $\bar{f}_c^i$ are elements of the corresponding matrix and vectors of the actuator (3.5), $\Omega_{max}^i$ and $\Omega_{min}^i$ are the maximal and minimal values of the accelerations of the i-th link. The feedback gains synthesized in this way have to ensure the compensating movements such that the accelerations does not exceed certain limit, fixed in advance. As a consequence, the induced inertial forces will not cause an undesirable motion of unpowered d.o.f., i.e. displacement of ZMP out of a prescribed area.

### 3.2 Synthesis of Global Control with Respect to ZMP Position

If decentralized control defined by (3.9), applied at the mechanism's joints, it is not sufficient to ensure tracking of internal nominal trajectories with addition of the appropriate behavior of unpowered subsystem, an additional feedback has to be introduced at one of powered joints to ensure satisfactory motion of the complete mechanism. The task of this feedback is to reduce the destabilizing effect of the coupling action upon the unpowered subsystems.

Because a predominant role in the system stability is played by the unpowerd d.o.f., it is necessary to reduce the destabilizing coupling effects acting upon them. Because the unpowered subsystem can not compensate for its own deviation from the nominal state, one of the powered subsystems has to be chosen to accomplish it. As a coupling of the subsystems $S^j$ is a function of control input to the i-th subsystem $S_a^i$, it is clear that a feedback from subsystem $S^j$ to the inputs $\Delta u^i$ of the subsystem $S_a^i$ should be introduced.

With bipeds, where the unpowered d.o.f. are formed in contact of the feet and ground, it is possible to measure the ground reaction force using force sensors (three at least) to determine actual acting point of total vertical reaction force. For the known motion of the whole mechanism, the ground reaction force (or forces in double-support phase) is defined by its intensity, direction and position of acting point on the foot. If force sensors A, B and C are introduced (Fig. 3.1) and the system is performing gait, the measured values of vertical reaction forces $R_A$, $R_B$ and $R_C$ correspond to their nominal values, and the nominal position, of ZMP can be determined. Measurement of vertical reaction forces $R_A$, $R_B$ and $R_C$, when the mechanism is performing the gait in the presence of disturbances, enables determination of the actual position of ZMP. If the nominal ZMP position corresponds to point 0, it can be written

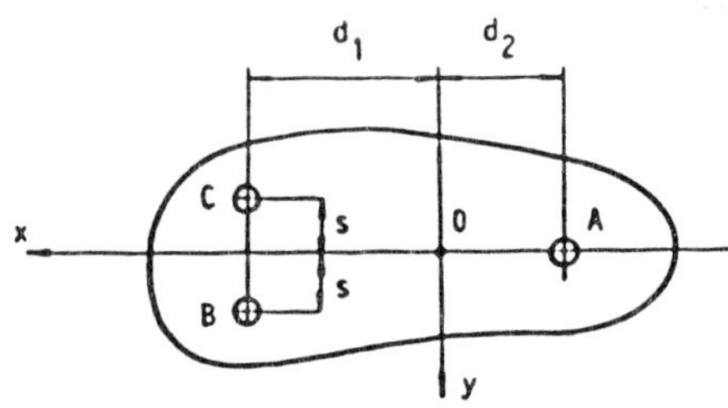


Fig. 3.1. Force sensors ob the robot foot

$$s(\Delta R_B - \Delta R_C) = M_x = R_z \cdot \Delta y$$

$$d_1(\Delta R_B + \Delta R_C) - d_2 \Delta R_A = M_y = R_z \cdot \Delta x \qquad (3.10)$$

where $\Delta R_A$, $\Delta R_B$ and $\Delta R_C$ are deviations of the corresponding measured forces from their nominal values; $R_z$ is the total resultant vertical reaction force; $\Delta x$ and $\Delta y$ are the displacements of the actual position of ZMP from its nominal position. These displacements can be computed from (3.10), provided the sensors dispositions and vertical reaction forces are known. The actual position of the ZMP is the best indicator of the overall biped behavior, so that we are going to use it to achieve a stable motion.

Our aim is to synthesize such control which will ensure a stable gait. The primary task of the feedback with respect to ZMP position is to prevent its excursion out of the allowable region, or, to prevent the system from falling down by rotation about the foot edge. If this is fulfilled, a further requirement imposed is to ensure that the actual ZMP position is as close as possible to its nominal.

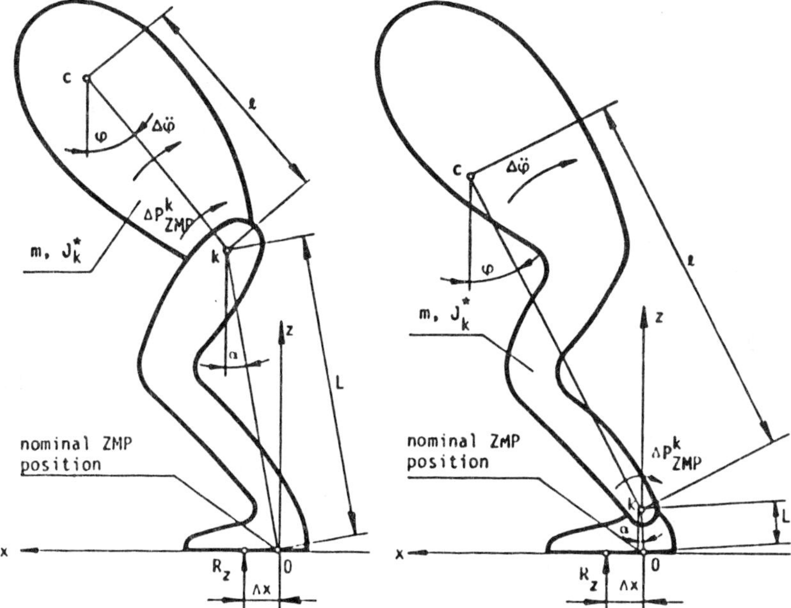

Fig. 3.2. Selection of joint for ZMP displacement compensation

Our further considerations will be restricted to biped motion in the sagittal plane, what means that ground reaction force position will deviate only in the direction of x axis by $\Delta x$. Fig. 3.3. illustrates the case when the vertical ground reaction force $R_z$ deviates from the nominal position ) by $\Delta x$; thus, the moment

$$R_z \cdot \Delta x = M^x_{ZMP}$$ is a measure of the mechanism overall behavior.

In the same way, we can consider the mechanism motion in the frontal plane, and $R_z \cdot \Delta y = M^y_{ZMP}$ is a measure of the mechanism behavior in the direction of y axis. Let us assume the correction of the $R_z$ acting point in one direction is done by the action at only one joint, arbitrarily selected in advance. A basic assumption introduced for the purpose of simplicity is that the action at the chosen joint will not cause a change in the motion at anyother joint. If we consider only this action, the system will behave as if composed of two rigid links connected at joint k, as presented in Fig. 3.3. In other words, the servo systems are supposed to be sufficiently stiff. In Fig. 3.3. two situations are illustrated, when the joint which has to compensate the ZMP displacement is the hip (case a) and ankle joint (case b) of supporting leg. In both cases, this joint is denoted by k, and all links above and below it are considered as a single rigid body. The upper link is of total mass m and inertia moment $J^*_k$ for the axis of joint k. Of course, numerical values are different for both cases. Furthermore, the distance from the ground surface to k is denoted by L,

## Table 3.1. Kinematic and dynamic parameters of the mechanism

| Link | Mass [kg] | Moment of inertia [kgm²] | | | Distance of the axes centres of joints from the link centre [m] | Joint unit axes |
|---|---|---|---|---|---|---|
| | | $J_x$ | $J_y$ | $J_z$ | | |
| 1 | 2 | 3 | 4 | 5 | 6 | 7 |
| 1 | 0.0 | 0.0 | 0.0 | 0.0 | $\vec{r}_{1,1} = (0,\ 0,\ 0.0001)^T$;  $\vec{r}_{1,2} = (0,\ 0,\ -0.0001)^T$ | $\vec{e}_1 = (1,\ 0,\ 0)^T$ |
| 2 | 1.53 | 0.00006 | 0.00055 | 0.00045 | $\vec{r}_{2,2} = (0,\ 0,\ 0.030)^T$;  $\vec{r}_{2,3} = (0,\ 0,\ -0.070)^T$ | $\vec{e}_2 = (0,\ 1,\ 0)^T$ |
| 3 | 0.0 | 0.0 | 0.0 | 0.0 | $\vec{r}_{3,3} = (0,\ 0,\ 0.0001)^T$;  $\vec{r}_{3,4} = (0,\ 0,\ -0.0001)^T$ | $\vec{e}_3 = (1,\ 0,\ 0)^T$ |
| 4 | 3.21 | 0.00393 | 0.00393 | 0.00038 | $\vec{r}_{4,4} = (0,\ 0,\ 0.210)^T$;  $\vec{r}_{4,5} = (0,\ 0,\ -0.210)^T$ | $\vec{e}_4 = (0,\ 1,\ 0)^T$ |
| 5 | 8.41 | 0.01120 | 0.01200 | 0.00300 | $\vec{r}_{5,5} = (0,\ 0,\ 0.220)^T$;  $\vec{r}_{5,6} = (0,\ 0,\ -0.220)^T$ | $\vec{e}_5 = (0,\ 1,\ 0)^T$ |
| 6 | 0.0 | 0.0 | 0.0 | 0.0 | $\vec{r}_{6,6} = (0,\ 0,\ 0.0001)^T$;  $\vec{r}_{6,7} = (0,\ 0,\ -0.0001)^T$ | $\vec{e}_6 = (0,\ 1,\ 0)^T$ |
| 7 | 0.0 | 0.0 | 0.0 | 0.0 | $\vec{r}_{7,7} = (0,\ 0,\ 0.0001)^T$;  $\vec{r}_{7,8} = (0,\ 0,\ -0.0001)^T$ | $\vec{e}_7 = (1,\ 0,\ 0)^T$ |
| 8 | 6.96 | 0.00700 | 0.00565 | 0.00625 | $\vec{r}_{8,8} = (0,\ 0.135,\ 0.1)^T$;  $\vec{r}_{8,9} = (0,\ -0.135,\ 0.1)^T$  $\vec{r}_{8,15} = (0,\ 0,\ -0.05)^T$ | $\vec{e}_8 = (1,\ 0,\ 0)^T$ |
| 9 | 0.0 | 0.0 | 0.0 | 0.0 | $\vec{r}_{9,9} = (0,\ 0,\ -0.0001)^T$;  $\vec{r}_{9,10} = (0,\ 0,\ 0.0001)^T$ | $\vec{e}_9 = (1,\ 0,\ 0)^T$ |
| 10 | 0.0 | 0.0 | 0.0 | 0.0 | $\vec{r}_{10,10} = (0,\ 0,\ -0.0001)^T$;  $\vec{r}_{10,11} = (0,\ 0,\ 0.0001)^T$ | $\vec{e}_{10} = (0,\ 0,\ 1)^T$ |
| 11 | 8.41 | 0.01120 | 0.01200 | 0.00300 | $\vec{r}_{11,11} = (0,\ 0,\ -0.220)^T$;  $\vec{r}_{11,12} = (0,\ 0,\ 0.220)^T$ | $\vec{e}_{11} = (0,\ -1,\ 0)^T$ |
| 12 | 3.21 | 0.00393 | 0.00393 | 0.00038 | $\vec{r}_{12,12} = (0,\ 0,\ -0.210)^T$;  $\vec{r}_{12,13} = (0,\ 0,\ 0.210)^T$ | $\vec{e}_{12} = (0,\ -1,\ 0)^T$ |
| 13 | 0.0 | 0.0 | 0.0 | 0.0 | $\vec{r}_{13,13} = (0,\ 0,\ -0.0001)^T$;  $\vec{r}_{13,14} = (0,\ 0,\ 0.0001)^T$ | $\vec{e}_{13} = (0,\ -1,\ 0)^T$ |
| 14 | 1.53 | 0.00006 | 0.00055 | 0.00045 | $\vec{r}_{14,14} = (0,\ 0,\ -0.070)^T$ | $\vec{e}_{14} = (1,\ 0,\ 0)^T$ |
| 15 | 0.0 | 0.0 | 0.0 | 0.0 | $\vec{r}_{15,16} = (0,\ 0,\ 0.0001)^T$;  $\vec{r}_{15,16} = (0,\ 0,\ -0.0001)^T$ | $\vec{e}_{15} = (0,\ 1,\ 0)^T$ |
| 16 | 30.85 | 0.15140 | 0.13700 | 0.02830 | $\vec{r}_{16,16} = (0,\ 0,\ 0.34)^T$;  $\vec{r}_{16,17} = (0,\ 0.2,\ -0.06)^T$;  $\vec{r}_{16,19} = (0,\ -0.2,\ -0.06)^T$ | $\vec{e}_{16} = (1,\ 0,\ 0)^T$ |
| 17 | 2.07 | 0.00200 | 0.00200 | 0.00022 | $\vec{r}_{17,17} = (0,\ 0,\ -0.154)^T$;  $\vec{r}_{17,18} = (0,\ 0,\ 0.154)^T$ | $\vec{e}_{17} = (1,\ 0,\ 0)^T$ |
| 18 | 1.14 | 0.00250 | 0.00425 | 0.00014 | $\vec{r}_{18,18} = (0,\ 0,\ -0.132)^T$ | $\vec{e}_{18} = (1,\ 0,\ 0)^T$ |
| 19 | 2.07 | 0.00200 | 0.00200 | 0.00022 | $\vec{r}_{19,19} = (0,\ 0,\ -0.154)^T$;  $\vec{r}_{19,20} = (0,\ 0,\ 0.154)^T$ | $\vec{e}_{19} = (-1,\ 0,\ 0)^T$ |
| 20 | 1.14 | 0.00250 | 0.00425 | 0.00014 | $\vec{r}_{20,20} = (0,\ 0,\ -0.132)^T$ | $\vec{e}_{20} = (-1,\ 0,\ 0)^T$ |

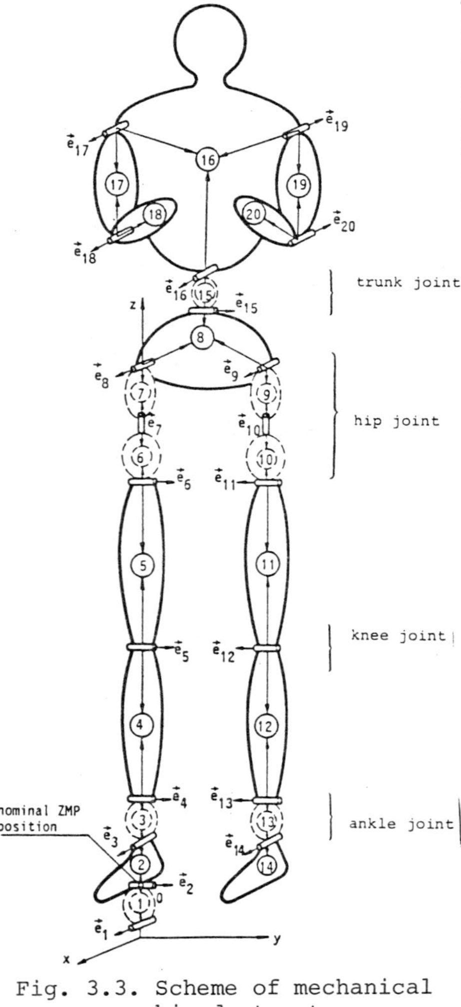


Fig. 3.3. Scheme of mechanical biped structure

from k to c (c is the mass center of the upper link) by $\ell$ , whereas $\Delta P^k_{ZMP}$ stands for correctional additional torque, applied to joint k. In Fig. 3.3. the upper (compensating) link is presented as a single link above joint k. In fact, in both cases presented, the compensating link includes also the other leg which is in swing phase, and which is not drawn in the figure. The inertia moment $J^*_k$ has to be calculated in such a way to include all the links which are found further onward with respect to the selected compensating joint. In this analysis, all the joints except the k-th one are considered "frozen", and, as a consequence, the lower link, representing the sum of all the links below the k-th joint, is also considered as rigid body, which is standing on the ground surface and does not move.

The procedure by which the correctional amount of global control with respect to ZMP position is synthesized is as follows. Assume the mechanism performs the gait such that a displacement of the ground reaction force $\vec{R}$ in the x direction occurs, so $M^x_{ZMP} = R_z \cdot \Delta x$ . Then, the quantity $\Delta P^k_{ZMP}$ is to be determined on the basis of the value $M^x_{ZMP}$ and of the known mechanism and gait characteristics. It is supposed the additional torque $\Delta P^k_{ZMP}$ will cause change in acceleration of the compensating link $\Delta\ddot{\varphi}$, while velocities will not change due to the action of $\Delta P^k_{ZMP}$, $\Delta\dot{\varphi} \approx 0$. From the equation of planar motion of considered system of two rigid bodies (Fig. 3.3.) which is driven by $\Delta P^k_{ZMP}$, and under assumption that terms $(\dot{\varphi}\,\Delta\dot{\varphi})$ and $(\Delta\dot{\varphi})^2$ from expression for normal component of angular acceleration of the upper link are neglected, it follows that

$$\Delta P^k_{ZMP} = \frac{M^x_{ZMP}}{1 + \dfrac{m \cdot \ell \cdot L \cdot \cos\varphi\,\cos\alpha}{J^*_k} + \dfrac{m \cdot \ell \cdot L \cdot \sin\varphi\,\sin\alpha}{J^*_k}} \tag{3.11}$$

The control input to the actuator of the compensating joint which has to realize $\Delta P^k_{ZMP}$ can be computed from the model of the actuator deviation from the nominal. Thus,

$$\begin{bmatrix} \Delta\dot{q}^k \\ \Delta\ddot{q}^k_T \\ \Delta\dot{i}^k_R \end{bmatrix} = \begin{bmatrix} 0 & 1 & 0 \\ 0 & a^k_{22} & a^k_{23} \\ 0 & a^k_{32} & a^k_{33} \end{bmatrix} \begin{bmatrix} \Delta q^{ki} \\ \Delta\dot{q}^k \\ \Delta\dot{i}^k_R \end{bmatrix} + \begin{bmatrix} 0 \\ \bar{f}^k_c \\ 0 \end{bmatrix} (\Delta P^k_c + \Delta P^k_{ZMP}) + \begin{bmatrix} 0 \\ 0 \\ \bar{b}^k_c \end{bmatrix} (\Delta u^k + \Delta u^k_{ZMP}) \tag{3.12}$$

This model differs from (3.5) by terms $\Delta P^k_{ZMP}$ and $\Delta u^k_{ZMP}$. From the second equation of (3.12) the change of rotor current is

$$\Delta i^k_R = \frac{\Delta\ddot{q}^k_T - a^k_{22} \cdot \Delta\dot{q}^k - \bar{f}^k_c(\Delta P^k_c + \Delta P^k_{ZMP})}{a^k_{23}} \tag{3.13}$$

Here, the subscript "T" is used for the acceleration $\Delta\ddot{q}^k$ from (3.12). It denotes the total change of link acceleration which consists of two parts. The first part is "regular" change of acceleration due to the control already applied to each powered joint defined by (3.8) and corresponds to $\Delta P^k_c$. The second part is direct consequence of the compensation torque $\Delta P^k_{ZMP}$. Thus,

$$\Delta\ddot{q}^k_T \approx \Delta\ddot{q}^k + \Delta\ddot{q}^k_{ZMP} \approx \Delta\ddot{q}^k + \frac{\Delta P^k_{ZMP}}{J^*_k} \tag{3.14}$$

the supporting foot. The mechanism rotation about z axis is supposed to be prevented by sufficiently large friction between the mechanism sole and ground surface.

Nominal motion is synthesized using prescribed synergy method. The compensating movements are executed by the trunk: in the frontal plane about $\vec{e}_{15}$ and $\vec{e}_{16}$. In Fig. 3.4. is given stick diagram of the nominal biped gait in the sagittal plane. "0" denotes the nominal position of the ZMP under the supporting foot, the other leg is being in the swing phase.

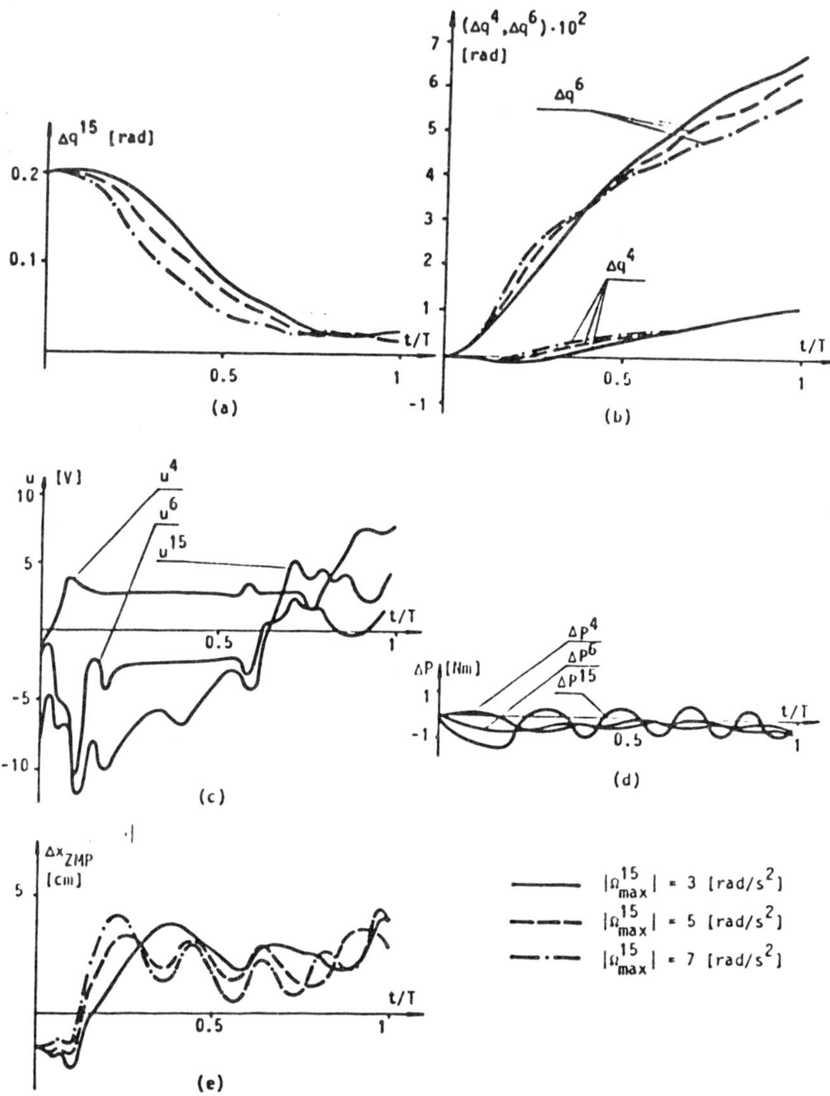



Fig. 3.5. Walk simulation without feedback with respect to ZMP position, $\Delta q^{15}(0) = 0.2$ [rad]

where $\Delta\ddot{q}^k(t)\approx(\Delta\dot{q}^k(t)-\Delta\dot{q}^k(t-\Delta t))/\Delta t$. Then, from the third equation of the (3.12) we have

$$\Delta u^k_{ZMP}=\frac{\Delta\dot{i}^k_R-a^k_{32}\cdot\Delta\dot{q}^k-a^k_{33}\cdot\Delta i^k_R}{\bar{b}^k_c}-\Delta u^k \qquad (3.15)$$

here $\Delta u^k$ is the control defined by (3.8), while $\Delta i^k_R$ stands for $\Delta\dot{i}^k_R(t)\approx(\Delta i^k_R(t)-\Delta i^k_R(t+\Delta t))/\Delta t$.

Equation (3.15) defines the control input to the k-th actuator which has to produce $\Delta P^k_{ZMP}$. Taking into account that $\Delta P^k_{ZMP}$ is derived by introducing certain simplifications, an additional feedback gains $k^{Gk}_{ZMP}\in R^1$ has to be introduced into (3.15). Thus, (3.15) becomes

$$\Delta u^k_{ZMP}=k^{Gk}_{ZMP}\left(\frac{\Delta\dot{i}^k_R-a^k_{32}\cdot\Delta\dot{q}^k-a^k_{33}\cdot\Delta i^k_R}{\bar{b}^k_c}-\Delta u^k\right) \qquad (3.16)$$

In this way, the additional feedback introduced and correctional input to selected powered mechanism's subsystem have only the purpose of maintaining the ZMP position. It is quite possible that the feedback introduced could even spoil the tracking of the internal nominal; trajectory of joint k, but the stability of the overall system would be preserved, what is the most important task for a locomotion system. Which joint (ankle, hip, ...) is the most suitable for this purpose it cannot be stated in advance, because the answer is dependent on the particular task imposed.


3.3 Example

The scheme of biped structure used for the walk simulation is presented in Fig. 3.3. and its mechanical parameters are given in Table 3.1. The joint with more than one d.o.f. has been modeled as a set of simple rotational joints connected with light links and with no length ($\vec{r}_{i,k}=0$). These links are called fictious links, and in Fig. 3.3. are represented with dashed line. For example, simple rotational joints with the unit rotational axes $\vec{e}_3$ and $\vec{e}_4$ connected to the fictious link 3, constitute the ankle joint of the right leg. In similar way are represented hip and trunk joint. Other joints possess one d.o.f. only.

As in the single support phase the mechanism as a whole can rotate about foot edges in the frontal and sagittal plane, these two d.o.f. were modelled as a simple rotational joints with axes $\vec{e}_1$ and $\vec{e}_2$ below

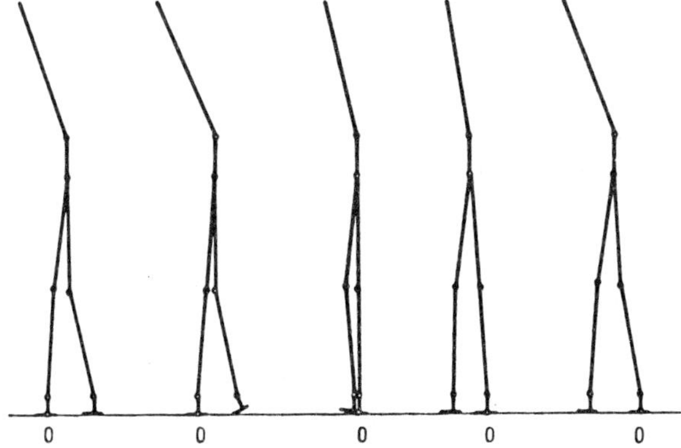

Fig. 3.4. Stick diagram of the nominal gait

The motion was simulated for one half-step period, and for the single support phase, only. Duration time of simulated motion was T=0.75 [s]. The perturbed motion of the system around the nominal trajectory has been simulated, where, trunk angular displacement from the nominal trajectory in the frontal plane, of $\Delta q^{15}(0) = 0.2\,[rad]$ at the initial moment was adopted as disturbance. Each gait is simulated using three different quantities of $\Omega^i_{max}$ (i=4 for ankle joint, i=15 for trunk) defined by $k^G_{i5}$. They are

$$\left|\Omega^i_{max}\right| = 3\,[rad/s^2]\,, \quad \left|\Omega^i_{max}\right| = 5\,[rad/s^2] \quad \text{and} \quad \left|\Omega^i_{max}\right| = 7\,[rad/s^2]$$

In the Fig. 3.5. is given example when ZMP displacement is compensated by ankle joint. . The trunk inclination for 0.2 [rad] was adopted as initial disturbance, and $k^{Gk}_{ZMP} = 0.5$. Trunk convergence to its nominal value is very fast. The ankle the hip joint slightly diverge for any value of $\Omega^{15}_{max}$, but absolute value of deviation are very small. Thus, we can practically say that ankle and hip joints track nominal trajectories well.

The most interesting is the diagram in Fig. 3.5. e), illustrating the ZMP behaviour. Maximal average deviation is about 1 [cm] what can be considered very succesfull. Behaviour of the other joints, especially of the ankle, is not spoiled much by such very "strong" keeping ZMP position under control.


## 4. STABILITY ANALYSIS OF BIPED GAIT

To analyze stability of the locomotion mechanisms agregation-decomposition method via Lyapunov vector functions in bounded regions of state space which originally has been developed for manipulation robots. As it is valid for the mechanism with all joints powered, this method cannot be directly applied to the locomotion mechanisms containing unpowered d.o.f. Because of that, we modify the subsystems modelling by incorporeting the models of unpowered d.o.f. into the composite subsystems models. In this way, the complete mechanism is considered in stability analysis.


### 4.1 Modelling of Composite Subsystems

The mathemathical model of the complete system S consists of two parts: the model of mechanical structue $S^M$ and the model of actuators $S^i_a$. These models are:

$$S^M: \quad P = H\,(q)\cdot\ddot{q} + h\,(q,\dot{q}) \tag{4.1}$$

$$S^i_a: \quad \dot{x}^i_c = A^i_c x^i_c + b^i_c N(u^i) + f^i_c P^i_c \tag{4.2}$$

The notation is same as before. The machanical structure of n d.o.f. is powered by m actuators. Since (n-m) joints are unpowered, the driving torques $P^i$ around the axes of these joints are assumed to be zero, i.e. the vector of driving torques P has following form $P = (P^1_c, P^1_c, \ldots, P^m_c, 0, \ldots, 0)^T$. In order to apply method for stability analysis we shall rearrange this model in another way. The model of the $\ell$-th unpowered joint follows from (4.1):

$$-H_{\ell\ell}\ddot{q}^\ell_N = \sum_{\substack{j=1 \\ j\neq\ell}} H_{\ell j}\ddot{q}^j + h_\ell(q,\dot{q}) \tag{4.3}$$

where $\ddot{q}_N^\ell \in R^1$ is the angle of the $\ell$-th unpowered joint, $H_{\ell j}$ are the members of matrix $H(q)$, and $h_\ell$ is the member of vector h. The subscript N denotes unpowered d.o.f. However, instead of this model, let us describe the motion of the system around the axis of the $\ell$-th unpowered joint as a motion as an inverted pendulum. The equation of inverted pendulum motion in plane is

$$\ddot{q}_N^\ell = \frac{M}{I_0 + M\rho^2} g \sin q_N^\ell + \frac{1}{I_0 + M\rho^2} P_N^\ell \qquad (4.4)$$

where M and $I_0$ are mass and inertia moment of the pendulum (in our case the pendulum corresponds to the whole system) $\rho$ is the distance from the supporting point to the pendulum mass centre, $P_N^\ell \in R^1$ is the resultant generalized force acting on the pendulum. If angle $q_N^\ell$ is small we can introduce the approximation $\left(\sin q_N^\ell\right) \approx q_N^\ell$. If the term multiplying $P_N^\ell$ by $\bar{f}_N^\ell$, and $x_N^\ell = \left[q_N^\ell, \dot{q}_N^\ell\right]^T$ is adopted as state vector, then (4.4) can be written in the matrix form

$$\begin{bmatrix} \dot{q}_N^\ell \\ \ddot{q}_N^\ell \end{bmatrix} = \begin{bmatrix} 0 & 1 \\ C_o^{\ell *} & 0 \end{bmatrix} \begin{bmatrix} q_N^\ell \\ \dot{q}_N^\ell \end{bmatrix} + \begin{bmatrix} 0 \\ \bar{f}_N^\ell \end{bmatrix} P_N^\ell \qquad (4.5)$$

what in compact form is

$$\dot{x}_N^\ell = A_N^\ell x_N^\ell + f_N^\ell P_N^\ell$$

Since we want the models (4.5) and (4.1) to coincide, we shall define the force $P_N^\ell$ as

$$P_N^\ell = \frac{-H_{\ell\ell}^{-1}}{f_N^\ell} \left[ \sum_{\substack{j=1 \\ j \neq \ell}}^{n} H_{\ell j} \ddot{q}^j + h_\ell\left(q, \dot{q}\right) \right] - \frac{C_o^{\ell *}}{f_N^\ell} q_N^\ell \qquad (4.6)$$

In this way we ensure that (4.5) is an exact model of the system motion about the axis of unpowered joint.

$$\begin{bmatrix} \begin{bmatrix} \dot{x}_N^\ell \end{bmatrix} \\ \begin{bmatrix} \dot{x}_c^k \end{bmatrix} \end{bmatrix} = \begin{bmatrix} \begin{bmatrix} A_N^\ell \end{bmatrix} & 0 \\ 0 & \begin{bmatrix} A_c^k \end{bmatrix} \end{bmatrix} \begin{bmatrix} \begin{bmatrix} x_N^\ell \end{bmatrix} \\ \begin{bmatrix} x_c^k \end{bmatrix} \end{bmatrix} + \begin{bmatrix} \begin{bmatrix} f_N^\ell \end{bmatrix} & 0 \\ 0 & \begin{bmatrix} f_c^k \end{bmatrix} \end{bmatrix} \begin{bmatrix} P_N^\ell \\ P_c^k \end{bmatrix} + \begin{bmatrix} 0 \\ \begin{bmatrix} b_c^k \end{bmatrix} \end{bmatrix} N\left(u^k\right) \qquad (4.7)$$

The subscript N corresponds to the unpowered and subscript c to the powered d.o.f. Here, $x_N^\ell \in R^{n_N^\ell}$ and $x_c^k \in R^{n_c^k}$ are the state vectors of the $\ell-$th unpowered $x_N^\ell = \left(q_N^\ell, \dot{q}_N^\ell\right)$ k-th powered d.o.f. $x_c^k = \left(q_c^k, \dot{q}_c^k, i_R^k\right)$; $i_R^k$ is the rotor current of the corresponding DC motor, whereas $n_N^\ell = 2$ and $n_c^k = 3$ are their orders. $A_N^\ell \in R^{n_N^\ell \times n_N^\ell}$ and $A_c^k \in R^{n_c^k \times n_c^k}$, $f_N^\ell \in R^{n_N^\ell}$ and $f_c^k \in R^{n_c^k}$, $P_N^\ell \in R^1$ and $P_c^k \in R^1$ are the system matrices, force distribution vectors, and generalized forces of unpowered and powered d.o.f., respectively. $A_N^\ell$ and $f_N^\ell$ are defined by (4.5). Taking into account the form of the actuator matrix $A_c^k$, and the form of unpowered d.o.f. (4.5), expression (4.7) can be written as

$$
\begin{bmatrix} \begin{bmatrix} \dot{q}_N^\ell \\ \ddot{q}_N^\ell \end{bmatrix} \\ \begin{bmatrix} \dot{q}_c^k \\ \ddot{q}_c^k \\ \dot{i}_R^k \end{bmatrix} \end{bmatrix} = \begin{bmatrix} \begin{bmatrix} 0 & 1 \\ c_o^* & 0 \end{bmatrix} & \begin{matrix} 0 & 0 & 0 \\ 0 & 0 & 0 \end{matrix} \\ \begin{matrix} 0 & 0 \\ 0 & 0 \\ 0 & 0 \end{matrix} & \begin{bmatrix} 0 & 1 & 0 \\ 0 & a_{2,2}^k & a_{2,3}^k \\ 0 & a_{3,2}^k & a_{3,3}^k \end{bmatrix} \end{bmatrix} \begin{bmatrix} \begin{bmatrix} q_N^\ell \\ \dot{q}_N^\ell \end{bmatrix} \\ \begin{bmatrix} q_c^k \\ \dot{q}_c^k \\ i_R^k \end{bmatrix} \end{bmatrix} + \begin{bmatrix} 0 & 0 \\ \bar{f}_N^\ell & 0 \\ 0 & 0 \\ 0 & \bar{f}_c^k \\ 0 & 0 \end{bmatrix} \begin{bmatrix} P_N^\ell \\ P_c^k \end{bmatrix} + \begin{bmatrix} 0 \\ 0 \\ 0 \\ 0 \\ \bar{b}_c^k \end{bmatrix} N(u^k) \qquad (4.8)
$$

where $a_{i,j}^k$ are the elements of matrix $A_c^k$, or, in a compact form as

$$
\dot{x}_Z^k = A_Z^k \cdot x_Z^k + f_Z^k \cdot P_Z^k + b_Z^k \cdot N(u^k) \qquad \forall k \in J
$$

where $x_Z^k \in R^{n_Z^k}$ is the state vector of the composite subsystem, $A_Z^k \in R^{n_Z^k \times n_Z^k}$, $f_Z^k \in R^{n_Z^k \times 2}$, $b_Z^k \in R^{n_Z^k}$ are the subsystem matrix, the matrix of force distribution and vector of control distribution, respectively. Thus, $n_Z^k = n_N^\ell + n_c^k$, $x_Z^k = (x_N^{\ell T}, x_C^{kT})^T$ and $P_Z^k = (P_N^\ell, P_C^k)^T$. Obviously, (4.8) defines only the k-th composite subsystem model. Set J is defined as $J=\{j, j=2m-n+1, \dots ,m\}$. It is assumed that k-th powered joint is associated with $\ell$ – th unpowered joint.

In the stability analysis, it is required that all decoupled subsystems are exponentially stable. If the subsystem correspond to joints of kinematic chain, their coupling are represented by moments around the joint axis. In fact, decoupling means an investigation of the subsystem model without the term which corresponds to the generalized force. In case of a composite subsystem this term is $\left( f_Z^k \cdot P_Z^k \right)$, i.e. the decoupled composite subsystem can be written as

$$
\dot{x}_Z^k = A_Z^k x_Z^k + b_Z^k N\left(u^k\right) \qquad (4.9)
$$

The interaction between these d.o.f. is, in fact, the only way to control the motion of the unpowered d.o.f. In order to preserve the integrity of the decoupled composite model, some additional elements should be introduced into matrix $A_Z^i$ in the places which represent the influence of powered d.o.f. on the unpowered d.o.f. and vice versa. Then, the model of the composite subsystem is of the final form

$$
\begin{bmatrix} \begin{bmatrix} \dot{q}_N^\ell \\ \ddot{q}_N^\ell \end{bmatrix} \\ \begin{bmatrix} \dot{q}_c^k \\ \ddot{q}_c^k \\ \dot{i}_R^k \end{bmatrix} \end{bmatrix} = \begin{bmatrix} \begin{bmatrix} 0 & 1 \\ c_o^* & 0 \end{bmatrix} & \begin{bmatrix} D_1^{1k} & D_1^{2k} & D_1^{3k} \end{bmatrix} \begin{matrix} 0 & 0 & 0 \end{matrix} \\ \begin{bmatrix} D_2^{1k} & D_2^{2k} \end{bmatrix} \begin{matrix} 0 & 0 \end{matrix} & \begin{bmatrix} 0 & 1 & 0 \\ 0 & a_{2,2}^k & a_{2,3}^k \\ 0 & a_{3,2}^k & a_{3,3}^k \end{bmatrix} \end{bmatrix} \begin{bmatrix} \begin{bmatrix} q_N^\ell \\ \dot{q}_N^\ell \end{bmatrix} \\ \begin{bmatrix} q_c^k \\ \dot{q}_c^k \\ i_R^k \end{bmatrix} \end{bmatrix} + \begin{bmatrix} 0 & 0 \\ \bar{f}_N^\ell & 0 \\ 0 & 0 \\ 0 & \bar{f}_c^k \\ 0 & 0 \end{bmatrix} \begin{bmatrix} P_N^\ell - \dfrac{D_1^{1k} \cdot x_C^k}{\bar{f}_N^\ell} \\ P_C^k - \dfrac{D_2^{1k} \cdot x_N^\ell}{\bar{f}_c^k} \end{bmatrix} + \begin{bmatrix} 0 \\ 0 \\ 0 \\ 0 \\ \bar{b}_c^k \end{bmatrix} N(u^k) \qquad (4.10)
$$

or

$$
\dot{x}_Z^k = A_Z^{k*} x_Z^k + f_Z^k P_Z^{k*} + b_Z^k N\left(u^k\right)
$$

The vector $D_1^k = \begin{bmatrix} D_1^{1k} & D_1^{2k} & D_1^{3k} \end{bmatrix}$ represents the influence of the powered d.o.f. on the unpowered one, whereas $D_2^k = \begin{bmatrix} D_2^{1k} & D_2^{2k} \end{bmatrix}$ represents an opposite effect. Since the vectors $D_1^k$ and $D_2^k$ are chosen arbitrarily, $D_1^k \cdot \left[ x_k \right]^T$ and $D_2^k \cdot \left[ x_n^\ell \right]^T$ will be subtracted from the $\left( f_z^k \, P_z^k \right)$, i.e. $P_z^{k*} = \left( P_N^{\ell*}, P_c^{k*} \right)$,

$P_N^{\ell*} = P_N^\ell - \left[ \left( D_1^k \cdot x_c^k \right) / \bar{f}_N^\ell \right]$, $P_c^{k*} = P_c^k - \left[ \left( D_2^k \cdot x_N^1 \right) / \bar{f}_c^k \right]$. The composite subsystem model formed in this way is suitable for stability investigation and enables a stability analysis of the system having joints without actuators. It should be emphasized that the models of "composite" subsystems (4.10) are exact, i.e. they contain no approximations. The model (4.10) coincides with the original model of the $\ell$ – th unpowered joint (4.3) and the model of the k-th powered joint with the actuator (4.2 ) which is driving the k-th joint. We only rearranged the model in order to obtain it in a convenient form. The mathematical model of the mechanism part which consists of composite subsystems is

$$\dot{x}_z = \hat{A}_z^* x_z + f_z P_z^* + b_z N(u_z) \tag{4.11}$$

where $x_z \in R^{N_z}$ is state vector; $x_z = \left( x_z^{(2m-n+1)T}, \ldots, x_z^{mT} \right)^T$, $\hat{A}_z^* \in R^{N_z \times N_z}$, $\hat{A}_z^* = \text{diag} \left\{ A_z^{k*} \right\}$

is the system matrix, while $b_z = \text{diag} \left\{ b_z^k \right\}$ and $f_z = \text{diag} \left\{ f_z^k \right\}$, $b_z \in R^{N_z \times (n-m)}$, $f_z \in R^{N_z \times 2(n-m)}$,

are the distribution matrices of control force; $N(u_z) \in R^{n-m}$ and $P_z^* \in R^{2(n-m)}$ are the corresponding control and force ( defined by (4.10)), $N_z$ is the order of the model formed of composite subsystems,

$$N_z = \sum_{k=2m-n+1}^{m} n_z^k \tag{4.12}$$

Thus, the mathematical model of a complete biped mechanism S with composite subsystems included, can be obtained by uniting the model of composite subsystems (4.11), (including (n-m) powered d.o.f) and the rest (2m-n) powered d.o.f.

$$S: \quad \dot{x} = Ax + FP + BN(u) \tag{4.13}$$

where $x \in R^N$, $x = (x_c^{1T}, \ldots, x_c^{(n-m)T}, x_z^T)^T$ is the system state vector $P = (P_{c_{N \times n}}^1, P_c^2, \ldots$

$P_c^{2m-n}, P^{2m-n+1*T}, \ldots, P_z^{m*T})^T$. Matrices $A \in R^{N \times N}, B \in R^{N \times m}$ and $F \in R^{N \times n}$ are

$$A = \begin{bmatrix} \hat{A}_c & 0 \\ 0 & \hat{A}_z \end{bmatrix}, \quad B = \begin{bmatrix} \hat{b}_c & 0 \\ 0 & b_z \end{bmatrix}, \quad F = \begin{bmatrix} \hat{f}_z & 0 \\ 0 & f_z \end{bmatrix}, \quad N = N_z + \sum_{i=1}^{2m-n} n_i \quad \hat{A}_c = \text{diag} \left[ A_c^i \right], \quad \hat{b}_c = \text{diag} \left[ f_c^i \right],$$

$\forall i \in I_2$, $I_2 = \left\{ i, i = 1, \ldots, 2m-n \right\}$.

The complete system S (4.13) is composed of m subsystems:(2m-n) subsystems correspond to the powered joints modelled as in (4.2), and (n-m) composite subsystems modelled as in (4.11). In fact, all the subsystems can be written in the same form:

$$\dot{x}^i = A^i x^i + b^i N(u^i) + f^i \hat{P}_i(x), \qquad \forall i \in I_1 \tag{4.14}$$

where $x^i$ stands for $x_c^i$ if $i = 1,2, \ldots, 2m-n$, and for $x_z^i$ if $i = 2m-n+1, \ldots, m$. The same holds for $A^i, b^i, f^i$ and $u^i$, while $\hat{P}_i$ stands for $P_c^i$ if $i = 1,2, \ldots, 2m-n$, and for $P_z^{i*}$ if $i = 2m-n+1, \ldots, m$.

The order of subsystems (4.14) are denoted by $n_i$ ( though, it might be either $n_i$, or $n_z^i$, depending on i ).

4.2. Stability analysis

Let us consider the overall system model S defined as in (4.14) , which can be considered as a set of  m  subsystems $S^i$ (either of the composite or powered joints ) which are coupled through the term $\left(f^i \cdot \hat{P}_i\right)$ ,

$$\dot{x}^i = A^i x^i + b^i N(u^i) + f^i \hat{P}_i(x) , \qquad \forall i \in I_1$$

Let us assume the nominal trajectory of the state vector $x^\circ(t)$, $\forall t \in T$ is given in such a way that is satisfies  $x^\circ(0) \in X^I$, $x^\circ(t) \in X^F$ , $\forall t \in T_s$ and $x(t) \in X^t(t)$ , $\forall t \in T$. Further, let us assume the nominal trajectory c has been selected in such a way that we can find a nominal  (programed ) control $u^\circ(t)$, which is a function of time, and which satisfies

$$\dot{x}^{\circ i} = A^i x^{\circ i} + b^i N(u^{\circ i}) + f^i \hat{P}_i^\circ(x^\circ) , \qquad \forall i \in I_1, \; \forall t \in T \qquad (4.15)$$

where $x^\circ(t) = \left(x^{\circ 1T}(t), x^{\circ 2T}(t), \dots, x^{\circ mT}(t)\right)^T$ , $u^\circ = \left(u^{\circ 1}, u^{\circ 2}, \dots, u^{\circ m}\right)^T$.

Here , $\hat{P}_i^\circ(x^\circ)$ denotes nominal values of $\hat{P}_i(x)$. Because the subsystems (4.14) include the composite subsystems, this means that the nominal trajectory $x^\circ(t)$ satisfies the composite subsystems. In other words, we assume that the nominal trajectory $x^\circ(t)$ and the corresponding nominal control $u^\circ(t)$, satisfying (4.15), can be determined.

However, due to the perturbation actions uopon the system, a deviation of the system state from its nominal trajectory must appear. The model of deviation from the nominal trajectory can be written ( according to (4.14) and (4.15) ) as

$$\Delta \dot{x}^i = A^i \Delta x^i + b^i N(t, \Delta u^i) + f^i \Delta \hat{P}_i(t, \Delta x, x^\circ(t)) , \quad \forall i \in I_1 \qquad (4.16)$$

where $\Delta x^i = x^i - x^{\circ i}(t)$ , $\Delta u^i = u^i - u^{\circ i}(t)$ , $\Delta \hat{P}_i = \hat{P}_i - \hat{P}_i^\circ(x^\circ)$. Now, the problem is to stabilize the model of deviation (4.16) from the nominal trajectory $x^\circ(t)$, i.e. we have to synthesize the control $\Delta u^i$ such that the model of deviation from $x^\circ(t)$ (4.16) is stabilized. The aim is to ensure practical stability of the system around the nominal trajectory $x^\circ(t)$, such that for each $\Delta x(0) \in X^I - x^\circ(0)$ it is fulfilled $\Delta x(t) \in X^F - x^\circ(t)$ , $\forall t \in T_s$, and $\Delta x(t) \in X^t(t) - -x^\circ(t)$ , $\forall t \in T$.

Let us synthesize a decentralized control. To do this let consider an approximate model of deviation in its decoupled form (i.e. the model in which the coupling terms between subsystems ($f^i \Delta \hat{P}_i$) are neglected ):

$$\Delta \dot{x}^i = A^i \Delta x^i + b^i N(t, \Delta u^i) , \qquad \forall i \in I_1 \qquad (4.17)$$

The decoupled model of system (4.17) represents a set of decoupled linear subsystems which can be stabilized by simple linear feedback control

$$\Delta u^i = -k_i^{LT} \Delta x^i , \qquad \forall i \in I_1 \qquad (4.18)$$

where $k_i^L \in R^{n_i}$ , is the vector of local feedback gains selected such that the subsystem

$$\Delta \dot{x}^i = (A^i - b^i k_i^{LT}) \Delta x^i = \tilde{A}^i \Delta x^i , \qquad \forall i \in I_1 \qquad (4.19)$$

(where  $\tilde{A}^i$ is a closed-loop subsystem matrix ) is exponentially stable. In (4.19) we have neglected the amplitude saturation upon the input $N(t, \Delta u)^i$. If this nonlinearity is taken into account , it can be shown that subsystem (4.19) is exponentially stabilized in the finite region $X_i$ in the state space, with a desired stability degree $\Pi_i$. If decoupled subsystems (4.19) are considered, it is obvious that this model will be exponentially stable in the region

$$X = X_1 \times X_2 \times \ldots \times X_n \tag{4.20}$$

We shall analyze stability of the complete system (4.16) if a decentralized control (4.18) is applied. Let us express the subsystems characteristics by the Lyapunov functions, which together with their derivatives along solutions for decoupled subsystems have to satisfy

$$\Pi_{i1}\|\Delta x^i\| \langle V_i(\Delta x^i) \langle \Pi_{i2}\|\Delta x^i\| \tag{4.21}$$

$$-\Pi_{i3}\|\Delta x^i\| \langle \dot{V}_i(\Delta x^i) \langle -\Pi_{i4}\|\Delta x^i\| \tag{4.22}$$

along solution of (4.19)

for $\forall i \in I_1$, $\Pi_{ik} \rangle 0$ are real numbers, for $k = 1,2,3,4$, $V_i \rangle 0$, $V_i : R^{n_i} \to R^1$. The analysis concerning the stability on finite regions using aggregation-decomposition method can be conservative. Therefore, it was shown that functions $V_i$ should be chosen in such a way to be the best estimates of the degree of exponential stability $\Pi_1$ of the decoupled subsystems. Thus, we should select such Lyapunov function $V_i$ which satisfies:

$$\dot{V}_i(\Delta x^i) = \left(\text{grad } V^i\right)^T \Delta x^i \leq -\Pi_{i4}\Pi_{i2}^{-1} V_i \leq -\Pi_i V_i \ , \quad \forall i \in I_1 \tag{4.23}$$

where $\dot{V}_i$ is taken along the trajectory of decoupled subsystem (4.19). Let us select the Lyapunov function in the form

$$V_i = \left(\Delta x^{iT} H^i \Delta x^i\right)^{1/2} \ , \quad \forall i \in I_1 \tag{4.24}$$

where matrix $H^i \in R^{n_i \times n_i}$ (symmetric and positive definite) can be derived as the solution of the Lyapunov matrix equation

$$\tilde{A}^{iT} H^i + H^i \tilde{A}^i = -G^i \tag{4.25}$$

where $G^i \in R^{n_i \times n_i}$ is an arbitrarily defined, symmetric and positive definite matrix. If we select $G^i$ to be equeal to $\Pi_i H^i$, then the selected Lyapunov function (4.24) obviously satisfies (4.23). Since the control signal is of limited amplitude, the condition (4.23) can be satisfied only in the finite region of initial conditions $x_i(0) \in X_i$, i.e. the decoupled system is asymptotically stable in the region $X$, defined by (4.20). The region $X_i$ can be estimated via Lyapunov functions by regions $\tilde{X}_i$ with an adequate choice of $V_{io}$

$$\tilde{X}_i = \left\{\Delta x^i : V_i(\Delta x^i) \langle V_{io} \text{ and } \Delta x^i \in X_i\right\} \ , \quad \forall i \in I_1, \ \tilde{X}_i \subseteq X_i \tag{4.26}$$

where $V_{io} > 0$ are positive numbers. Then, the region

$$\tilde{X}(0) = \tilde{X}_1 \times \tilde{X}_2 \times \ldots \times \tilde{X}_m \ , \qquad \tilde{X}(0) \subseteq R^N \tag{4.27}$$

is the best estimate of the region of asymptotic stability $X$ of the set of decoupled subsystems (4.19). However, in (4.19) we have neglected the coupling terms $\left(f^i \cdot \Delta \hat{P}_i\right)$.

Now it should be investigated how the coupling influences the stability of the overall system S. Since $\lim\limits_{\Delta x \to 0} \Delta \hat{P}_i \to 0$ the coupling influence can be estimated by the $\xi_{ij}$ $\left(\xi_{ij} \geq 0 \text{ for } i \neq j\right)$ which satisfy

$$(\text{grad } V_i)^T f^i \Delta \hat{P}_i(t, \Delta x) \leq \sum_{j=1}^m \xi_{ij} V_j \ , \quad \forall i \in I_1 \ , \ \forall t \in T \ , \ \forall \Delta x \in \tilde{X} - x^\circ(t) \tag{4.28}$$

A sufficient condition that the whole system S is asymptotically stable in the region $\tilde{X}(0)$ is

$$Gv_o < 0 \tag{4.29}$$

where $V_o$ is the $m \times 1$ vector, and $V_o = (V_{1o}, \ldots, V_{mo})^T$, $V_o \in R^m$ and the elements of the $m \times m$ matrix $G$ are defined as

$$G_{ij} = -\Pi_i \delta_{ij} + \xi_{ij},$$ 
(4.30)

where $\delta_{ij}$ is the Kronecker symbol.

It is necessary to point out that (4.29) is only a sufficient, but not necessary condition. If this condition is not fulfilled, then $\tilde{X}(0)$ is an estimate of the region of the overall system stability. Then, it is possible to estimate the region $\tilde{X}(t)$ which contains the system state during the tracking of the nominal trajectory $x^\circ(t)$ by

$$\max_{i \in I_1} (V_i(\Delta x^i(t))/V_{io}) \langle \max_{i \in I_1} (V_i(\Delta x^i(0))/V_{io}) \exp(-\beta t)$$ 
(4.31)

where $\beta > 0$ can be computed from

$$\beta = \min_{i \in I_1} (-V_{io}^{-1} \sum_{j=1}^{m} G_{ij} V_{jo}) = \min_{i \in I_1} (\beta_i)$$ 
(4.32)

where $\beta_i = -V_{io}^{-1} \sum_{j=1}^{m} G_{ij} V_{jo}$

Inequality (4.31) is an estimation of shrinkage of the region $\tilde{X}(t)$ which contains a solution of system S. Now the practical stability of the system can be checked. If

$$X^I \subseteq \tilde{X}(0) \quad \text{and} \quad \tilde{X}(t) \subseteq X^t(t), \quad \forall t \in T, \quad \tilde{X}(t) \subseteq X^F(t), \quad \forall t \in T_s$$ 
(4.33)

is satisfied, then it can be stated that the system S is practically stable around $x^\circ(t)$. If the local linear feedback controllers defined by (4.18), are not sufficient to stabilize the system, and additional control input should be introduced. We may introduce the global control in the form ($\Delta \hat{P}_i^*$ instead $\Delta P_c^{i*}$ is used)

$$\Delta u_i^G = k_{i4}^G \Delta \hat{P}_i^* + k_{i5}^G$$ 
(4.34)

where $k_{i4}^G$ and $k_{i5}^G$ are the scalar gains which are defined in (4.4.10). Here, $\Delta \hat{P}_i^*$ represents a value which corresponds to the coupling $\Delta \hat{P}_i$. By measuring forces at the contact point between the sole of the supporting leg and the ground, we get information on the effects of coupling upon the unpowered joint $\Delta P_N^\ell$. Therefore, we can establish a global control from the unpowered joint to the one of the powered joints (i.e. to its actuator) and by this to compensate for the effects of coupling upon the unpowered joint. If a global control is introduced, the stability analysis can be perfomed as described above. However, the numbers $\xi_{ij}^*$ estimating coupling are now defined to satisfy the following (instead of (4.28)):

$$(\text{grad } V_i)^T f^i \Delta \hat{P}_i + (\text{grad } V_i)^T b^i \Delta u_i^G \leq \sum_{j=1}^{m} \xi_{ij}^* V_j, \quad \forall i \in I_1, \forall t \in T, \quad \forall \Delta x \in \tilde{X} - x^\circ(t) \quad (4.35)$$

The next step is to check conditions (4.29), i.e. to test whether the system with applied local and global control is asymptotically stable in the region $\tilde{X}(0)$. Then, the numbers $\xi_{ij}$ in (4.30) have to be replaced by numbers $\xi_{ij}^*$. If the global control is properly selected, then the numbers $\xi_{ij}^*$ have to satisfy

$$\xi_{ij}^* \leq \xi_{ij}, \quad \forall i, j \in I_1$$

Therefore, the fulfillment of stability test has to be easier if the global control is introduced, than if only the local control is applied.

### 4.3. Example

The scheme of adopted locomotion mechanism is same as in Fig. 2.4. Each powered joint is modelled as one subsystem; the composite subsystem comprises the models of one powered and one unpowered joint. The inactive d.o.f. are not included into subsystem modelling. To make the examples of stability analysis easier to follow, a redrown scheme of the same mechanism is presentedd in Fig. 4.1., with only those d.o.f. which will be included in the stability analysis. All the joints represented by the unit rotational axes $\vec{e}_i'$ $(i = 1, \ldots, 9)$, and the corresponding links are re-enumerated. Let us note that the link representing the upper body comprises the trunk and both hands. We shall investigate system stability in the sagittal plane only, so that there is only one unpowered d.o.f. Thus, the mechanism which we are to consider here has nine d.o.f. $(n = 9)$, eight of them $(m = 8)$ being powered. The elements of matrices of the actuator models and their distribution per joints are given in Table 4.1

Table 4.1. Actuator parameters

| Actuator \ Term | $a_{2,2}$ | $a_{2,3}$ | $a_{3,2}$ | $a_{3,3}$ | $b_3$ | $f_2$ | used at joint |
|---|---|---|---|---|---|---|---|
|  | -4.0 | 0.13 | $-10^5$ | -450 | 2000 | $-7 \cdot 10^{-4}$ | 2, 3, 6, 7 |
| $M_2$ | -1.928 | 4.03 | -6800 | -264 | 400 | -0.179 | 4, 5 , 8, 9 |

The nominal trajectories are synthesized using prescribed synergy method. The control input to the i-th actuator consist of two parts

$$u^i = u^{oi} + \Delta u^i \tag{4.36}$$

where $u^{oi}$ is the nominal control input to the i-th actuator while $\Delta u^i$ is the corrective input to the same actuator, synthesized at the level of peturbed regimes. The control low (3.8) holds for the subsystems $i = (1, 2, \ldots, 2m-n)$, and a similar control is derived for the composite subsystems, taking into account that $\Delta \hat{P}_i^*$ for composite subsystems are $(2 \times 1)$ vectors.

In (3.9), the part depending only on local states of the i-th joint corresponds to the local and the rest to the global control. The global control is introduced in the form of feedback with respect to both the driving torques $\Delta \hat{P}_i^*$, and the bang- bang part $k_{i5}^G$. Here, $\Delta \hat{P}_i^*$ represents the force feedback (i.e. the measured moments about joints). An additional feedback respecting ZMP position, defined by (3.16), is also available.

Let us determine the stability region $X_i$ of the decoupled subsystem. Consider first the local control (4.5.9), (4.11) which has to stabilize the decoupled subsystem. If we assume that the complete state vector $\Delta x^i$ is measurable, the closed-loop subsystem is given by (4.19). It is clear that in the case of a stable subsystem, the poles have to be at the left-hand side of the complex plane. If we denote the modulus of their real part by $\left| \sigma_p^i \right|$, the subsystem will be exponentially stable with a stability degree defined as

$$\Pi_i = \min_{p=1,2,3} \left| \sigma_p^i \right| \tag{4.37}$$

which can be guaranteed only if the control inputs are within the limits

$$\left| k_i^{LT} \Delta x^i \right| < u_m^{-i} = u_m^i - \max_{t \in T} \left| u^{oi}(t) \right| \tag{4.38}$$

The actuator velocity-torque characteristucs limit the values of the state coordinates. According to this characteristics we can write

$$\left| \bar{k}_i^2 \Delta \dot{q}^i + \bar{k}_i^3 \Delta i_R^i \right| \le \bar{k}_m^i \rightarrow \left| k_i^{-T} \Delta x^i \right| \le \bar{k}_m^i \tag{4.39}$$

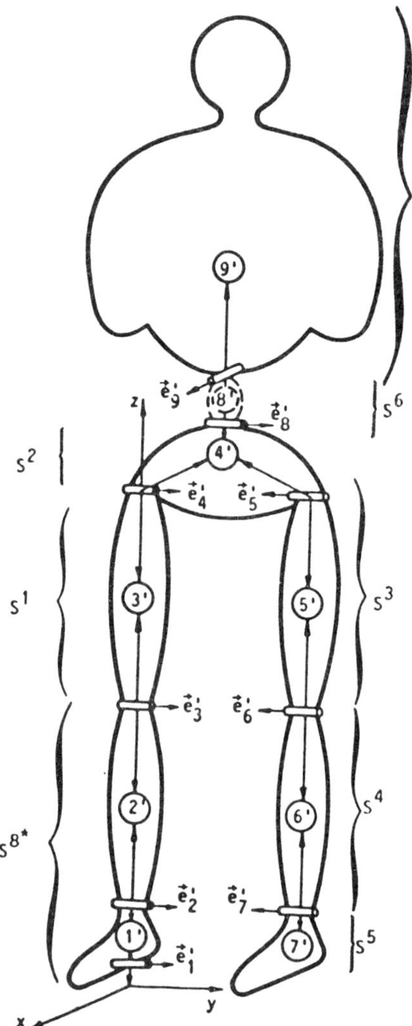



Fig.4.1. Simplified scheme of
        mechanical biped
        structure with dispo-
        sition of modelled
        subsystems

where $\overline{k}_i = (0, \overline{k}_i^2, \overline{k}_i^3)^T$ and $\overline{k}_m^i$ are defined by the

motor characteristics. Further, the regions of allowable angle deviations for each d.o.f are introduced. In this way, the stability regions are constrained, for both powered and composite subsystems.

We may define a finite region $X_i$ ( according to (4.20)) in the state space $R_i^n$, in which the subsystem $S^i$ is exponentially stable with a stability degree $\Pi_i$

$$X_i = \left\{ \Delta x^i, \left| k_i^{LT} \Delta x^i \right| < \left| \overline{u}_m^i \right| \wedge \left| k_i^{-T} \Delta x^i \right| \leq \overline{k}_m^i \right\}$$

$$(4.40)$$

Now we have to investigate the stability of the whole system. For this purpose, the Lyapunov subsystem functions have to be chosen according to (4.24) taking into account relation (4.23) which has to be satisfied in the region $X_i$. $\widetilde{X}_i$ will be an estimate of $X_i$

$$\widetilde{X}_i = \left\{ \Delta x^i : V_i (\Delta x^i) \leq V_{io} \right\}, \qquad \forall i \in I_1$$

To investigate the asymptotic stability of the overall system, the values $\xi_{ik}^*$, which estimate the subsystem coupling, have to be determined according to (4.35). This expression for the composite subsystem is of the form

$$(\text{grad } V_i)^T \left[ f_z^i \dot{\Delta} P_z^{i*} (t, \Delta x) - b_z^i (k_{i4}^G \cdot \Delta \hat{P}_i^* + k_{i5}^G) \right] \leq$$

$$\leq \sum_{k=1}^m \xi_{ik}^* V_k, \quad i = 2m\text{-}n+1, \ldots, m$$

where global control by both $\Delta P_N^\ell$ and $\Delta P_c^i$ is introduced. If for $\xi_{ij}^*$ thus defined, the condition (4.29) is satisfied, it can be claimed that region $\widetilde{X}$ , defined by (4.27) is an estimate of the region of the overall system stability.

We will form the composite subsystem model of the models of unpowered d.o.f. , and ankle joint. First, let us denote the models of powered subsystems: the subsystem model $S^1$ corresponds to the model of joint 3 powered by the actuator, $S^2$ corresponds to joint 4, $S^3$ to joint 5, $S^4$ to joint 6, $S^5$ to joint 7, $S^6$ to joint 8, $S^7$ to joint 9. As the last model of powered subsystem, $S^8$, is adopted the model of powered subsystem which will be included into the composite subsystem. Thus, to $S^8$ corresponds the model of joint 2 with the model of the corresponding actuator. According to this, the model of composite subsystem will be denoted as $S^{8*}$ and it will comprise the models of unpowered subsystem and $S^8$ . The composite subsystem matrices $A_z^{8*}$ and $f_z^8$ and vector $b_z^8$ are defined as

$$A_z^{8*} = \begin{bmatrix} 0 & 1 & 0 & 0 & 0 \\ 0.882 & 0 & -80 & -10 & 0 \\ 0 & 0 & 0 & 1 & 0 \\ 300 & 100 & 0 & -3 & 0.13 \\ 0 & 0 & 0 & -100000 & -450 \end{bmatrix} \quad b_z^8 = \begin{bmatrix} 0 \\ 0 \\ 0 \\ 0 \\ 2000 \end{bmatrix}, \quad f_z^8 = \begin{bmatrix} 0 & 0 \\ 0.01387 & 0 \\ 0 & 0 \\ 0 & 0.0007 \\ 0 & 0 \end{bmatrix}$$

Obviously, the vectors $D_1^8$ and $D_2^8$ from (4.5.8) are $D_1^8 = [-80, -10, 0]$ and $D_2^8 = [300, 100]$. The Lyapunov functions of all subsystems are selected in the form of (4.24). The matrices $H^i$ are selected to satisfy (4.25) and they are obtained as

$$H^8 = \begin{bmatrix} 100422.00 & 33545.10 & 8660.65 & -98.68 & 0.02 \\ 33545.10 & 11425.23 & -3273.52 & -335.46 & -0.07 \\ 8660.65 & -3273.52 & 183099.94 & 8965.84 & 1.95 \\ -98.68 & -335.46 & 8965.84 & 1097.767 & 0.086 \\ 0.02 & -0.07 & 1.95 & 0.086 & 0.0009 \end{bmatrix}$$

The Lyapunov matrices corresponding to the models of powered subsystems $S^i$ are

$$H^i = \begin{bmatrix} 62777.42 & 2291.71 & 0.56 \\ 2291.71 & 161.15 & 0.02 \\ 0.56 & 0.02 & 0.00011 \end{bmatrix} \quad i = 1, 4, 5 \qquad H^i = \begin{bmatrix} 32912.207 & 408.621 & 4.535 \\ 408.621 & 6.482 & 0.065 \\ 4.535 & 0.065 & 0.00092 \end{bmatrix} \quad i = 2, 3, 6, 7$$

The regions of joints angle deviations (the superscripts correspond to the subsystems model numbers ), in which stability is investigated are (in radians)

$$\Delta q^1 = \pm 0.044, \quad \Delta q^2 = \pm 0.0422, \quad \Delta q^3 = \pm 0.0126, \quad \Delta q^4 = \pm 0.03,$$

$$\Delta q^5 = \pm 0.03, \quad \Delta q^6 = \pm 0.099, \quad \Delta q^7 = \pm 0.01, \quad \Delta q_z^1 = \pm 0.01, \quad \Delta q_z^2 = \pm 0.077$$

where $\Delta q_z^1$ and $\Delta q_z^2$ correspond to the joints comprising the composite subsystem i.e. the unpowered and powered d.o,f (ankle joint with axis of rotation $\vec{e}_2$ ).

Constants $V_{io}$ which define estimates of stability regions $\widetilde{X}_i$ are computed to be

$$V_{30} = 0.65, \qquad V_{20} = 1.0399, \quad V_{30} = 0.4256, \quad V_{40} = 0.1545,$$

$$V_{50} = 0.75166, \quad V_{60} = 0.7395, \quad V_{70} = 0.1814, \quad V_{80} = 0.3291$$

Constant $V_{8o}$ corresponds to composite subsystem. The results of stability analysis are presented in Table 4.2. Three types of control law are investigated:
a) The complete feedback structure defined by (3.8) plus the global control with the respect to ZMP displacement defined by (3.16).
b) The local control is introduced ($k_{i1}^L, k_{i2}^L$ and $k_{i3}^L$ from 3.8) plus global control with respect to ZMP position (3.16).
c) Only local control from (3.8) is introduced

   To save space and make comparison easier, all three cases are presented together. The first row correspond to case a), the second to b), and third one to c). The first and the second set of three rows correspond to the knee and the hip of the supporting leg, the third, fourth and the fifth to the hip, knee and ankle of ther leg in swing phase, while the sixth and seventh set correspond to the trunk motion in the frontal and saggital plane. The last set of three rows corresponds to the composite subsystem.

Table 4.2.  Results of stability analysis (composite system consisting of ankle joint and unpowered joint)

$$
G = \begin{bmatrix}
-2402.97 & 0 & 0 & 0 & 0 & 0 & 0 & 0 \\
-2360.45 & 0 & 0 & 0 & 0 & 0.195 & 0 & 0 \\
-2360.45 & 0 & 0 & 0 & 0 & 0.195 & 0 & 0 \\
0 & -120.65 & 0 & 0 & 0 & 0 & 0 & 0 \\
0 & -120.43 & 0 & 0 & 0 & 0 & 0 & 0 \\
0 & -120.43 & 0 & 0 & 0 & 0 & 0 & 0 \\
0 & 0 & -76.15 & 0 & 0 & 0 & 0 & 0 \\
0 & 0 & -73.88 & 0 & 0 & 0 & 0 & 0 \\
0 & 0 & -73.88 & 0 & 0 & 0 & 0 & 0 \\
0 & 0 & 0 & -5114.02 & 0 & 0 & 0 & 0 \\
0 & 0 & 0 & -4761.15 & 0 & 0 & 0 & 0 \\
0 & 0 & 0 & -4761.15 & 0 & 0 & 0 & 0 \\
0 & 0 & 0 & 0 & -789.58 & 0 & 0 & 0 \\
0 & 0 & 0 & 0 & -764.16 & 0 & 0 & 0 \\
0 & 0 & 0 & 0 & -764.16 & 0 & 0 & 0 \\
0 & 0 & 0 & 0 & 0 & -67.56 & 0 & 0 \\
0 & 0 & 0 & 0 & 0 & -66.40 & 0 & 0 \\
0 & 0 & 0 & 0 & 0 & -66.40 & 0 & 0 \\
0 & 0 & 0 & 0 & 0 & 0 & -32.84 & 0 \\
0.323 & 0.1 & 0 & 0 & 0 & 0.309 & -28.86 & 0.114 \\
0.323 & 0.1 & 0 & 0 & 0 & 0.309 & -28.86 & 0.114 \\
13.04 & 11.62 & 0 & 0 & 0 & 6.14 & 0 & -218.33 \\
33.537 & 24.44 & 2.745 & 0 & 0 & 23.78 & 0 & -177.82 \\
37.065 & 26.65 & 8.138 & 8.872 & 1.278 & 26.89 & 11.38 & -170.84
\end{bmatrix}
$$

$$
G \cdot v_0 = \begin{bmatrix}
-1563.62 & -125.46 & -32.41 & -790.28 & -593.50 & -49.96 & -5.96 & -46.74 \\
-1535.81 & -125.24 & -31.44 & -735.75 & -574.39 & -49.10 & -4.66 & +7.48 \\
-1535.81 & -125.24 & -31.44 & -735.75 & -574.39 & -49.10 & -4.66 & +23.35
\end{bmatrix}^T
$$

$$
\eta = \begin{bmatrix}
2402.97 & 120.65 & 76.15 & 5114.01 & 789.58 & 67.56 & 32.84 & 142.03 \\
2360.23 & 120.43 & 73.88 & 4761.14 & 764.16 & 66.40 & 25.66 & - \\
2360.23 & 120.43 & 73.88 & 4761.14 & 764.16 & 66.40 & 25.66 & -
\end{bmatrix}^T
$$

To derive final conclusion about the system stability, thee product $G \cdot v_0$ has to be observed. If this product is negative, the stability under the given conditions is proved. Vector $\eta$ represents shrinkage of the bounds of the regions . $\widetilde{X}(t)$

## 5. INTELLIGENT CONTROL OF BIPED ROBOTS

This section demonstrates the suitability of fuzzy logic for building lookup tables for tuning parameters of legged robot control systems.

The simple mechanical model of two-legged mechanism was chosen as an example model. The reason for this choice is that this mechanism, in spite of its mechanical simplicity, belongs to a class of robotic mechanisms that require introduction of different feedback loops in order to implement the dynamic control scheme, including feedback loop according to dynamic reaction force that acts between the mechanism's foot and the ground. If the decentralized control scheme is adopted, considered mechanism requires, besides feedforward compensation and local controllers, introducing global control loops (cross-coupling effects compensation in perturbed regime) and reaction force feedback in order to preserve dynamic equilibrium of the complete system. As in the past period the simulation experiments and experiments on real walking systems were extensively done on the basis of the traditional approach of model-based control, an attempt to make a hybridization of dynamic control scheme by introducing fuzzy-logic controller in control scheme with partially calculated dynamic model was a challenging task.

Regardless of an example that represents minimal configuration of anthropomorphic robot, the obtained results certify the usefulness of this approach, where the fuzzy logic controller is not the simple alternative to the traditional model-based control. Moreover, if the walking system becomes more complicated, it is reasonable to expect even more advantages of this fuzzy–model based control. The important result is the analysis of the numerical complexity of different control schemes versus trajectory tracking accuracy. This analysis shows that for the same tracking accuracy the schemes that include the fuzzy controller have less numerical complexity.


5.1 Model-based dynamic control

According to problem complexity, and some rough knowledge about biological solutions of walk control, it is clear that several stages in the control synthesis could be the most appropriate strategy. We propose the next four stages of control synthesis:

- At the first stage of control synthesis, we prescribe the motion (gait pattern) for the part of the system, and then calculate the compensation movements for the remaining part of the system (mechanism) in order to satisfy the dynamic equilibrium of the overall system. At this stage, nominal driving torques are calculated, too. This is, in fact, a stage of nominal (feedforward) dynamics, or open-loop control.

- in the next stage of control synthesis, based on the centralized feedforward introduced at the first stage, classical local PID controllers around mechanism joint are applied. That means that we look at completely decoupled system under ideal, unperturbed conditions and we try to stabilize every joint separately (decentralized control).

- for disturbances that cannot be stabilized by use of local control only, it is necessary to include some supplementary feedback loops to handle both the strong coupling between the subsystems and ground reaction forces that act at foot–ground contact surfaces and can cause the complete system to overturn around the foot edges. A conventional way to do this is introducing global control to handle the strong coupling between the subsystems (third stage of control synthesis), and reaction force feedback to stabilize the influence of ground reaction forces (fourth stage of control synthesis). These two last control feedback loops can be realized in two ways:

  - since the coupling among subsystems is represented by generalized forces which can be measured directly during gait, it is possible to introduce torque feedback loops as the global control. For this realization we need force/torque sensors mounted at every joint and force sensor on the foot (last link) of the mechanism for the reaction force control.

  - the second way for global control realization is on-line calculation of the coupling among subsystems.

However, both strategies suffer from some drawback. First, the dynamic model may become a very complex system of nonlinear differential equations. Thus, an important question in control design is to what extent it is necessary to model the robot dynamics. The more complex model allows to accomplish better performance characteristics, but at the same time it requires the more expensive controller hardware. In order to cope with the complexity of the model, several computer-based techniques have been developed for automatic generation of procedures for fast computation of either the complete model or its simplified forms in which some terms are neglected. The second problem follows from the fact that the model used in robot control is always more or less approximation of the real robot behaviour. There are always unmodeled effects whose incorporation would significantly increase the time needed for a precise calculation of the inverse dynamics. A solution of the problem could be in the utilization of force transducers, e.g. joint force sensors. Since they measure total dynamic forces, the joint force sensory feedback is robust to parameter variations and model uncertainties. However, application of joint torque sensors is related to numerous technical problems. Implementation of force transducers usually requires special design of the robot joints. Further, joint torque sensors reduce structural stiffness of the mechanism.

An alternative for attacking the problem of model complexity and uncertainty is offered by knowledge-based control and approximate reasoning techniques. Application of approximate reasoning in automatic control has attracted many researchers investigating the possibilities for automatic control of processes that are ill defined, or have too complex mathematical description, or where the control is performed in environment that is not a priori known, or the control objectives themselves are defined in vague terms. In this field of research, fuzzy logic-based controllers (FLC), inspired by works of Zadeh, have received enormous popularity during the last decade.

In the text to follow we will adopt the decentralized model-based control procedure. The decentralized approach to robot control is intended to decouple the robotic system into a set od independent subsystems which can be stabilized by local servos. In this paper, the decentralized control of the general form:

$$u_i = u_i^0 + \Delta u_i^{Lf} + \Delta u_i^G + \Delta u_i^F \tag{5.1}$$

is considered, where:

- $i$ – joint index, $i = 1, 2, \cdots, n$;
- $u_i$ – $i$-th joint control voltage;
- $u_i^0$ – feedforward signal, computed for the prescribed (synthesized) trajectory;
- $\Delta u_i^{Lf}$ – local control signal, initially determined as output of classical PID controller, and then modified according to the change of local feedback gains caused by fuzzy controller;
- $\Delta u_i^G$ – global control term;
- $\Delta u_i^F$ – control signal to stabilize effects of foot-ground contact.

In the following subsections, we will discuss synthesis of all mentioned control loops in more details.

### 5.2 Fuzzy logic based tuners

Fuzzy controllers of various types have been developed during the last two decades. The fuzzy controller is usually located at the error channel and is composed by a fuzzy algorithm that relates and converts significant observed variables to control actions. The fuzzy rules employed depend on the type of system under control as well as on the heuristic functions used. In robotics, fuzzy controllers were applied, for example, to the dynamic control of a robot arm and to navigation problems for autonomous mobile robots.

Here we implemented fuzzy-logic based controller as an adaptive local controller. In every joint of the walking mechanism we used a fuzzy controller in order to, according to adopted rules, change gains of local controllers to achieve better nominal trajectory tracking.

### 5.3 Case study

In order to verify the described hybrid approach, a simulation case study with a simplified biped mechanism has been made. In this section, parameters of the robot and the control system as used in the simulation experiments are described.

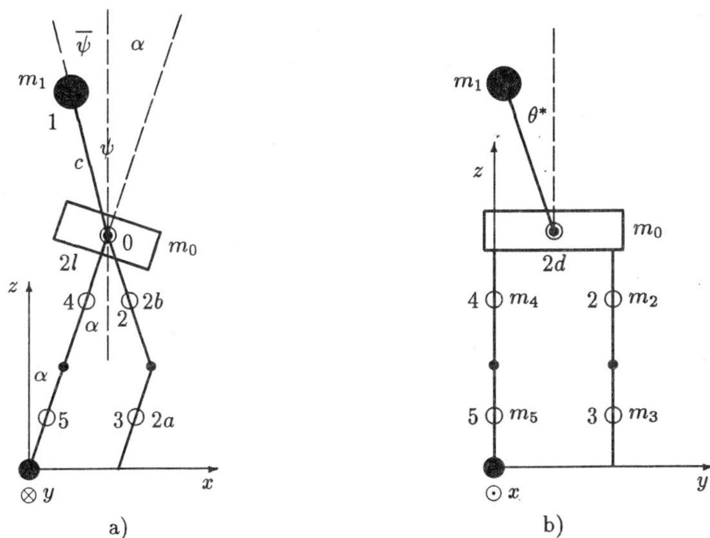


Figure 5.1: Considered mechanism in frontal and in sagittal plane

A six-link mechanism represented on Fig. 5.1 is considered. A "sliding" gait is adopted. Its specificity is that both legs of the model are always in kinematical contact with the ground, but the whole weight is always supported by only one leg. One of the legs is always extended, and the shanks are always parallel. The pelvic part $O$ of the system is attached to the leg which is extended. In that case the position of the legs and the pelvic part can be represented by one coordinate only - angle $\alpha$ between the extended leg and the vertical direction. The upper portion of the model presents a concentric mass on a rigid massless stick (inverted pendulum). With respect to the pelvic part $O$ this pendulum has two degrees of freedom, one in the sagittal (angle $\psi$) and one in the frontal (angle $\theta$) plane. Definition of angle $\psi$ can be seen from Fig. 5.1a). Fig. 5.1b) shows a value for angle $\theta$ only for $\psi = 0$; for $\psi \neq 0$ projection of angle $\theta$ to the vertical plane $\theta^*$ is shown in Fig. 5.1b). For the sake of numerical simplicity, in all calculations angle $\overline{\psi}$, also presented in Fig. 5.1a) is used.

Kinematic and dynamic parameters of the mechanism are listed in Table 5.1. All numerical values are in SI units.

For the prescribed gait it is adopted that angle $\alpha$ changes according to the law:

$$\alpha = \frac{\alpha_m}{2}(1 - \cos\omega t), \quad \omega = \frac{2\pi}{T} \tag{5.2}$$

where $\alpha_m$ is maximum angular amplitude, and $T$ is half period of the step.

For the upper portion of the system, nominal trajectory should be calculated, taking into account that gait repeatability conditions:

$$[\theta(0) \quad \psi(0) \quad \dot{\theta}(0) \quad \dot{\psi}(0)]^T = [-\theta(T) \quad \psi(T) \quad -\dot{\theta}(T) \quad \dot{\psi}(T)]^T \tag{5.3}$$

where $T$ is half-period of one step, must be satisfied.

Centralized dynamic model of the mechanical part of the system should be written in the form:

$$P = H(q)\ddot{q} + h(q, \dot{q}). \tag{5.4}$$

| link | name | shape | length | mass | moment of inertia |
|------|------|-------|--------|------|-------------------|
| 0 | pelvic | thin parallelepiped | $0.21 \times 0.3$ | 6.75 | 0.0127 |
| 1 | body | concentrated mass on a long massles stick | 0.865 | 5 | – |
| 2 | right thigh | long, narrow stick | 0.49 | 1.9 | 0.038 |
| 3 | right lower leg | long, narrow stick | 0.465 | 1.3 | 0.0234 |
| 4 | left thigh | long, narrow stick | 0.49 | 1.9 | 0.038 |
| 5 | left lower leg | long, narrow stick | 0.465 | 1.3 | 0.0234 |

Table 5.1: Kinematic and dynamic parameters of the mechanism

Three DC motors are included into system, and they realize angles $\alpha$, $\theta$ and $\psi$. Their model should be written in the form:

$$S_i : \dot{x}_i = A_i x_i + b_i u_i + P_i \tag{5.5}$$

where $A$-matrix is of dimensions $2 \times 2$, i. e. second order model should be applied, and in the model of the complete $i$-th subsystem (mechanical part + actuators) joint position and velocity should be the state variables. Accordingly, we have:

$$x_1 = [\alpha \ \dot{\alpha}]^T, \quad x_2 = [\theta \ \dot{\theta}]^T, \quad x_3 = [\overline{\psi} \ \dot{\overline{\psi}}]^T \tag{5.6}$$

and for the centralized system we have:

$$x = [\alpha \ \dot{\alpha} \ \theta \ \dot{\theta} \ \overline{\psi} \ \dot{\overline{\psi}}]^T. \tag{5.7}$$

### 5.3.2 Selection of control parameters

As second-order model for actuators (5.5) was considered, where joint position and velocity are state variables, it was suitable to implement local state feedback instead of classical PID controllers. Local feedback was introduced in the form:

$$u_i^L = k_i^p \Delta x_i + k_i^v \Delta \dot{x}_i, \tag{5.8}$$

and for the closed-loop system it was demanded to have a damping factor $\zeta = 0.7$ (slightly under-damped system) and $\omega_n = 5$. By linearization of the nonlinear system for a typical step, position and velocity gains $k_i^p$ and $k_i^v$ were determined for every joint.

Although this model is weakly coupled (mainly degrees of freedom $\alpha$ and $\psi$ are coupled), global control is implemented, as in more complicated mechanism model would be necessary. Global control was implemented by on-line calculation of dynamic forces, and $K_i^G = 0.5$, $i = 1, 2, 3$ was adopted.

Motions in $\theta$ and $\psi$ directions of concentrate mass that represents body were chosen for ZMP displacement compensation. Two additional compensating moments for actuators that realize angles $\theta$ and $\psi$ were calculated in order to force ZMP back to its nominal position. As ZMP must be at foot-ground contact, instead of point contact, in these calculations it was assumed that there exist massless feet of given dimensions.

Fuzzy controller in form of a lookup-table implemented in every joint is according to, and its role is to adjust gains $k_i^p$ and $k_i^v$ of classically determined state feedback.

Prior to submitting to the inference logic for determination of suggested changes in local gains, the inputs $\Delta q$ and $\Delta \dot{q}$ (deviations of state coordinates from their nominal values) are subjected to a nonlinear transformation to obtain the normalized values $\Delta q'$, $\Delta \dot{q}'$ in the closed interval $[-1, +1]$.

The normalized input error space is partitioned into fuzzy regions (primary fuzzy sets) and for each of the regions a set of gain-tuning rules is assigned. The result of evaluation of the rules for given $\Delta q'$, $\Delta \dot{q}'$ are the two fuzzy sets $\Delta \tilde{K}^p$, $\Delta \tilde{K}^v$, which are also defined in the normalized universe $[-1, +1]$. The obtained fuzzy changes are the input to a defuzzification interface which produces the crisp values that are further converted into actual gain changes by applying appropriate nonlinear output transformations.

The universe of discourse for each of the normalized inputs is partitioned into three fuzzy intervals, labeled as *negative, zero* and *positive*, characterized by triangle-shaped grade membership functions.

In the reference, a rather simple heuristics for synthesizing gain-tuning rules is used. A single rule has the form:

$$\text{Rule } r : \text{ if } \Delta q' \text{ is } \tilde{A}_r \text{ and } \Delta \dot{q}' \text{ is } \tilde{B}_r \text{ then } \Delta K' \text{ is } \tilde{C}_r \tag{5.9}$$

where $\tilde{A}_r, \tilde{B}_r, \tilde{C}_r \in \{negative, zero, positive\}$.

The gain tuning rules are schematically presented in the state-action diagram in Table 5.2.

| Position error / Velocity error | negative | zero | positive |
|---|---|---|---|
| positive | zero | zero | positive |
| zero | positive | negative | positive |
| negative | positive | zero | zero |

Table 5.2: Gain tuning rules

Given $\Delta q'$, $\Delta \dot{q}'$, the result of evaluating the individual rule is the fuzzy set $\Delta \tilde{K}_r$ characterized by the grade of membership function

$$\mu_{\Delta \tilde{K}_r}(\Delta K') = \mu_{\tilde{A}_r}(\Delta q') \wedge \mu_{\tilde{B}_r}(\Delta \dot{q}') \rightarrow \mu_{\tilde{C}_r}(\Delta K') \tag{5.10}$$

and the result of evaluating the rule base is the union $\Delta \tilde{K}$ of individual $\Delta \tilde{K}_r$, characterized by

$$\mu_{\Delta \tilde{K}}(\Delta K') = \bigvee_r \mu_{\Delta \tilde{K}_r}(\Delta K') \tag{5.11}$$

The implemented algorithm for evaluating the control rules and defuzzification strategy follows the recommendations by Ying and others. According to these recommendations, the operators "$\wedge$" and "$\rightarrow$" are implemented as minimum operators, whereas the operator "$\vee$" is implemented as bounded sum.

The crisp output $\Delta K'$ is generated as weighted average of those values for which the output primary fuzzy sets attain their maxima, with normalized grades of membership serving as the weighting factors. The obtained value $\Delta K'$ is interpreted as the normalized relative change in gain. So, for the next integration interval, the new gain value is calculated according the expression:

$$K(t + \Delta t) = \min(\max(K(t) \cdot e^{\beta \Delta K'}, K_0), K_{max}) \tag{5.12}$$

where parameter $\beta$ determines the maximum relative rate of change, and $K_0$ and $K_{max}$ are minimum and maximum allowed values for gain $K$.

In our control scheme, both gains $K^p$ and $K^v$ change according to the same set of rules, and parameter $\beta$ is chosen to be $\beta_p = \log 1.2 = 0.1823$ for the position gain, and $\beta_v = 0.5\beta_p$ for the

| dZMP | $K^G$ | Effects included in feedforward | Classical controller | | | Fuzzy controller | | |
|---|---|---|---|---|---|---|---|---|
| | | | av.err. | max.err | Nflops | av.err. | max.err | Nflops |
| dx=0 dy=0 | 0 | Actuators+gravity | 0.0158 | 0.6945 | 312 | 0.0112 | 0.6512 | 379 |
| | | Same+self-inertia | 0.0130 | 0.6410 | 326 | 0.0105 | 0.6327 | 392 |
| | | Same+full inertia | 0.0128 | 0.6411 | 356 | 0.0104 | 0.6328 | 423 |
| | | Complete model | 0.0126 | 0.6414 | 411 | 0.0102 | 0.6328 | 478 |
| | 0.5 | Actuators+gravity | 0.0156 | 0.6945 | 319 | 0.0110 | 0.6512 | 386 |
| | | Same+self-inertia | 0.0128 | 0.6410 | 346 | 0.0102 | 0.6327 | 412 |
| | | Same+full inertia | 0.0126 | 0.6474 | 399 | 0.0101 | 0.6355 | 466 |
| | | Complete model | 0.0124 | 0.6480 | 509 | 0.0099 | 0.6356 | 576 |
| dx=0.06 dy=0.02 | 0 | Actuators+gravity | 0.0154 | 0.6945 | 372 | 0.0113 | 0.6512 | 439 |
| | | Same+self-inertia | 0.0132 | 0.6410 | 386 | 0.0106 | 0.6327 | 453 |
| | | Same+full inertia | 0.0128 | 0.6411 | 415 | 0.0103 | 0.6328 | 483 |
| | | Complete model | 0.0127 | 0.6414 | 471 | 0.0101 | 0.6328 | 538 |
| | 0.5 | Actuators+gravity | 0.0151 | 0.6945 | 379 | 0.0111 | 0.6512 | 446 |
| | | Same+self-inertia | 0.0130 | 0.6410 | 406 | 0.0105 | 0.6327 | 472 |
| | | Same+full inertia | 0.0128 | 0.6474 | 460 | 0.0102 | 0.6356 | 527 |
| | | Complete model | 0.0126 | 0.6480 | 570 | 0.0100 | 0.6356 | 636 |
| dx=0.20 dy=0.05 | 0 | Actuators+gravity | 0.0165 | 0.6945 | 372 | 0.0113 | 0.6512 | 440 |
| | | Same+self-inertia | 0.0144 | 0.6410 | 386 | 0.0107 | 0.6327 | 454 |
| | | Same+full inertia | 0.0135 | 0.6411 | 415 | 0.0106 | 0.6328 | 484 |
| | | Complete model | 0.0131 | 0.6414 | 471 | 0.0105 | 0.6328 | 539 |
| | 0.5 | Actuators+gravity | 0.0163 | 0.6945 | 379 | 0.0110 | 0.6512 | 447 |
| | | Same+self-inertia | 0.0141 | 0.6410 | 406 | 0.0106 | 0.6327 | 474 |
| | | Same+full inertia | 0.0138 | 0.6475 | 460 | 0.0105 | 0.6356 | 528 |
| | | Complete model | 0.0133 | 0.6481 | 570 | 0.0103 | 0.6357 | 637 |

Table 5.3: Tracking accuracy with different feedforward complexity

velocity gain. These values correspond to maximal relative change of 20% per integration interval for position gain.

In order to reduce the computational burden, the values of $e^{\beta \Delta K'}$ for both position and velocity gains are precalculated for equidistant values of $\Delta q'$, $\Delta \dot{q}'$ and stored in a lookup table. When the table has $2^n \cdot 2^n$ entries, $2n$ comparisons are needed to find an entry that corresponds to given errors $\Delta q$, $\Delta \dot{q}$.

## 5.4 Simulation results and discussion

In this section simulation results of mechanism's behaviour with and without fuzzy-controller in different conditions will be compared. Main gait parameters we varied were maximal angular amplitude of the step $\alpha_{max}$ and half-period of the step $T$, so that gait speeds varied from $2.56km/h$ ($\alpha_{max} = 20^0$, $T = 1[s]$) to $5.82km/h$ ($\alpha_{max} = 30^0$, $T = 0.7[s]$). When calculating feedforward compensation, we used different simplified models of system dynamics:

1. actuator models + gravity;

2. actuator models + gravity + self-inertia;

3. actuator models + gravity + self-inertia + full-inertia;

4. actuator models + gravity + self-inertia + full-inertia + velocity terms (the complete model).

We also calculated the control signal in different forms: with and without global term, with and without the fuzzy controller. We examined three values of ZMP deviations: no deviation, small deviation ($5cm$ along $x-$axis and $2cm$ along $y-$axis) and large deviation ($20cm$ along $x-$axis and $5cm$ along $y-$axis).

In the following subsections, we will display our results when $\alpha_{max} = 30^0$ and $T = 0.7[s]$ were adopted, but similar results were obtained for all other combination of mentioned gait parameters. We compared cases when local fuzzy controllers were implemented, to the same cases without the fuzzy controller. $K^G$ is the gain of the global control loop (5.1).

### 5.4.1 Trajectory tracking accuracy

In the Table 5.3, average tracking error (mean square error for all joints) and maximum tracking error that occurred during the path are displayed, for classical controllers versus fuzzy local controller, with ($K^G = 0.5$) and without ($K^G = 0$) global controller. Number of floating point operations (Nflops) per integration interval for considered control laws is included in the Table, too.

We can see that average errors are 15% to 50% smaller when the fuzzy controller is implemented, with a couple of percentage smaller maximal errors.

### 5.4.2 Dynamic equilibrium maintenance

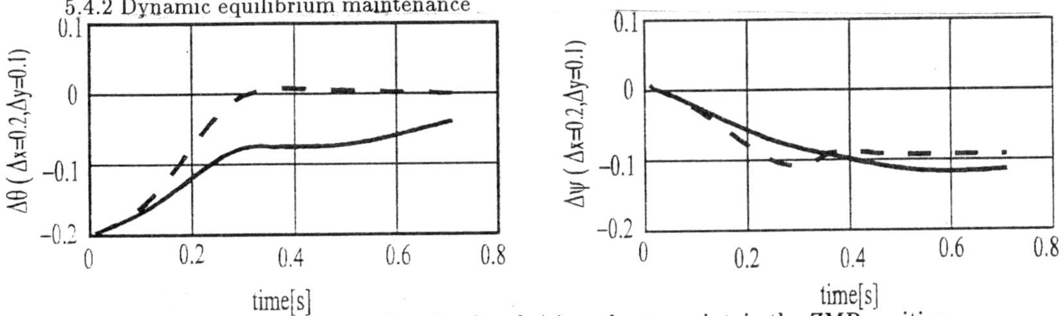

Figure 5.2: Deviations of angles $\theta$ and $\psi$ in order to maintain the ZMP position

Feedback loop for ZMP position regulation has been realized in classical way – shifting from nominal position of ZMP influences two powered degrees of freedom that realize angles $\theta$ and $\psi$. The purpose of these feedback loops is to maintain the ZMP position on its nominal trajectory.

From Fig. 5.2. can be seen that deviations of angles $\theta$ and $\psi$ from their nominal trajectories are less in case of fuzzy controller than in the classical case (full line represents classical case and dashed line fuzzy controller).

### 5.4.3 Numerical complexity

From Table 5.3. it can be seen that the implementation of fuzzy controller does not significantly increase the numerical complexity. But, more important are the diagrams 5.3, that represent average tracking error and maximum tracking error versus numerical complexity for control schemes that include the fuzzy controller and for classical control schemes. This diagrams clearly show that for same tracking error, the fuzzy controllers need less floating point operations, and if the number of floating operations is the same, then the fuzzy controllers give better tracking characteristics, without spoiling any other system characteristics.

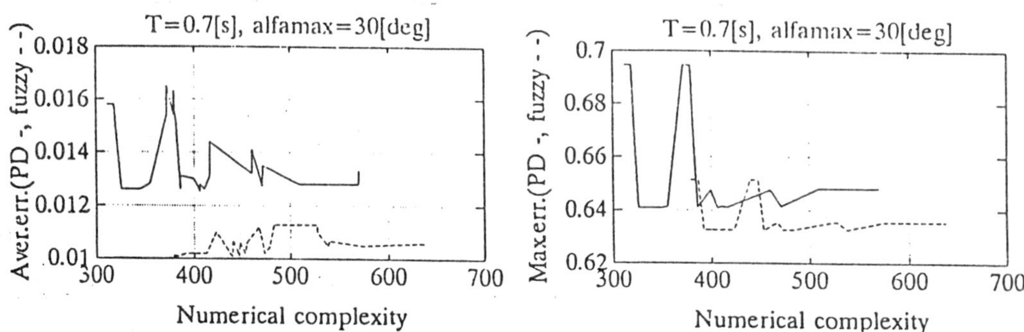


Figure 5.3: Average and maximal error in tracking the nominal trajectory in the $x$−direction for legs of the mechanical model

# References


[1] M. Vukobratović and D. Juričić, "Contribution to the synthesis of biped gait," *IEEE Trans. on Biomedical Engineering*, vol. BME-16, pp. 1–6, January 1969.

[2] M. Vukobratović, "How to control artificial anthropomorphic systems," *IEEE Trans. on Systems, Man, and Cybernetics*, vol. SMC-3, pp. 497–507, September 1973.

[3] M. Vukobratović, *Legged locomotion robots and anthropomorphic mechanisms, research monograph.* Belgrade: Mihailo Pupin Institute, 1975.

[4] M. Vukobratović and D. Stokić, *Control of Manipulation Robots.* Vol. 2 of *Scientific fundamentals of robotics*, Springer Verlag, 1982.

[5] B. Borovac, M. Vukobratović, and D. Stokić, "Stability analysis of mechanisms having unpowered degrees of freedom," *Robotica*, vol. 7, pp. 349–357, 1989.

[6] M. Vukobratović, B. Borovac, D. Surla, and D. Stokić, *Biped locomotion.* Vol. 7 of *Scientific fundamentals of robotics*, Springer-Verlag, 1990.

[7] M. Vukobratović and O. Timčenko, "Experiments with nontraditional hybrid control technique of biped locomotion robots," *Journal of intelligent and robotic systems*, vol. 16, pp. 25–43, 1996.

[8] L. A. Zadeh, "Outline of a new approach to the analysis of complex systems and decision processes," *IEEE Transactions on systems, man, and cybernetics*, vol. 3, pp. 28–44, January 1973.

[9] H. Ying, W. Siler, and J. J. Buckley, "Fuzzy control theory: a nonlinear case," *Automatica, the journal of IFAC*, vol. 26, pp. 513–520, May 1990.

# BALLISTIC LOCOMOTION OF A BIPED

## DESIGN AND CONTROL OF TWO BIPED MACHINES


**A.M. Formal'sky**

**Moscow Lomonossov State University, Moscow, Russia**


## ABSTRACT


This article contains two parts.

1. Direct method of anthropomorphic biped locomotion design is developed. The designed walk consists of the alternating phases of single and double support. During the single-support motion the control torques are zeros, therefore this motion is called ballistic. The double-support phase is instantaneous. At the instant of double support the impulsive control torques are applied in the joints. They are described by $\delta$-functions. The problem of ballistic locomotion design is formulated as a boundary-value problem for the system of equations describing the single-support motion.

2. Two bipeds were designed at the Institute of Mechanics, Moscow Lomonossov State University: one with telescopic legs and another with anthropomorphic kinematic scheme. The design of the bipeds, control systems, and adaptive algorithms for controlling the vehicle locomotion in the sagittal plane are described.

# 1. BALLISTIC LOCOMOTION OF A BIPED

## INTRODUCTION

The problem of control and dynamics of two-legged walk has been studied theoretically by many investigators. They are, for instance, Beletskii, Berbyuk, Bordyug, Bolotin, Farnsworth, Frank, Gubina, Hemami, Larin, McGeer, Mochon, McMahon, Morecki, Moreinis, Novozhilov, Schiehlen, Seireg, Townsend, Vukobratovich, Zatsiorskii.

Most researchers investigate the dynamics of two-legged walk using the inverse or semi-inverse approach. They prescribe the motion of the biped, fully or partly, and then, using the motion equations, find the forces applied to the biped, evaluate the consumed energy.

Direct method of anthropomorphic biped locomotion design is used in the present theoretical investigation. The designed walk consists of the alternating phases of single and double support. Each single-support motion terminates with an impact of the transferred leg onto the surface. The subsequent double-support phase is instantaneous. At the instant of double support, there is a change in the support from one leg to another. Then the new single-support phase begins. During the single-support motion the control torques are zeros, therefore this motion is called ballistic. At the instant of double support the impulsive control torques are applied in the joints. They are described by $\delta$-functions. The velocities of the links undergo the jumps at this instant. The problem of ballistic locomotion design is formulated as a boundary-value problem for the system of equations describing the single-support motion. We investigate it both analytically and numerically.

The first publication of author on the ballistic locomotion of a biped is the article "Motion of anthropomorphic biped under impulsive control" in the book "Some questions of robots mechanics and biomechanics", 1978, Institute of Mechanics, Moscow University, p.17-34 (in Russian). See also the monograph "Locomotion of anthropomorphic mechanisms", 1982, Moscow, "Nauka", 386 p. (in Russian) and papers in the journal "Mechanics Solids".

## MOTION EQUATIONS OF A BIPED

### Model Description

Consider the mathematical model of anthropomorphic biped walk in sagittal plane. The investigated model of biped contains the torso $OC$ and two identical legs $OBA$ and $ODE$. Each leg consists of the thigh ($OB$ and OD) and the shin ($BA$ and $DE$). The scheme of the biped is shown in Figure 1. All these five links are massive and absolutely rigid. We neglect the friction in the hip and knee joints considering them as ideal. Note, that in human joints the friction is very small.

The position of the considered biped can be described in the plane $XY$ by seven generalized coordinates: $x$, $y$, $\psi$, $\alpha_1$, $\alpha_2$, $\beta_1$, $\beta_2$ (Fig. 1).

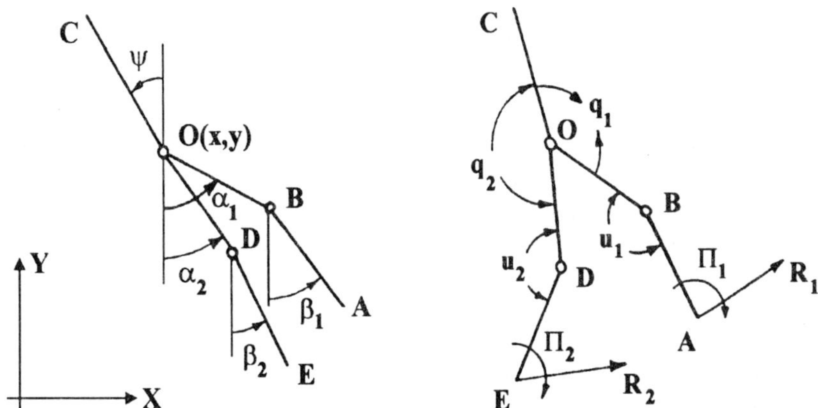


*Fig. 1: The scheme of the biped*          *Fig. 2: The general forces*

Let $q_1$ and $q_2$ be the torques of the forces acting between the trunk and thighs, $u_1$ and $u_2$ be the torques of the forces in the knee joints $B$ and $D$, $\Pi_1$ and $\Pi_2$ be the torques in the ankle joints $A$ and $E$, $R_1(R_{1x}, R_{1y})$ and $R_2(R_{2x}, R_{2y})$ be the forces applied to the leg tips $A$ and $E$ (Fig. 2). Similarly to the human walk, the walk modeled here consists of alternating phases of single and double support. In the double-support phase both legs are on the bearing surface (on the ground), the forces $R_1$ and $R_2$ are the support reactions, and they are nonzero. During the single-support motion, one of reactions $R_1$, $R_2$ is zero.

### Planar Motion Equations of Five-Link Biped

We can obtain the equations of the planar motion of the described biped by the second Lagrange method. Omitting the intermediate calculations, we write the equations in the following matrix form

$$B(z)\,\ddot{z} + gF\,\|\sin z_i\| + D(z)\,\|\dot{z}_i^2\| = C(z)Q \tag{1}$$

where

$$z = \|z_i\| = \|x,\, y,\, \psi,\, \alpha_1,\, \alpha_2,\, \beta_1,\, \beta_2\|^{*}$$

$$\|\sin z_i\| = \|0,\ 1,\ \sin\psi,\ \sin\alpha_1,\ \sin\alpha_2,\ \sin\beta_1,\ \sin\beta_2\|^*$$

$$\|\dot{z}_i^2\| = \|0,\ 0,\ \dot{\psi}^2,\ \dot{\alpha}_1^2,\ \dot{\alpha}_2^2,\ \dot{\beta}_1^2,\ \dot{\beta}_2^2\|^*$$

$$Q = \|u_1,\ u_2,\ q_1,\ q_2,\ \Pi_1,\ \Pi_2,\ R_{1x},\ R_{1y},\ R_{2x},\ R_{2y}\|^*$$

The asterisk denotes transpose. The symmetrical, positive definite matrix of kinetic energy $B(z)$ is of the size $(7 \times 7)$, matrices $F$, $D(z)$ and $C(z)$ are of the sizes $(7 \times 7)$, $(7 \times 7)$ and $(7 \times 10)$ respectively and $g$ is the gravity acceleration.

To describe the motion during the single- or double-support phase this system must be complemented by constraint equations, defining the conditions for fixation of one or both feet on the support.

### Single-Support Motion

In Figure 3 the scheme of the biped standing on one leg is shown.

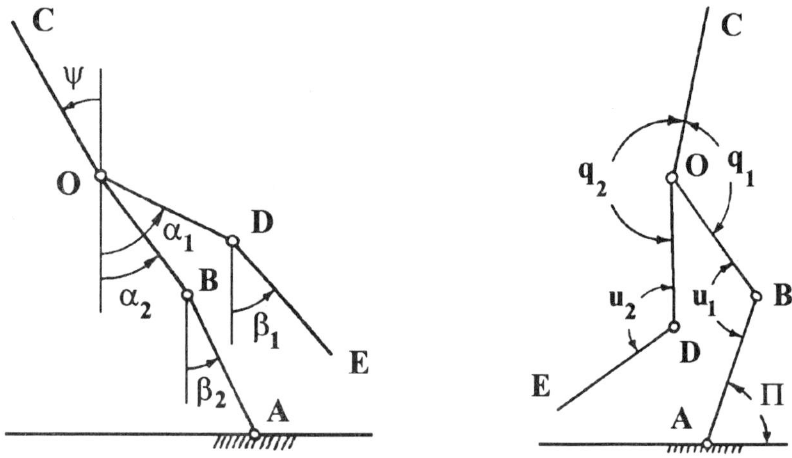

*Fig. 3: The general coordinates of the biped in single-support phase*      *Fig. 4: The general forces*

The tip $A$ is motionless on the bearing surface. We can assume that it is connected to the surface by an ideal joint. But during the locomotion the bearing surface does not keep the supporting leg. Therefore the ground reaction in the point $A$ must be directed upwards. In the single-support phase, the biped has five degrees of freedom and five general coordinates: $\psi$, $\alpha_1$, $\alpha_2$, $\beta_1$, $\beta_2$ (Fig. 3).

We can describe the biped motion during the single-support phase by system (1). But it must be complemented by two constraint equations, defining the condition for fixation of the tip $A$ on the bearing surface. However, it is possible to exclude the reaction force in supporting leg from system (1). We write now the equations of single-support motion excluding this reaction force in matrix form too

$$H(\zeta)\ddot{\zeta} + gL\|\sin\zeta_i\| + M(\zeta)\,\|\dot{\zeta}_i^2\| = N(\zeta)W \qquad (2)$$

where

$$\zeta = \|\zeta_i\| = \|\psi,\ \alpha_1,\ \alpha_2,\ \beta_1,\ \beta_2\|^*$$

$$\|\sin\zeta_i\| = \|\sin\psi,\ \sin\alpha_1,\ \sin\alpha_2,\ \sin\beta_1,\ \sin\beta_2\|^*$$

$$\|\dot{\zeta}_i^2\| = \|\dot{\psi}^2,\ \dot{\alpha}_1^2,\ \dot{\alpha}_2^2,\ \dot{\beta}_1^2,\ \dot{\beta}_2^2\|^*$$

$$W = \|u_1,\ u_2,\ q_1,\ q_2,\ \Pi\|^*$$

Here we denote by $\Pi$ the torque in the ankle joint $A$ (Fig. 4). No force is applied to the tip $E$ of the leg being transferred. The symmetrical, positive definite matrix of the kinetic energy $H(\zeta)$ and matrices $L$, $M(\zeta)$, $N(\zeta)$ are of the sizes $(5 \times 5)$. Having solved the equations (2) we can check whether the supporting leg loses contact with the surface or slips.

## PROBLEM STATEMENT

### *Reasons*

When formulating this problem the following considerations were taken into account. Some authors (Bernstein, Bogdanov and Gurfinkel, Gurfinkel and Fomin, Mochon and McMachon, McGeer, Vitenzon) suppose that in many motions muscle activity alternates with some period of relaxation. Apparently, the motions of that kind are less energy-consuming. During human walk the considerable efforts are acting in the double-support motion on the whole (Vitenzon). The motion of the leg being transferred, for instance, is very close to that of a free pendulum (Gurfinkel and Fomin). Therefore we believe that in the single-support motion of our model there is no active torques in joints, but they are acting in double-support phase. Of course, during the single-support phase the ground reaction in supporting leg is nonzero. But no active forces are acting, and we call this single-support motion ballistic.

Thus we consider a ballistic, in other words, free single-support motion, when active forces are zeros, that is $W(t) = 0$. The equations of ballistic single-support motion can be obtained from (2)

$$H(\zeta)\ddot{\zeta} + gL\|\sin\zeta_i\| + M(\zeta)\,\|\dot{\zeta}_i^2\| = 0 \tag{3}$$

### Single-Support Phase

At the beginning of the step $(t = 0)$ let the biped be in the initial configuration shown in Figure 5 left (position $i$). It is described by some vector

$$\zeta(0) = \|\psi(0),\ \alpha_1(0),\ \alpha_2(0),\ \beta_1(0),\ \beta_2(0)\,\|^* \tag{4}$$

Assume that in this configuration the front and hind legs are both on the surface. For $t > 0$ the front leg is supporting and hind leg is being transferred (see Figs. 3, 4).

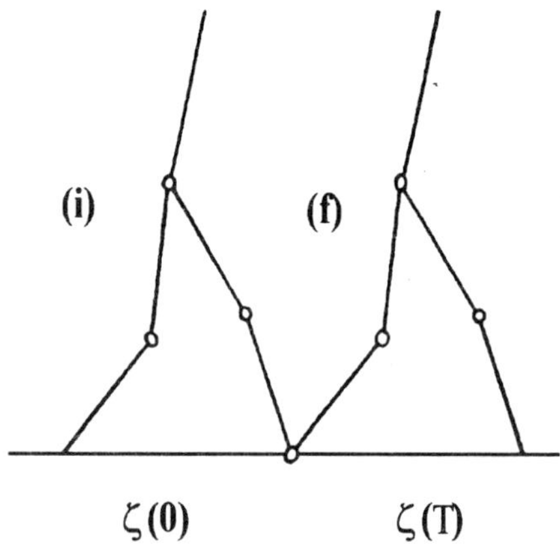


*Fig. 5: The boundary configurations of the biped in single-support phase*

We want to transfer the biped into the final configuration shown in Figure 5 right (position $f$) in a fixed time $t = T$. It is described by vector

$$\zeta(T) = \|\psi(T),\ \alpha_1(T),\ \alpha_2(T),\ \beta_1(T),\ \beta_2(T)\,\|^* \tag{5}$$

We assume that the final configuration coincides with the initial one, but the legs are swapped. The final configuration is described by equality

$$\zeta(T) = P\zeta(0) \tag{6}$$

The symmetric matrix $P$ has only five nonzero elements

$$P = \begin{Vmatrix} 1 & 0 & 0 & 0 & 0 \\ 0 & 0 & 1 & 0 & 0 \\ 0 & 1 & 0 & 0 & 0 \\ 0 & 0 & 0 & 0 & 1 \\ 0 & 0 & 0 & 1 & 0 \end{Vmatrix} \tag{7}$$

It is easily to see that $P = P^{-1}$. Therefore, we can to rewrite the equality (6) so

$$\zeta(0) = P\zeta(T)$$

We can write the expression (6) in scalar form

$$\psi(T) = \psi(0),$$

$$\alpha_1(T) = \alpha_2(0), \quad \alpha_2(T) = \alpha_1(0), \tag{8}$$

$$\beta_1(T) = \beta_2(0), \quad \beta_2(T) = \beta_1(0),$$

If in the single-support phase there is no active forces, the biped can be transferred from the given initial configuration to the final one by selection of initial values for angular velocities of links only. Thus it is required to find the suitable vector $\dot{\zeta}(0)$ of angular velocities. In other words, the problem of ballistic single-support motion design is formulated mathematically as a boundary-value problem for the equation (3). It is required to find the solution $\zeta(t)$ of this equation under boundary conditions (4) and (5).

The problem as stated above leaves no means to ensure that the transferred leg tip moves above the support, the legs bend "knee forward", the torso does not fall down, the reaction force is directed upwards. It is necessary to check these conditions in the solution of the boundary-value problem.

We formulated above the first part of the problem statement. After the single-support phase comes the double-support one and the second part of the problem is the following.

### Double-Support Phase

During the human double-support motion, there is a transition of the support from one leg to another. The double support time in human locomotion is less than 20 per cent of the whole step period. In our study the double support time is assumed infinitely small, that is, the double-support phase is regarded as instantaneous.

Assume that $T$ is the instant when the double-support phase occurs. At that instant a constraint is imposed on the transferred leg, that is, its tip $E$ becomes stationary with respect to the surface. This results in an impulsive reaction (impact), and the velocities of the biped links get instantaneously changed. In addition to this constraint let us apply impulsive efforts in the joints, i.e.

$$Q(t) = I\delta(t - T) \tag{9}$$

where $\delta$ - function is nonzero for $t = T$ only and

$$I = \left\| I_{u_1}, I_{u_2}, I_{q_1}, I_{q_2}, I_{\Pi_1}, I_{\Pi_2}, I_{R_{1x}}, I_{R_{1y}}, I_{R_{2x}}, I_{R_{2y}} \right\|^*$$

is vector of the intensities of impulsive actions (weights of $\delta$-functions), that is, of the torques in the joints and reaction forces. We hope that under impulsive control (9) the desired link velocities can be achieved just before the beginning of the next single-support phase.

The relations between the velocity jumps and intensities of impulsive efforts can be obtained easily from equation (1)

$$B(z(T))[\dot{z}] = C(z(T))I \tag{10}$$

Here $z(T)$ is the known configuration of the biped at the instant $T$ of the double-support phase, $[\dot{z}] = \dot{z}(T + 0) - \dot{z}(T - 0)$ - vector of velocity jumps. The matrix algebraic equation (10) is obtained by integrating of the equation (1) during the null interval $(T - 0, T + 0)$. The second and third terms in the left part of equation (1) have a finite values, so its integration during null interval, is zero.

Let the boundary-value problem formulated above be solved. Then the velocities vector $\dot{z}(0)$ and $\dot{z}(T)$ at the start and the end of the single-support phase are known. We assume that the bearing surface is a plane. Let the gait of the biped be regular, that is its single-support motions coincide on all the steps. Then the equality

$$\dot{z}(T + 0) = \dot{z}(0)$$

holds. Let $\dot{z}(T - 0)$ denotes the velocities vector at the end of the single-support phase. This vector is known from the solution of boundary-value problem. Hence the vector of velocity jumps $[\dot{z}]$ can be computed.

If an active leg tip allows to choose the values $I_{R_1}(I_{R_{1x}}, I_{R_{1y}})$, $I_{R_2}(I_{R_{2x}}, I_{R_{2y}})$, then the impulsive torques and forces to be applied can be calculated from the equation (10). This relation is composed of seven equations and ten unknowns variables of vector $I$. An infinite number of solutions exists in this situation. We can choose the unique solution by minimizing some functional of the components of impulsive forces and (or) torques, for example, the sum of its absolute values. Thus from the relation (10) we can find vector $I$ required to produce desired link velocities at the beginning of the next single-support phase.

Thus in our problem statement the biped locomotion is decomposed. We can design separately the single-support motion by solving the boundary-value problem. Then we can find the forces (torques) in double-support phase.

If passive leg tips are used, the impulsive forces during the double-support phase, $I_{R_1}$ and $I_{R_2}$, must be produced by the ground. In this case we decompose the instantaneous double-support phase into three instantaneous parts (sub-phases) as shown in Figure 6

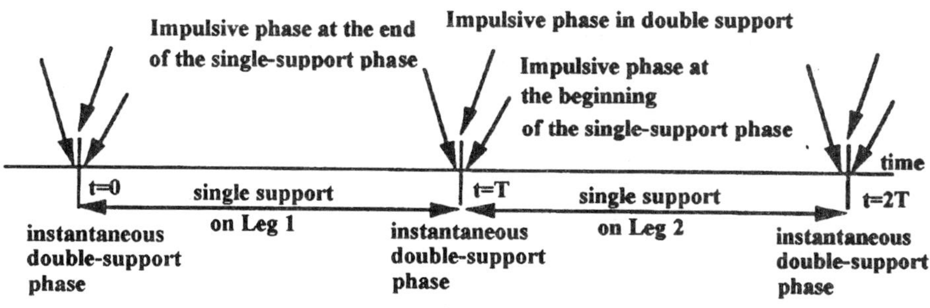


*Fig. 6: Three parts (sub-phases) of each instantaneous double-support phase*

The first sub-phase is impulsive single-support phase with supporting leg 1. In the instant of this sub-phase we change the velocity of the biped from the vector-value $\dot{z}(T - 0)$ to some vector-value $\dot{z}_1$. Both vectors are satisfied to the constraint equations, defining the conditions for fixation of the leg 1 tip on the support. The corresponding impulsive torques and forces are calculated by the following matrix algebraic equation

$$B(z(T))(\dot{z}_1 - \dot{z}(T-0)) = C(z(T))I_1 \qquad (11)$$

In the unknown vector $I_1$ the reaction force $I_{R_2}$ ($I_{R_{2x}}$, $I_{R_{2y}}$) is zero ($I_{R_2} = 0$), because the leg 1 is on the support and leg 2 in transfer.

The second sub-phase is double-support phase. In the instant of this sub-phase we change the velocity of the biped from vector-value $\dot{z}_1$ to some vector-value $\dot{z}_2$. Vector $\dot{z}_2$ is satisfied to the constraint equations, defining the conditions for fixation of both legs tips on the support. The impulsive torques and forces for this sub-phase are calculated by the following matrix algebraic equation

$$B(z(T))(\dot{z}_2 - \dot{z}_1) = C(z(T))I_2 \qquad (12)$$

In the unknown vector $I_2$ all components are nonzero generally.

The third sub-phase is impulsive single-support phase with supporting leg 2. In the instant of this sub-phase we change the velocity of the biped from vector-value $\dot{z}_2$ to the known vector-value $\dot{z}(T+0)$. The corresponding impulsive torques and forces are calculated by the following matrix algebraic equation

$$B(z(T))(\dot{z}(T+0) - \dot{z}_2) = C(z(T))I_3 \qquad (13)$$

In the unknown vector $I_3$ the reaction force $I_{R_1}$ ($I_{R_{1x}}$, $I_{R_{1y}}$) is zero ($I_{R_1} = 0$), because the leg 2 is on the support and leg 1 in transfer.

The configuration of the biped is unchanged during these three sub-phases, because they are instantaneous.                                                                    We consider the equations (11), (12), (13) and aforenamed constrains as a global system with unknown variables $I_1$, $I_2$, $I_3$, $\dot{z}_1$, $\dot{z}_2$. The vectors $\dot{z}_1$ and $\dot{z}_2$. are two intermediate velocities. The number of system equations is less than the number of unknown scalar variables. Therefore, the system has an infinite number of solutions. We can choose the single solution by minimizing some functional of the components of impulsive forces and (or) torques. In the solution the vertical components of the reaction forces and of the velocities of the leg tips must not be directed downwards.

## SEVEN-LINK BIPED MODEL

A seven-link model with massless feet added is considered as well (Fig. 7)

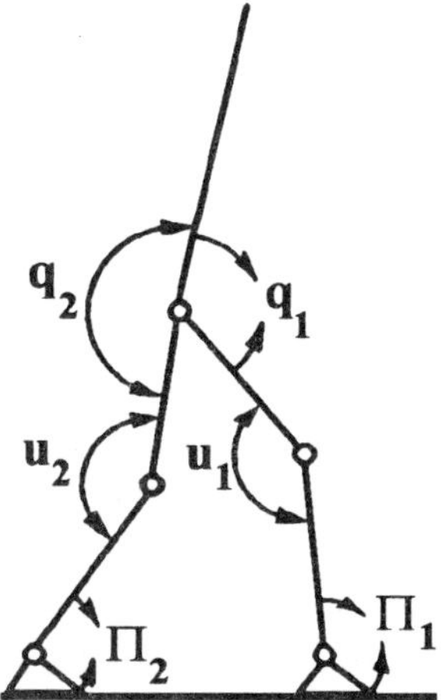


*Fig. 7: A seven-link model with massless feet*

The statement of the problem for seven-link model is similar to the above problem statement for the five-link model of the biped. The problem of single-support motion design is formulated mathematically as a boundary-value problem.

During the single-support motion the foot of the supporting leg is motionless *i.e.,* in equilibrium. We assume that the point of reaction force application (the zero torque point) to the supporting leg moves along the sole from the heel to the toe uniformly in the time. Each foot is massless and its motion equations are the conditions of equilibrium. Therefore, torque in the ankle joint must compensate the torque of the reaction force and is nonzero. The torques in all other joints of the biped during the single-support motion are zeros as for the five-link model. Thus the motion of the seven-link model with feet can not be completely ballistic.

We investigate the boundary-value problem for five-link and seven-link model formulated above both analytically and numerically.

## SYMMETRY PROPERTIES OF THE BALLISTIC MOTION

The system (3) of ballistic single-support motion equations is conservative. Therefore, the energy integral exists:

$$E = 0,5\dot{\zeta}^{*}H(\zeta)\dot{\zeta} + V(\zeta) = const$$

Here $V(\zeta)$ is potential energy.

Now we describe the symmetry properties of the system (3).

*$1°$. If function $\zeta(t)$ is solution of the system (3), then function $-\zeta(t)$ is solution of this system as well.*

The configuration $-\zeta(t)$ is symmetric to configuration $\zeta(t)$ with respect to the vertical axis passing through the ankle joint of the supporting leg.

*$2°$. If function $\zeta(t)$ is solution of the system (3), then function $\zeta(-t)$ is solution of this system as well.*

General mechanical conservative systems with an even Lagrange function have this property. The stick-diagram of the motion $\zeta(-t)$ can be obtained, if the configurations of the stick-diagram $\zeta(t)$ are considered in the reverse sequence. In other words, if forward walking of our five-link model corresponds to solution $\zeta(t)$, then backward walking corresponds to solution $\zeta(-t)$. It is easy to demonstrate the property $2°$ by substituting the function $\zeta(-t)$ into the system (3).

The system (3) is autonomous one. Therefore, along with solution $\zeta(t)$ the system (3) has solution $\zeta(T+t)$ . Here $T$ is arbitrary number. Thus from property $2°$ we have the following one.

*$3°$. If function $\zeta(t)$ is solution of the system (3), then function $\zeta(T-t)$ is solution of this system as well.*

From $1°$ and $3°$ the next assertion follows

*$4°$. If function $\zeta(t)$ is solution of the system (3), then function $-\zeta(T-t)$ is solution of this system as well.*

The property $4°$ means that if $\zeta(t)$ is some ballistic motion of our five-link model in the single-support phase, then $-\zeta(T-t)$ is ballistic motion of this model as well. In other words, if function $\zeta(t)$ is solution of formulated above boundary-value problem (3) - (5), then function $-\zeta(T-t)$ is solution of this problem too.

Let be

$$\zeta(0) = -\zeta(T) \tag{14}$$

*i.e.*, the boundary configurations are symmetric. It follows from property $4^{\circ}$ that if solution $\zeta(t)$ of the boundary-value problem (3) - (5) exists and is unique for these symmetric configurations, then

$$\zeta(t) \equiv -\zeta(T - t) \tag{15}$$

The stick-diagram of the solution satisfying to the equality (15) is symmetrical with respect to the vertical axis passing through the ankle joint of the supporting leg. From the identity (15) we have $\zeta(T/2)=0$. This means that at instant $T/2$ all five links of the biped are on this vertical axis. If in the interval $0<t<T/2$ the transferred leg bends "knee forward", then in the interval $T/2<t<T$ it bends "knee backward". In Figure 8 the stick-diagram of symmetrical solution of nonlinear boundary-value problem (3) - (5) is shown

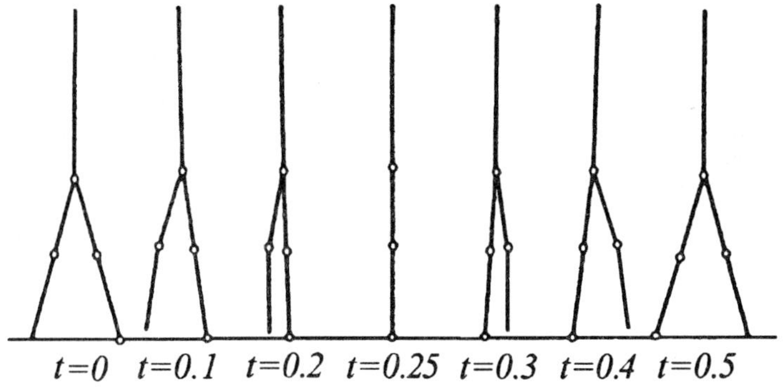


*Fig. 8: Symmetric solution of nonlinear boundary-value problem with $\Delta x = 0.45\,m$, $T = 0.5\,s$ and $\psi(0) = \psi(T) = 0$.*

This solution is obtained numerically for five-link model with anthropomorphic parameter values. The step length $\Delta x$, its duration $T$, the torso inclination at $t = 0$ and $t = T$ are respectively equal

$$\Delta x = 0.45\,m, \quad T = 0.5\,s, \quad \psi(0) = \psi(T) = 0 \tag{16}$$

At instants $t = 0$ and $t = T$ the legs are straight.

We can prove the next assertion.

$5^{\circ}$. *The equality $\zeta(T/2)=0$ exists only for symmetric solution $\zeta(t)$ satisfying condition (15). It is possible to obtain this symmetric solution by extending on the interval $[0,T]$ the solution with boundary conditions $\zeta(0)$ and $\zeta(T/2)=0$.*

The properties $1^\circ$ - $5^\circ$ are very helpful for numerical investigations of boundary-value problem (3) - (5).

The gait shown in Figure 8 is not like human gait. But for the conditions (16) we have found numerically an asymmetric solution $\zeta_1(t)$ of nonlinear boundary-value problem (3) - (5) too. In Figure 9 the stick-diagram of this asymmetric solution is shown

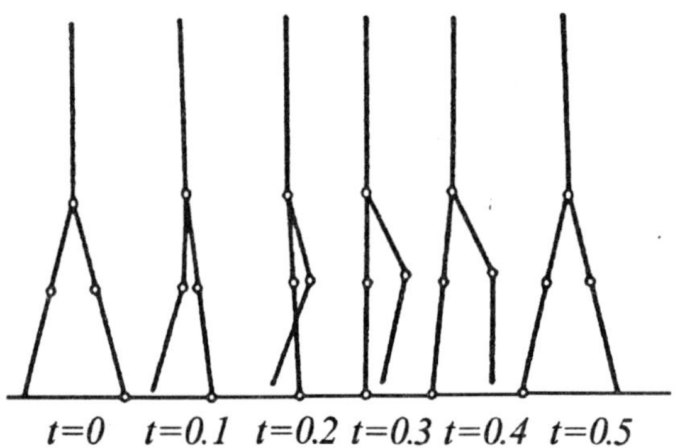


*Fig. 9: Asymmetric solution of boundary-value problem*

It seems that the gait corresponding to this solution $\zeta_1(t)$ is like human gait.

It follows from property $4^\circ$ that function $\zeta(t) = -\zeta_1(T - t)$ is the solution of boundary-value problem too. The backward walking of the biped corresponds to this solution. Thus for conditions (16) the nonlinear boundary-value problem (3) - (5) has at least three solutions. In vicinity of point (16) this problem has three solutions as well.

## SOLUTION OF LINEARIZED BOUNDARY-VALUE PROBLEM

Linearize the system (3) around the equilibrium $\zeta = 0$

$$H(0)\ddot{\zeta} + gL\zeta = 0 \qquad (17)$$

The linear stationary system (17) is conservative. Therefore, using the linear nonsingular transformation with constant matrix $R$

$$\zeta = Rp \qquad p = \|p_i\| \qquad (i=1,...,5) \qquad (18)$$

we can reduce this system to the canonical Lagrange form

$$\ddot{p} + \Omega p = 0 \tag{19}$$

where $\Omega$ is diagonal matrix

$$\Omega = \begin{Vmatrix} \lambda_1 & 0 & 0 & 0 & 0 \\ 0 & \lambda_2 & 0 & 0 & 0 \\ 0 & 0 & \lambda_3 & 0 & 0 \\ 0 & 0 & 0 & \lambda_4 & 0 \\ 0 & 0 & 0 & 0 & \lambda_5 \end{Vmatrix} \tag{20}$$

Here $\lambda_i$ $(i=1,...,5)$ are the roots of the characteristic equation

$$\det\|H(0)\lambda - gL\| = 0 \tag{21}$$

Two roots are positive and three negative

$$\lambda_i = \omega_i^2 \quad (i=1,2); \qquad \lambda_i = -\omega_i^2 \qquad (i=3,4,5) \tag{22}$$

Thus we can rewrite the system (19) in the following scalar form

$$\ddot{p}_i + \omega_i^2 p_i = 0 \qquad (i=1,2) \tag{23}$$

$$\ddot{p}_i - \omega_i^2 p_i = 0 \qquad (i=3,4,5) \tag{24}$$

Note that the transformation matrix $R$ and eigen values $\lambda_i$ $(i = 1,...,5)$ can be calculated using standard computing procedures.

The vectors of initial and terminal conditions for system (19) or (23), (24) are the following

$$p(0) = R^{-1}\zeta(0), \qquad p(T) = R^{-1}\zeta(T) \tag{25}$$

Now we can formulate the boundary-value problem for simple equations (23), (24). It is required to find the solution $p(t)$ of equations (23), (24) under boundary conditions (25). The desired solution has the form

$$p_i(t) = \frac{p_i(T)\sin\omega_i t + p_i(0)\sin\omega_i(T-t)}{\sin\omega_i T} \qquad (i=1,2) \tag{26}$$

$$p_i(t) = \frac{p_i(T)\operatorname{sh}\omega_i t + p_i(0)\operatorname{sh}\omega_i(T-t)}{\operatorname{sh}\omega_i T} \qquad (i=3,4,5) \tag{27}$$

Solution (26), (27) of boundary-value problem (23) - (25) exists for arbitrary boundary conditions if and only if

$$\omega_i T \neq \pi k \qquad (i=1,2; \quad k=1,2,3,...) \tag{28}$$

This solution is unique. Using the transformation (18) we can obtain the desired solution in the original variables.

Note that the properties $1°$ - $5°$ are true for the linear system (19) too.

Thus it is possible to design the solution of linear boundary-value problem using the analytical formulas (26), (27). But to understand the properties of the biped gait it is necessary to carry out the numerical investigations. Numerical solutions of linear boundary-value problem with different step lengths $\Delta x$, its times $T$, boundary configurations (4), (5) are obtained for the model with anthropomorphic parameter values. We were using the display to estimate the pattern of the synthesized locomotion. It is possible to choose configurations (4), (5), times $T$ so that the corresponding gaits are in some sense human-like.


## NONLINEAR BOUNDARY-VALUE PROBLEM

Unlike the solution of linear boundary-value problem, solution of the nonlinear problem can be found using an iterative numerical procedure only. In Figures 10-12 the solution of nonlinear boundary-value problem (3) - (5) for

$$\Delta x = 0.7\,m, \quad T = 0.55\,s, \quad \psi(0) = \psi(T) = -0,075 \tag{29}$$

is shown

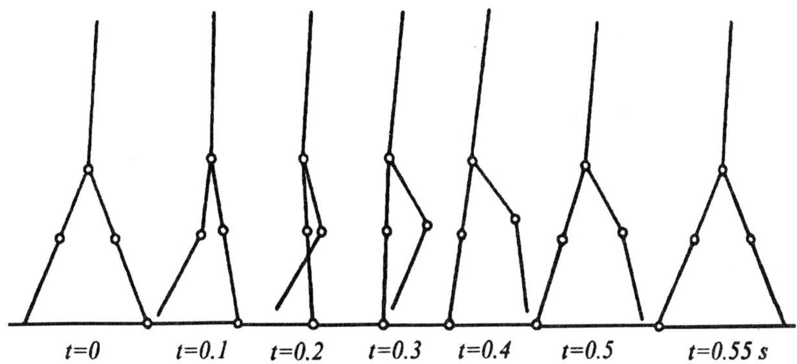



*Fig. 10: Stick-diagram of the gait*

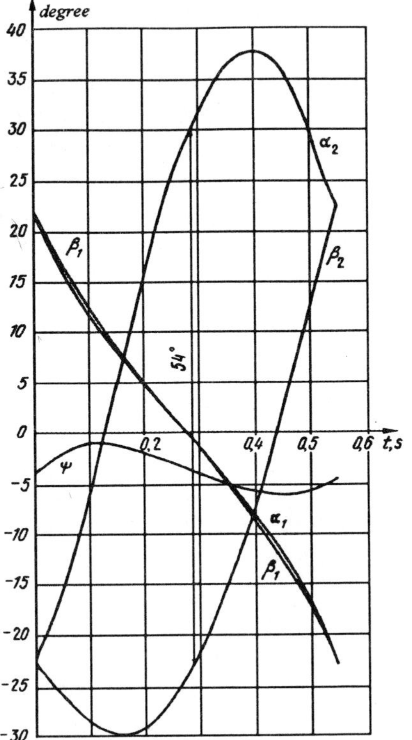

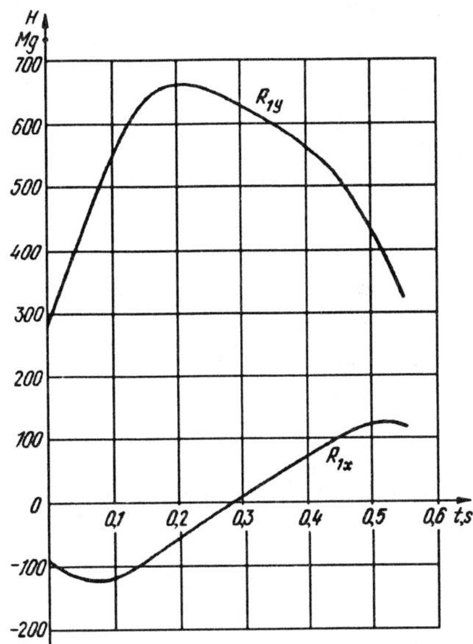

*Fig. 11: Time dependencies of the angles*

*Fig. 12: Time dependencies of the
ground reaction components in the
supporting leg*

The transferred leg tip moves above the support (see Fig. 10). The supporting leg is almost straight ($\alpha_1(t) \cong \beta_1(t)$). The trunk does not fall and oscillates near the vertical once per step. The transferred leg moves with knee forward ($\alpha_2(t) > \beta_2(t)$). The vertical component $R_{1y}$ of the ground reaction is positive. Its maximal value is less than biped weight $Mg$. The sign of the horizontal component $R_{1x}$ changes as in human gait.

## SIMULATION OF SEVEN-LINK MODEL WITH MASSLESS FEET

Figure 13 shows the stick-diagram of the walk of the biped model with massless feet.

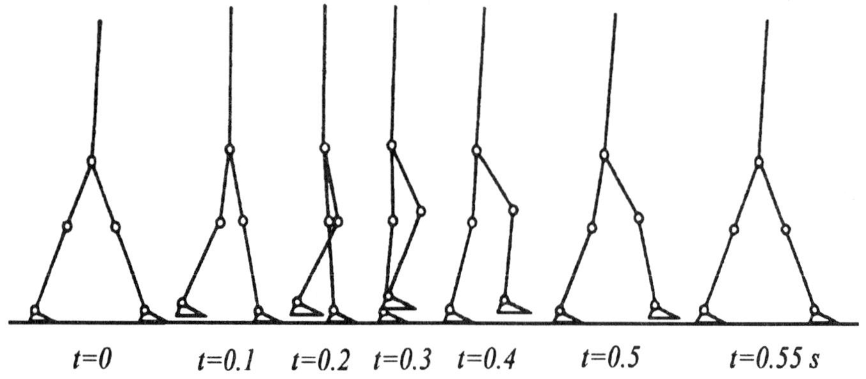


*Fig. 13: The gait of the biped with massless feet*

## CONCLUSION TO THE THEORY ON BALLISTIC LOCOMOTION OF ANTHROPOMORPHIC BIPED

The problem of ballistic locomotion design of anthropomorphic biped is formulated. In this problem statement the biped locomotion is decomposed. It is possible to design separately the single-support motion by solving the boundary-value problem (3) - (5). Then we can find the forces in double-support phase.

We investigate the boundary-value problem both analytically and numerically. It has some symmetry properties which are important to reveal the general pattern of the gait. In the case of linearized motion equations the solution is found analytically. It is unique for any boundary configurations (4) and (5). For the complete nonlinear boundary-value problem a numerical solution can be found using an iterative procedure. It should be noted that several solutions are possible for the same boundary configurations (4), (5) and the time $T$.

Having solved the boundary-value problem for the model with anthropomorphic parameter values, we use the display to estimate the pattern of the synthesized locomotion. At first, we look at the solutions for linearized equations of the five-link model (without feet), then at the solution for complete nonlinear equations of five-link model and finally at the solution for nonlinear equations describing the seven-link model (with massless feet).

We can choose the configurations (4), (5) and time $T$ so that the leg tips move above the support, the mechanism moves with knees forward, the torso doesn't fall and slightly oscillates near the vertical position once per step. It is necessary to point out that the reactions are directed upwards both in the single and in the double support. It is important to note that these "human" features of the gait are not inferred by the problem statement in itself. Hence these are the intrinsic features of ballistic motion. The designed ballistic gaits are in some sense human-like. This resemblance gives additional hints to suppose that human walk contains some intervals of ballistic movement as well.

For the model with feet we estimated the work of control forces performed during one step. It amounts near 70 J. This value is less that the energy consumption estimated by others authors for different (non-impulsive) controls.

# 2. DESIGN AND CONTROL OF TWO BIPED MACHINES

## INTRODUCTION

Several prototype two-legged walking vehicles and algorithms for their control have been designed, and many algorithms have been tested experimentally. Authors of these works are, for instance, Kato et al.; Katoh and Mori; Miura and Shimoyama; Furusho and Mashubushi; Furusho and Sano; Zheng and Sias; McGeer; Kajita, Yamaura and Kobayashi. Raibert developed a biped robot that ran based on his one-legged hopping machine (uniped). Unlike multilegged walking vehicles that can move in the static stability mode, bipeds with uncontrollable feet and unipeds can maintain dynamic stability only. This makes the control of bipeds difficult.

At the Institute of Mechanics, Moscow Lomonossov State University two biped vehicles were designed: one with telescopic legs and another with anthropomorphic kinematic scheme. The mass of each is about 7.5 kg, the height is approximately 0.75 m. We describe here the design of the bipeds, control systems, and adaptive algorithms for controlling the vehicle locomotion in a plane. The vehicle control is designed as tracking the commanded path. A part of the path is calculated in advance based on the mathematical model for the biped motion; the other part is built during walking based on information about the biped state.

## 2.1. BIPED WITH TELESCOPIC LEGS ACTUATED BY TWO DRIVES

At first we consider dynamic walking of a mechanism with telescopic legs and two drives. We describe its mechanical design and developed control algorithm. The first publication on this biped and its control is the article of A.A.Grishin, A.M.Formal'sky, A.V.Lensky and S.V.Zhitomirsky "Dynamic Walking of a Vehicle With Two Telescopic Legs Controlled by Two Drives" in the International Journal of Robotics Research, 1994, Vol. 13, No. 2, p. 137-147.

## MECHANICAL DESIGN

In Figure 1 the mechanism is shown. It consists of two telescopic legs and a trunk. The mass of the trunk is nearly 3.4 kg, and the length is 0.25 m. Each leg consists of two parts: the thigh and the shin, with masses of 1.5 kg and 0.55 kg, respectively. The shin can move along the thigh over the rails, and in this way the total length of the leg is changed. The shins are driven with a rope. The legs have passive (uncontrolled) feet that extend in the frontal plane. Thus the mechanism can fulfill planar walking only (in sagittal plane).

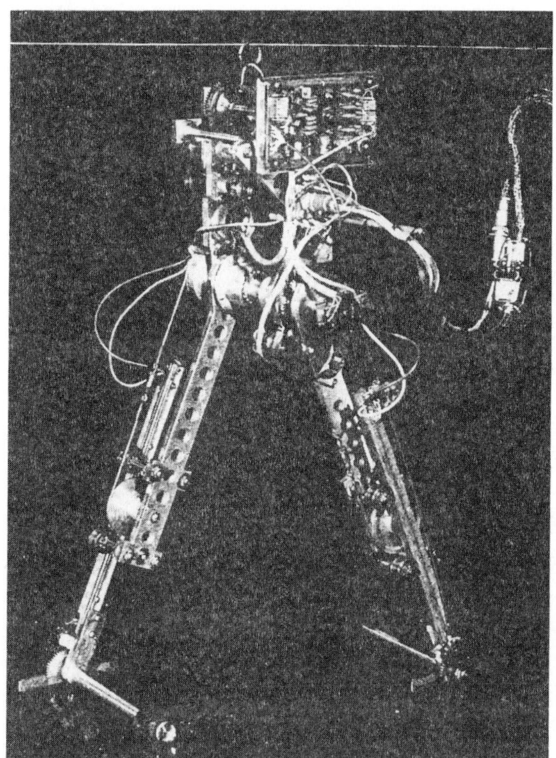

Fig. 1: Biped with two telescopic legs, actuated by two drives

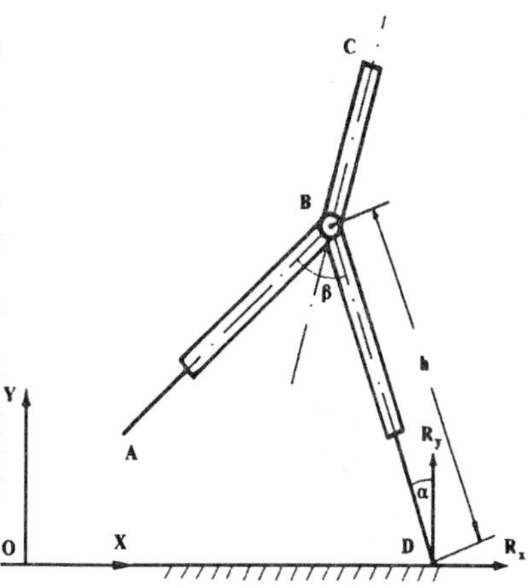

Fig. 2: The kinematic scheme of the biped standing on one leg (side view). The mechanism has three degrees of freedom. Coordinates: α, β, h

The mechanical design superimposes two constraints on the possible motions of all five links of the mechanism. First, both shins are linked together so that the sum of the lengths of both legs $H$ is constant ($H \cong 1\ m$). Thus an extension of one leg causes the respective retraction of another leg. Second, the longitudinal axis of the trunk is always in the middle of the angle formed by the legs. To implement this constraint, a drive is placed on the trunk; it turns the legs by the same angles with respect to the trunk but in opposite directions. The height of the biped standing on both legs with zero angle between them is about 0.75 m.

The schematics of the mechanism standing on one leg is shown in Figure 2 (side view). Here $BC$ is the trunk, $BA$ and $BD$ are the legs. Due to coupling of the leg motions,

$$BA + BD = H = const \tag{1}$$

This relation means that during a double-support phase, the point $B$ moves along an elliptical trajectory. So, in the double-support phase the mechanism has one degree of freedom, in single-support phase three.

Because of the kinematic constraints mentioned earlier, it is sufficient to have only two drives to control the biped. One of them - the telescoping drive - changes the length $h$ of one leg (and the length $H - h$ of another leg). The second drive - the swinging drive - controls the angle $\beta$ between the legs. We use $DC$ motors with a power of about $20\ W$. The gear ratio is $50$ for the swinging drive and $500\ m^{-1}$ for the telescoping drive.

Two potentiometers measure the length $h$ and the angle between legs $\beta$. Respective velocities $\dot{h}$ and $\dot{\beta}$ are taken from tachometers. Each shin is equipped with a single-component force sensor. The sensor enables evaluation of the vertical component $R_y$ of the foot force applied to the leg. Both feet have potentiometers that measure the angles of leg inclination with respect to support.

## EQUATIONS OF MECHANISM MOTION

The position of the biped in the plane $XOY$ is described by five coordinates. Let $x$ and $y$ be the coordinates of the center $B$ of the hip joint (see Fig. 2), $\alpha_1$ and $\alpha_2$ be the angles between the legs and the vertical counted counterclockwise, $h_1$ and $h_2$ be the lengths of the legs. In the presence of the two constrains described above (see equality (1)), the length $h_2$ and the angle $\psi$ of the inclination of the trunk $BC$ with respect to the vertical are expressed via the generalized coordinates as follows:

$$h_2 = H - h_1, \qquad \psi = (\alpha_1 + \alpha_2)/2 \tag{2}$$

In Figure 2 the variables $h$ and $\alpha$ correspond to $h_1$ and $\alpha_1$.

We obtain the motion equations of the described mechanism using second Lagrange method and write these equations in the following matrix form

$$B(z)\ddot{z} + b(z)g + D(z)\left\|\dot{z}_i \dot{z}_j\right\| = C(z)Q \tag{3}$$

where

$$z = \left\|x,\ y,\ \alpha_1,\ \alpha_2,\ h_1\right\|^*,$$

$$\left\|\dot{z}_i \dot{z}_j\right\| = \left\|\dot{\alpha}_1^2,\ \dot{\alpha}_2^2,\ \dot{\alpha}_1 \dot{\alpha}_2,\ \dot{h}_1 \dot{\alpha}_1,\ \dot{h}_1 \dot{\alpha}_2\right\|^*,$$

$$Q = \left\|R_{1x},\ R_{1y},\ R_{2x},\ R_{2y},\ M_1,\ M_2\right\|^*$$

Here $R_{1x}$, $\overset{*}{R}_{1y}$ are the components of the foot force $\boldsymbol{R}_1$ applied to the tip of the first leg; $R_{2x}$, $R_{2y}$ are the components of the foot force $\boldsymbol{R}_2$ applied to the tip of the second leg; $M_1 = \mu_1 - \eta_1$, $M_2 = \mu_2 - \eta_2$, where $\mu_1$ and $\mu_2$ are the torques of electromagnetic forces applied to the rotors of the telescopic and the stroke motors, respectively; $\eta_1$ and $\eta_2$ are the torques of the dissipation forces applied to the rotors of the respective motors. We assume that the dissipative forces are the forces of Coulomb friction, then

$$\eta_1 = \eta_{10} sign \dot{h}_1, \qquad \eta_2 = \eta_{20} sign(\dot{\alpha}_1 - \dot{\alpha}_2)$$

where $\eta_{10}$, $\eta_{20}$ are constants that define the friction force thresholds.

The symmetric matrix of kinetic energy $B(z)$ is a $5 \times 5$ matrix; $b(z)$ is its second column; the matrices $D(z)$ and $C(z)$ are $5 \times 5$ and $5 \times 6$ matrices, respectively; and $g$ is gravity acceleration. Here we will not write the entries of the matrices $B(z)$, $D(z)$ and $C(z)$.

The equation (3) should be confronted with equation (1) from the first part of this article.

In the supportless motion, $\boldsymbol{R}_1 = \boldsymbol{R}_2 = 0$. If the torques $M_1$ and $M_2$ are specified, system (3) with constrains (2) is complete. In the single-support or double-support motion system (3) must be complemented by the constraint equations. These equations define the conditions for fixation of one or both feet on the support

$$x + h_i \sin\alpha_i = x_i, \qquad y - h_i \cos\alpha_i = y_i \qquad (i=1,2) \tag{4}$$

Here $x_i$, $y_i$ are constants. For $i=1$ we get the condition for the fixation of the first leg, for $i=2$, for the second.

By differentiating relations (4) twice with respect to the time, we get the equations that complement the system (3) for the single- and double-support phases. The feet of the biped do not contain devices for the fixation on the support, therefore the constraints imposed on the ends of the legs are unilateral. So, for each designed trajectory, we should check that

$$R_{iy} \geq 0, \qquad |R_{ix}| \leq f R_{iy} \qquad (i=1,2) \tag{5}$$

where $f$ is the coefficient of Coulomb friction between the foot and the support.

If the motors are powered, by neglecting the inductance of the motor winding, we can express the torques of electromagnetic forces

$$\mu_1 = cu_1 - dn_1 \dot{h}_1, \qquad \mu_2 = cu_2 - dn_2(\dot{\alpha}_1 - \dot{\alpha}_2)$$

Here $u_1$ and $u_2$ are the voltages fed to the motors; $c$ and $d$ are the constants that describe the motor characteristics; $n_1$ and $n_2$ are the gear ratios for the telescopic and swinging drives, respectively (the coefficient $n_1$ has dimension $m^{-1}$). If the motors are off (the current is cut), then $\mu_i = 0$ ($i = 1,2$).

During biped motion, each transfer phase terminates with an impact when a leg is being placed on the support. The equations of impact are obtained from system (3) by substituting the vector column $[\dot{z}]$ of the jumps of the generalized velocities for the vector column $\ddot{z}$ of second derivatives. We omit the terms with limited magnitudes and describe unlimited external forces with δ-functions. Then we replace them by the intensities of these actions (weights of δ - functions) and obtain the equations of impact

$$B(z_0)[\dot{z}] = C(z_0)I \tag{6}$$

Here $z_0$ is the vector of generalized coordinates that describes the configuration of the mechanism at the time of impact, $I$ is the vector column of intensities of external actions. Because the torques $M_1$ and $M_2$ are limited, only the intensities $I_{R_{ix}}$ and $I_{R_{iy}}$ ($i = 1,2$) of the foot forces are nonzero in the column $I$.

The equation (6) should be confronted with equation (10) from the first part of this article.

The system (6) is not complete, since the values of $I_{R_{ix}}$ and $I_{R_{iy}}$ ($i = 1,2$) are unknown. To close the system, it is necessary to complement it with constraint conditions. We consider the impact as absolutely inelastic. Then the transferred leg should stay on the support. Using (4), this condition yields two constraint equations.

Commonly speaking, two results of the absolutely inelastic impact are possible. First, the second leg can stay on the support also. Then the system is complemented by another two constraint equations. This result is possible if the values $I_{R_{iy}}$ ($i = 1,2$) obtained by solving the full system are non-negative (see the first expression (5)).

As the second possible result of the impact, the supporting leg could lose the contact with the surface. In this case we suppose that $I_{R_{1x}} = I_{R_{1y}} = 0$ ($R_1 = 0$). Then the number of equations of the system is equal to the number of variables. This second result is possible, if the velocity of the leg tip after impact, calculated from these equations, direct upward.

When modeling the impact, each time we considered the two options. As a rule, one of then was possible while the other was not.

## NOMINAL REGIME

The nominal walking of the biped is designed with a mathematical model. The computer simulation uses the complete nonlinear equations of the planar motion of the mechanism, which are given above. The designed nominal walking regime consists of the alternating phases of single and double support. When the transferred leg hits the surface, the supporting leg does not lose the contact with the surface. So the double-support phase continues for a finite time.

The nominal walking regime should comply with the following requirements:

* The biped should fall neither forward nor backward.
* The foot of the transferred leg should pass over the support and may not touch the foot of the supporting leg.
* In walking, a reliable contact between the legs and the support should without slippage or loss contact.
* The power of drives should be sufficient to ensure the chosen walk pattern.

These demands define a certain domain of admissible walking patterns. The nominal regime should lie sufficiently far from the borders of the domain so that in the presence of disturbances, these requirements will still be satisfied.

Let us describe the design procedure for the nominal regime.

We want to synchronize changes in leg lengths and in the angle between them under possible variations of gait parameters. Therefore, we divide the step cycle into four time intervals (the single-support phase comprises three of them). The configurations at the intervals' ends are set in advance. The double-support motion interval $(0, T_0)$ is the first of the four (see Fig. 3). On this interval, the forward leg shortens, the backward leg extends, and the biped moves forward. The next interval $(T_0, T_1)$ is the initial part of the single-support phase. Here the supporting (forward) leg extends up to its maximum length, and the transferred leg shortens. This provides the difference in leg lengths necessary for the transfer. The angle between legs diminishes to zero, and the biped body moves forward due to inertia. The third interval $(T_1, T_2)$ corresponds to the middle part of the single-support phase. During this interval the supporting leg shortens, and the transferred leg moves forward. By the end of this interval, the mechanism's interior configuration (in terms of the controlled variables $h$ and $\beta$) is the desired configuration at the end of the single-support phase. The last interval $(T_2, T_3)$ is the final part of the single-support phase. On this interval the leg lengths, as well as the angle between the legs, do not change, and the whole mechanism turns around the point of support until it hits the supporting surface; i.e.,

$$h(t) \equiv h(T_3), \quad \beta(t) \equiv \beta(T_3); \quad T_2 \leq t \leq T_3 \tag{7}$$

Such a fixation of the final configuration helps to considerably reduce the error in biped configuration at the beginning of the next step.

When designing the periodic nominal regime on intervals $(T_0, T_1)$ and $(T_1, T_2)$ of the single-support phase, we compute the length $h(t)$ as time polynomials of the fifth order with unknown coefficients. The angle $\beta(t)$ is computed as a polynomial of the fourth order on the interval $(T_0, T_1)$ and of the fifth order on the interval $(T_1, T_2)$. The functions $h(t)$, $\beta(t)$ are smoothly combined at the point $T_1$ ("smoothly" means continuous up to the second derivative). To determine the polynomial coefficients, the following values are used:

* $h(T_3)$, $\beta(T_3)$: the mechanism configuration at the step end.
* $h(T_0)$, $\dot{h}(T_0)$: the length of the supporting leg and according velocity at the beginning of the single-support motion.
* $\beta(T_0)$, $\dot{\beta}(T_0)$ (calculated from four previous values).
* $h(T_1)$: maximal length of the supporting leg.
* The values $\beta(T_1)$, $\ddot{\beta}(T_1)$, $\dot{h}(T_1)$, $\dot{\beta}(T_2)$, $\dot{h}(T_2)$, and $\ddot{h}(T_2)$ are set to zero.
* Four parameters - $\ddot{h}(T_0)$, $\ddot{h}(T_1)$, $\ddot{\beta}(T_0)$, and $\ddot{\beta}(T_2)$ - are chosen.

The set of the above values enables us to determine the coefficients of all four polynomials.

In the single-support phase, the mechanism has three degrees of freedom. So, if the nominal values $h(t)$, $\beta(t)$, the angle between the supporting leg and the vertical $\alpha(T_0)$ and the angular velocity $\dot{\alpha}(T_0)$ are given, the single-support motion is uniquely determined by the equation (3). By solving these equations, we find the time dependencies of the angle $\alpha$, the ground reaction $R(R_x, R_y)$, and control voltage for telescoping and swinging motors $u_h$ and $u_a$. For them we can check whether the supporting leg loses contact with the surface or slips; i.e., whether the conditions (5) are satisfied. It is possible also to check whether the control voltages lie in the bounds

$$|u_h| \leq u^n, \qquad |u_a| \leq u^n \tag{8}$$

where $u^n = const$ is the maximal voltage of the motors.

By the solving the algebraic equations (6) for the velocity jumps and for the magnitudes of the foot force pulses, we can find the biped velocity after the transferred leg hits the surface (i.e., at the beginning of the double-support phase that follows the single-support one).

For the program $h(t)$, $\beta(t)$, $\alpha(t)$ designed for the single-support motion, we should "close" the nominal path by proper design of the double-support motion. If neither of the legs loses the contact with the support or slips in the double-support phase, the mechanism has one degree of freedom. Therefore, its double-support motion is completely defined, for instance, by time dependence of the length $h$. To ensure that the nominal regime is periodical, we should find a function $h(t)$ (the closing one), that satisfies the boundary conditions for $h$ and $\dot{h}$ at the beginning ($t = 0$) and the end ($t = T_0$) of the double-support phase. These boundary conditions are known, if the single-support motion is known. The time $T_0$ of the double support is not limited, and this simplifies design of the function $h(t)$.

We search this function such that the conditions (5) hold for each leg, and the voltages satisfy the conditions (8). The function $h(t)$ is considered in the form of second-degree polynomial.

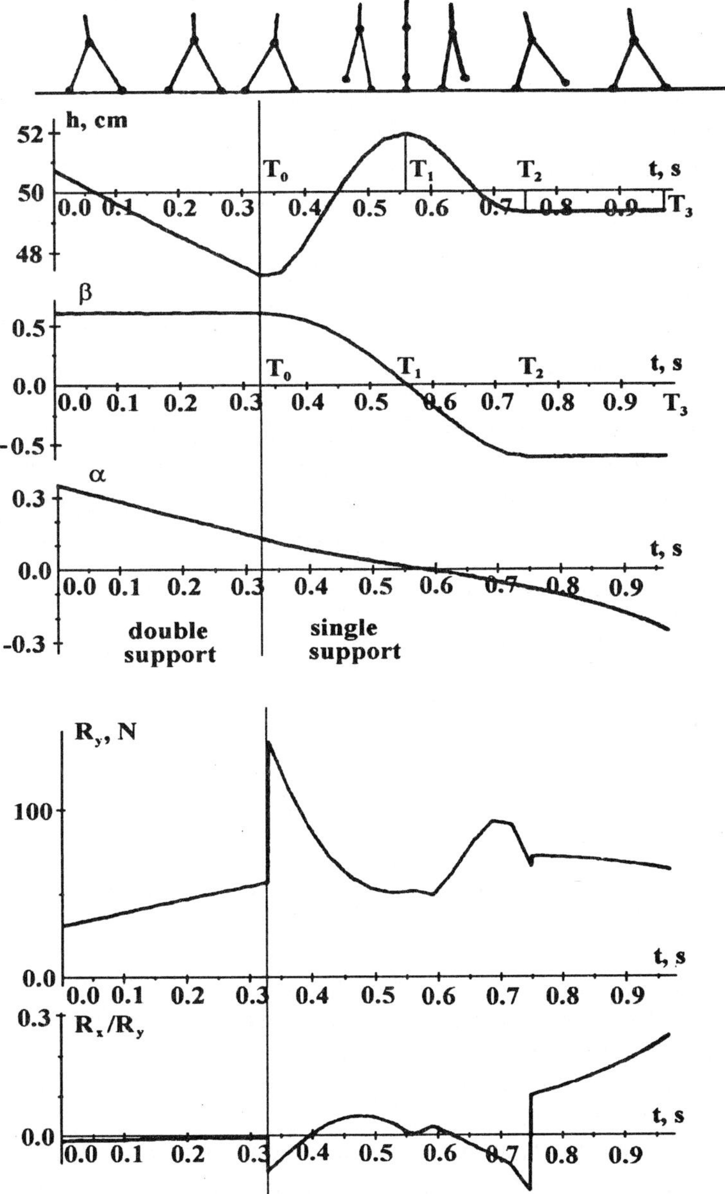


Fig. 3: Time dependencies of the configuration coordinates h, α, β, the ground reaction $R_y$, and the tangent $R_x / R_y$

The computed nominal regime used for the control of the biped walking with step length, *0.3 m*, and step duration, *0.97 s* is shown in Figure 3. Time dependencies of the three configuration coordinates $h$, $\alpha$, $\beta$ as well as the ground reaction $R_y$, and the tangent $R_x / R_y$, are plotted. The values $h$, $R_y$, and $R_x / R_y$ are displayed for the leg that supports the mechanism in the single-support motion. The vertical bar in Figure 3 divides the step cycle into double-support (to the left) and single-support (to the right) phases. One can see that equality (7) holds over the whole interval at the end of the single-support phase. As in the human walking , the plot of the reaction $R_y$ has two distinct maxima. The first (the greatest) maximum corresponds to the maximal vertical acceleration of the mass center. This acceleration develops when the supporting leg elongates (at the beginning of the single-support phase). The second maximum corresponds to the deceleration of the motion of the center of mass, when the leg shortens. In the single-support phase, the reaction $R_y$ is not lower than *65%* of the mechanism weight and $\left| R_x / R_y \right| < 0.25$. Figure 3 also shows the sequence of the mechanism configurations during one step in the corresponding instants.

We call the designed regime of locomotion and the respective functions $h(t)$, $\beta(t)$, the times $T_0$, $T_1$, $T_2$, $T_3$ etc., nominal. The nominal regime is a desired pattern of walking. In the experiments, the nominal functions $\beta(t)$ and $\dot\beta(t)$ are taken as the commanded functions $\beta_p(t)$ and $\dot\beta_p(t)$ over all single support phases. As it can be seen in Figure 3, at the double-support phase the nominal value of the angle $\beta$ is near constant. Therefore, during double-support motion the commanded angle $\beta_p$ is constant, which is close to the nominal one, and the velocity $\dot\beta_p$ is zero. However, the commanded values $h_p(t)$ and $\dot h_p(t)$ that go to the inputs of the servo system are equal to the nominal functions only on the single-support phase between the time $T_1$ of maximal extension of the supporting leg and the time of touching of the supporting surface by the transferred leg – that is, the beginning of the double-support phase. During the rest of the step cycle – in the double-support phase and the beginning of the single-support one, up to the time $T_1$ – the commanded values of $h_p(t)$ and $\dot h_p(t)$ are computed during walking. We describe below the method for their computation. To use nominal functions, it suffices to store the computed coefficients of the respective polynomials.

During the biped locomotion, the force sensor detects the collision of the transferred leg with the support. After the impact, neither of the legs loses contact with the surface, and the double-support phase begins (at $t = 0$). This corresponds to the results of mathematical modeling of the impact. Experiments show that when the biped walks, deviations from the nominal path are greatest just when the leg strikes into the support. Mechanism velocity after the impact varies widely.

## CONDITION FOR TRANSITION TO THE SINGLE-SUPPORT PHASE

If we linearize the system of the differential equations for the single-support motion in the vicinity of the vertical equilibrium state, we can separate the subsystem of equations for the angles $\alpha$ and $\beta$ from the rest. This fourth-order subsystem does not include the variations of the length $h$. Moreover, our numerical studies of the complete nonlinear system and of the linearized one show the following. The single-support motion, its duration, and the coefficients of the linear subsystem are such that the variation of the angle $\alpha$ with sufficient accuracy is described by a separate second-order equation

$$\tau^2 \ddot{\alpha} = \alpha , \tag{9}$$

where $\tau$ is a time constant (Fig. 4). For the biped under consideration, $\tau \approx 0.23\,\text{s}$. Equation (9) describes a linear approximation for the motion of a free inverted pendulum. This motion is ballistic motion.

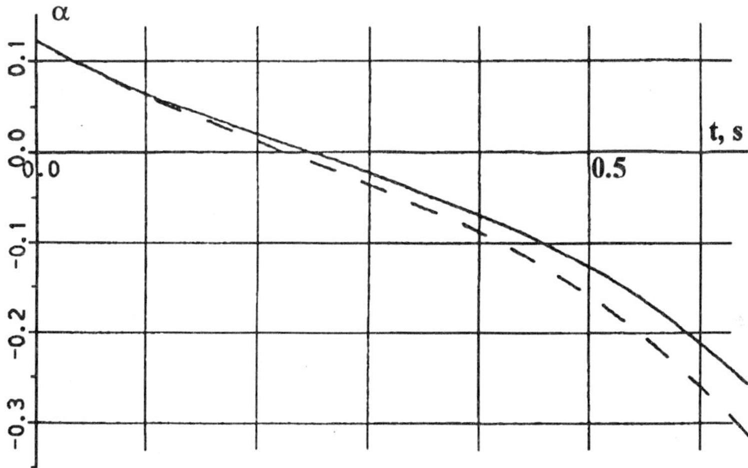


*Fig. 4: Numerical solution $\alpha(t)$ of complete nonlinear system (solid line) and of inverted pendulum equation (9) (dashed line) with the same initial conditions $\alpha(0)$ and $\dot{\alpha}(0)$.*

Thus, the telescoping and stroking drives weakly affect the changes in the angle $\alpha$. In other words, unlike $h$ and $\beta$ the coordinate $\alpha$ is weakly controllable. But we can influence the "ballistic" evolution of the angle $\alpha$ through the choice of the initial conditions $\alpha(T_o)$, $\dot{\alpha}(T_o)$. These conditions depend on the time of transition from the double-support to the single-support phase. Therefore, we can influence the evolution by choosing the time of transition. The motion of the inverted pendulum is unstable. So that this instability "will not manifest itself too much", the single-support motion should take as little time as possible. On the other hand, this time should be sufficient to move the transferred leg forward.

In the double-support phase, the front leg shortens (and the back leg lengthens), therefore $\dot{\alpha} < 0$. Thus, for the single-support phase, the initial value of the velocity is $\dot{\alpha}(T_o) < 0$.

Let $\alpha *$ be the nominal (negative) value of the angle $\alpha$ at the end of the single-support phase. If we want the angle $\alpha$, a variation of which is described by (9), to achieve the value $\alpha *$, the initial state $\alpha(T_o)$, $\dot{\alpha}(T_o)$ should lie in the phase plane $(\alpha, \dot{\alpha})$ to the left (lower) of the line

$$\alpha + \tau\dot{\alpha} = 0 \tag{10}$$

The time for change of $\alpha$ from its initial value to the final value $\alpha*$ must be greater that the nominal swing time $T_2 - T_0$ for the transferred leg. It could be shown easily that this inequality requires that the initial state must be to the right (higher) of the straight line

$$\alpha\mathbf{ch}\frac{T_2 - T_0}{\tau} + \tau\dot{\alpha}\mathbf{sh}\frac{T_2 - T_0}{\tau} = \alpha * \tag{11}$$

Let us replace equation (11) by a simpler one:

$$\alpha + \tau\dot{\alpha} = 2\alpha * \exp[-(T_2 - T_0)/\tau] \tag{12}$$

The greater the value of $(T_2 - T_0)/\tau$ the more accurate is the approximation. For the nominal regime described above, the time $T_2 - T_0 = 0{,}42$ s. If $\tau = 0.23$ s, then $(T_2 - T_0)/\tau = =1{,}83$ and $exp[(T_2 - T_0)/\tau] = 6.25$.

The parallel lines (10), (12) border a strip in the plane $\alpha$, $\dot{\alpha}$. The straight line $\pi$ that lies in the middle of the strip and is parallel to its boundaries is described by the equation

$$\alpha + \tau\dot{\alpha} = \alpha * \exp[-(T_2 - T_0)/\tau] \tag{13}$$

For the boundary conditions $\alpha(T_o)$, $\dot{\alpha}(T_o)$ lying on the line (13) (remember that $\dot{\alpha}(T_0) < 0$), the biped "overcomes" the vertical, but not rapidly, and the angle $\alpha$ reaches the value $\alpha*$ in the time greater than $T_2 - T_0$. The latter means that, if the mechanism achieves the prescribed posture with respect to the parameters $h$ and $\beta$ at time $T_2 - T_0$, then, for $(\alpha(T_o), \dot{\alpha}(T_o)) \in \pi$, this occurs before the transferred leg touches the supporting surface.

We find the initial time $T_0$ of the single-support phase from the condition that the trajectory of motion in the plane $(\alpha, \dot{\alpha})$ crosses the straight line (13). At this time, the telescoping drive begins to extend the front leg. The back leg simultaneously shortens. If the mechanism continues to move forward due to inertia, then the back leg loses contact with the support, and the single-support phase begins.

At the time $T_0$, the mechanism has certain coordinates $h(T_0)$ and $\beta(T_0)$ and velocities $\dot{h}(T_0)$, $\dot{\beta}(T_0)$. The variables $\beta(T_0)$ and $\dot{\beta}(T_0)$ usually are close to the nominal values, as the angle $\beta$ in the double-support phase varies little. Therefore, the nominal functions $\beta(t)$ and $\dot{\beta}(t)$ are taken as the commanded functions $\beta_p(t)$ and $\dot{\beta}_p(t)$ over all single support phases. However, $h(T_0)$ and $\dot{h}(T_0)$ can significantly differ from their nominal values. For the known $h(T_0)$ and $\dot{h}(T_0)$ we set the parameters $T_1$, $\dot{h}(T_0)$, $h(T_1)$, $\dot{h}(T_1) = 0$ and $\ddot{h}(T_1)$ to correspond to the precomputed nominal mode, and so we can compute the polynomial of the fifth degree $h(t)$ in real time. At time $T_1$, this polynomial smoothly matches the nominal one, which is stored in the computer. The constructed function $h(t)$ and its first derivative are fed to the servo system, as the commanded values for $T_0 < t < T_1$ (see (14)). Thus, for the double-support motion and for the initial part of the single-support one, at $T_0 < t < T_1$, the commanded trajectory $h_p(t)$ is computed during the locomotion of the biped so that it could, starting from the current state, "reach smoothly" the nominal walking regime. Such "smooth transition" is needed so that the drives do not develop forces that are too large and the legs of the vehicle do not lose the contact with the support.

## CONTROL SYSTEM

The commanded values $h_p(t)$, $\beta_p(t)$, $\dot{h}_p(t)$, $\dot{\beta}_p(t)$ for the leg length $h$, the angle $\beta$, and their first derivatives $\dot{h}$, $\dot{\beta}$ are calculated by computer. During walking, these commanded values are fed to the servo systems through digital/analog converters.

The servo system of the telescoping drive computes the control voltage $u_h$ at the single-support and the double-support phases in different ways. At the single-support phase, linear position and velocity feedback, combined with feedforward are used:

$$u_h = k_1[h_p(t) - h] + k_2[\dot{h}_p(t) - \dot{h}] + u_{hp}(t) \tag{14}$$

Here $k_1$, $k_2$ are the constant gains, $u_{hp}(t)$ is the commanded feedforward voltage. Feedforward $u_{hp}(t)$ increases accuracy of the commanded trajectory tracking. Part of $u_{hp}(t)$ is calculated in advance, when designing the nominal program, another part is calculated in the process of the walking. In the double-support case, the voltage $u_h$ is computed as the velocity feedback

$$u_h = k_3[\dot{h}_p(t) - \dot{h}] \tag{15}$$

where $k_3$ is the constant gain. The commanded speed $\dot{h}_p(t)$ is built as a piecewise linear function of time

$$\dot{h}_p(t) = \dot{h}(0) + [\dot{h}(T_0) - \dot{h}(0)]t / T^*, \quad \text{if} \quad t \le T^*$$

$$\dot{h}_p(t) = \dot{h}(T_0), \qquad\qquad\qquad \text{if} \quad t > T^* \tag{16}$$

Here $\dot{h}(0)$ is the velocity after the impact of the transferred leg on the support, $\dot{h}(T_0)$ is the nominal value for the speed $\dot{h}$ at the end of the double-support phase, $T^* = |\dot{h}(T_0) - \dot{h}(0)| / a$, where $a$ is the maximal acceleration for which the legs still stay on the support. In the experiments, we assumed that $a = 0.1 \; m/s^2$. The velocities $\dot{h}(0)$ and $\dot{h}(T_0)$ are negative, so the commanded speed $\dot{h}_p(t) < 0$. Therefore, according to program (16) in the double-support phase, the front leg shortens, the back leg extends according to (1) while the hip joint (point $B$ in Fig. 2) moves forward.

The swing servo system at both phases computes the control voltage $u_a$ as the linear position and velocity feedback:

$$u_a = \chi_1[\beta_p(t) - \beta] + \chi_2[\dot{\beta}_p(t) - \dot{\beta}] \tag{17}$$

where $\chi_1$, $\chi_2$ are constant gains. For the nominal regime, at the double-support phase the variations of the angle $\beta$ are small (see Fig. 3). So for the sake of simplicity, during this phase the constant commanded angle $\beta_p$, which is close to the nominal one, and the velocity $\dot{\beta}_p = 0$ go to the respective servo system (17).

The signals $h$, $\dot{h}$, $\beta$, $\dot{\beta}$ come to the inputs of servo systems from the respective potentiometers and tachometers. The output voltage of each servo system goes to the respective power amplifier and then to the motor.

We call the developed algorithm of walking control an adaptive algorithm, as the commanded values are "adjusted", at each step of the biped, to adapt for the state achieved when the transferred leg is put on the support..

Without modifications, the described algorithm enables the biped to start walking from the rest state, with the biped standing on the surface with the legs wide apart. In experiments, walking does begin in this way.

## EXPERIMENTS

The results of one experiment are illustrated in Figure 5. The mechanism starts from the rest state, makes seven steps (seven leg transfers), and halts. Figure 5 shows the time dependencies for the length $h$ of the supporting leg, the angle $\beta$ between the legs, and the angle $\alpha$ between the supporting leg and the vertical. Horizontal segments mark the single-support phases. The vertical lines bound the single-support phases. Other vertical lines mark the instants of completion of changes in commanded values $h_p(t)$, $\beta_p(t)$ at the ends of single-support phases. After these instants, equalities (7) hold.

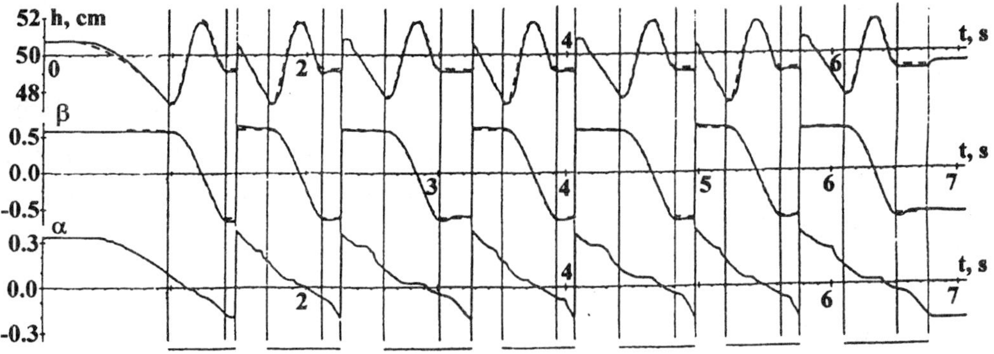

*Fig. 5: Experimental curves (solid line) and commanded values (dashed line)*

The legs interchange from step to step: the supporting one becomes the transferred, and vice versa. Because the plots in Figure 5 relate to the supporting leg, variables switch to the other leg at the beginning of the next step (i.e., at the beginning of the double-support phases). Along with functions $h(t)$ and $\beta(t)$, Figure 5 also displays their commanded values (see dashed lines) $h_p(t)$ and $\beta_p(t)$. As seen from the figure, the motion along the controlled coordinates $h$ and $\beta$ is close to the commanded one. At all the steps these coordinates reach the steady values before the transferred leg touches the support. The laboratory motion track has room for seven-eight steps of the biped vehicle. In experiments, the biped made seven steps to the end of the track many times. This walking was recorded on film.

## CONCLUSION

The design of the control law for walking of described above biped with telescopic legs is connected with two major difficulties. The first one is that the constraint imposed on the foot standing on the support is not bilateral. When the mechanism walks, the leg can rise over the surface or slip along it. Such an "unplanned" loss of the contact causes a deviation of motion from the program, which can result in the biped downfall. It seems that in the absence of the coupling (1) between the leg motions, it would be easier to satisfy conditions (5). The second difficulty is related to the fact that the biped motion in the single-support phase is unstable and difficult to control. Therefore, one should "correctly" choose the time for starting the single-support phase, and this time should be as short as possible.

## 2.2. ANTHROPOMORPHIC BIPED

Now we consider dynamic walking of a anthropomorphic mechanism. We describe its mechanical design and developed control algorithm. The description of this biped and its control algorithm is published for the first time in the article of A.A.Grishin, A.M.Formal'sky, A.V.Lensky and S.V.Zhitomirsky "Dynamic Walking of Two Biped Vehicles" in Proceedings of 9-th World Congress on the theory of Machines and Mechanisms, Politecnico di Milano, Italy, 1995, vol. 3, p. 2308-2312.

## MECHANICAL DESIGN

In Figure 6 the anthropomorphic mechanism is shown.

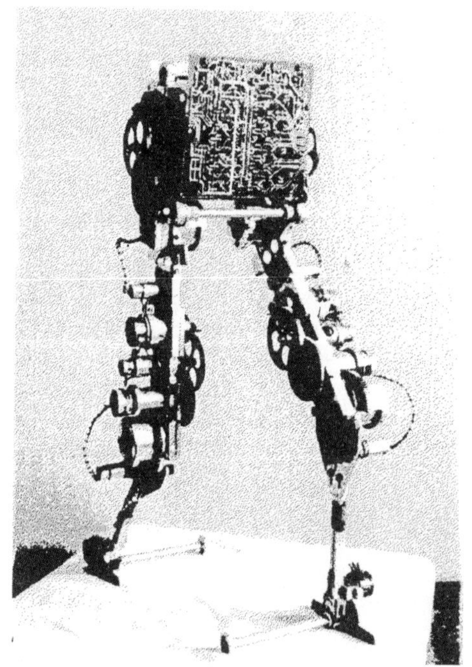

*Fig. 6: The five-link anthropomorphic mechanism actuated by four drives*

This five-link biped has a trunk and two two-link legs. The legs are attached to the trunk through the hip joints. Each leg consists of the thigh and the shin, linked together by the knee joint. The masses and the lengths of the links are closely the same as in the biped with telescopic legs. The legs equipped with passive feet extending in the frontal plane as well. So the mechanism also can move in sagittal plane only. The anthropomorphic mechanism is actuated by four DC drives. Two drives for the hip joints are located on the trunk and two drives for the knee joints are located on the thighs. The gear ratios are 50 for all four drives.

Four potentiometers measure the joint angles in the hips and the knees. Respective angular velocities are taken from tachometers. Each shin is equipped with a four-component force/torque sensor. But the designed control law uses only one component to evaluate the vertical component $R_y$ of the ground reaction applied to the leg. Each foot has a potentiometer to measure the angle of the leg inclination with respect to support.

During walking the commanded values $\varphi_{ip}(t)$ and their first derivatives $\dot{\varphi}_{ip}(t)$ are computed for all actuated joints ($i = 1, 2, 3, 4$). Here $\varphi_i$ are the internal joint angles (Fig. 7). These commanded values are fed to the digital servo system, which is described by the following formulas

$$u_i = k_i[\varphi_{ip}(t) - \varphi_i] + \chi_i[\dot{\varphi}_{ip}(t) - \dot{\varphi}_i] \qquad (i = 1, 2, 3, 4) \qquad (18)$$

Here $k_i$ and $\chi_i$ are constant gains. The signals $\varphi_i$ and $\dot{\varphi}_i$ go from the respective potentiometers and tachometers. The output of the servo system $u_i$ go to the respective power amplifiers and then to the motors. The expressions (18) are similar to the expressions (14) and (17).

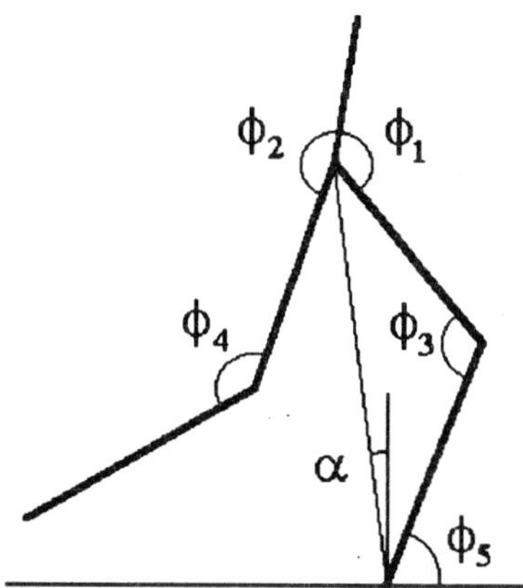


*Fig. 7: Kinematic scheme of the anthropomorphic biped*

## DETERMINATION OF A NOMINAL REGIME

We design the nominal walking of the biped using the mathematical model (1) from the first part of this article.

When designing the nominal regime, we divide the single-support phase into two time intervals: $(T_0, T_1)$ and $(T_1, T_2)$. Time $T_0$ is the beginning of the single-support phase. From the time $T_1$ up to $T_2$ the biped holds its final configuration

$$\varphi_i(t) \equiv \varphi_i(T_1) \qquad T_1 \leq t \leq T_2 \qquad (i = 1, 2, 3, 4) \qquad (19)$$

Hence in the nominal regime on the interval $(T_1, T_2)$ the biped is pivoting around the point of support until it hits the surface at the time $T_2$. Such a freezing of the final configuration helps to reduce considerably the error in biped configuration at the beginning of the next step. The conditions (19) are similar to the conditions (7) of a fixation of the final configuration for the biped with telescopic legs.

On the interval $(T_0, T_1)$ we compute the angles $\varphi_i$ ($i = 1, 2, 3, 4$) as the time polynomials with unknown coefficients. The knee angle $\varphi_4$ of the leg being transferred (see Fig. 7) is computed as a polynomial of the fifth order, other angles are computed as polynomials of fourth order. The functions $\varphi_i(t)$ are smoothly combined with constant values (19) at the point $T_1$ ($\dot{\varphi}_i(T_1) = 0$). To determine the polynomial coefficients, the following values are set:

* $\varphi_i(T_0)$, $\dot{\varphi}_i(T_0)$ ($i = 1, 2, 3, 4$), $\ddot{\varphi}_4(T_0)$: the joint angles and their derivatives at the beginning of the single-support phase.
* $\varphi_i(T_1)$, $\dot{\varphi}_i(T_1) = 0$ ($i = 1, 2, 3, 4$): the angles and the angular velocities at the instant $T_1$.
* $\varphi_i(t')$ ($i = 1, 2, 3, 4$): the angles at the some instant $t'$, that is closely the time $(T_1 - T_0)/2$.

The set of the above values enables to determine the coefficients of all four polynomials.

In the single-support phase, the anthropomorphic biped has five degrees of freedom. If the functions $\varphi_i(t)$ ($i = 1, 2, 3, 4$) are known along with the initial values of the angle between the vertical and the shin of supporting leg $\varphi_5(T_0)$ (see Fig. 7) and its derivative $\dot{\varphi}_5(T_0)$, then the single-support motion is uniquely determined by the motion equations. By solving these equations, we find the time dependencies of the angle $\varphi_5$, the ground reaction force $\boldsymbol{R}(R_x, R_y)$, and control voltages for all four drives. For them we can check whether the conditions (5) are satisfied, and control voltage lies within the limits ($u^n$ is the maximal voltage of the motors)

$$|u_i(t)| \leq u^n \qquad (i = 1, 2, 3, 4) \tag{20}$$

The constraints (20) are similar to the (8) ones for the biped with telescopic legs.

By trying various values of the parameters $\varphi_i(T_0)$, $\dot{\varphi}_i(T_0)$, $\ddot{\varphi}_4(T_0)$, $t'$, $\varphi_i(t')$, $T_1 - T_0$, $\varphi_i(T_1)$ ($i = 1, 2, 3, 4$), we can design the nominal regime for the single-support phase satisfying above-mentioned conditions.

## DOUBLE-SUPPORT PHASE

When the biped stands on the horizontal surface with known step length $S$, its configuration can be determined by the coordinates $x$, $y$ of the hip joints and the inclination angle $\psi$ of the body. When constructing the nominal regime we choose the same values for $S$ and $\psi$ at the beginning and the end of single-support phase. We consider these constants as program ones for the whole double-support phase. We also set beforehand the function $y = f(x)$, for example, $y = const$. Thus the trajectory of the mechanism at the double-support phase can be determined by the time-dependence of $x$-coordinate of the hip joints. We suppose that at the end of the single-support phase the value of $x$ is close to the nominal one. The control algorithm starts with this value and tries to move the biped forward with some nominal velocity $\dot{x}_n$. But after the impact the velocity of the biped $\dot{x}_r$ can differ considerably from the nominal one. Its value can be more or less depending on unpredictable circumstances of the impact, for example, on the magnitude of the friction forces in joints. If the difference between $\dot{x}_n$ and $\dot{x}_r$ is large enough, one of the legs can lose the contact with the support. Such an unexpected transition to the double-support phase results, as a rule, in the downfall of the biped. To avoid this situation, during the walking ground reaction forces in both legs are measured. If one of them decreased below some threshold, the control algorithm changes the desired velocity $\dot{x}$ and thereby, the commanded trajectory $\varphi_{ip}(t)$, $\dot{\varphi}_{ip}(t)$ ($i = 1, 2, 3, 4$). If the ground reaction are large enough, the control algorithm calculates the commanded trajectory on the basis of the nominal value $\dot{x}_n$. So the developed algorithm tries to maintain a contact with the support and to stabilize the mechanism's velocity at the same time.

The double-support phase continues until the control algorithm decides to begin the single-support phase.

## TRANSITION TO THE SINGLE-SUPPORT PHASE

Let $\alpha$ be the angle between the vertical and the straight line connecting the hip joint and ankle joint of supporting leg (see Fig. 3). Our numerical studies of the complete nonlinear system show that the variation of the angle $\alpha$ in the single-support case can be described with sufficient accuracy by the equation (9), as for the biped with telescopic legs. Thus we find the initial time $T_0$ of the single-support phase from the condition that the trajectory of motion in the plane $(\alpha, \dot{\alpha})$ crosses the straight line (13). The nominal regime, calculated for the single-support phase, is a desired pattern of walking. However, in the experiments the control algorithm forms the commanded values for the servo system which differ from the nominal ones. At the point $T_0$ we compute the commanded trajectory $\varphi_{ip}(t)$, $\dot{\varphi}_{ip}(t)$ $(i = 1, 2, 3, 4)$ in a way similar to the calculation of the nominal regime. Functions $\varphi_{ip}(t)$ are calculated in the form of polynomials of forth or fifth order using measured values of biped coordinates $\varphi_i(T_0)$ and velocities $\dot{\varphi}_i(T_0)$, and nominal values $\ddot{\varphi}_4(T_0)$, $t'$, $\varphi_i(t')$, $T_1 - T_0$, $\varphi_i(T_1)$ $(i = 1, 2, 3, 4)$.

The tracing of the commanded trajectory lasts until the transferred leg hits the support. The impact is detected reading the force sensor output. At this point the new step cycle begins.

## EXPERIMENTAL RESULTS

The results of one experiment are shown in Figure 8.

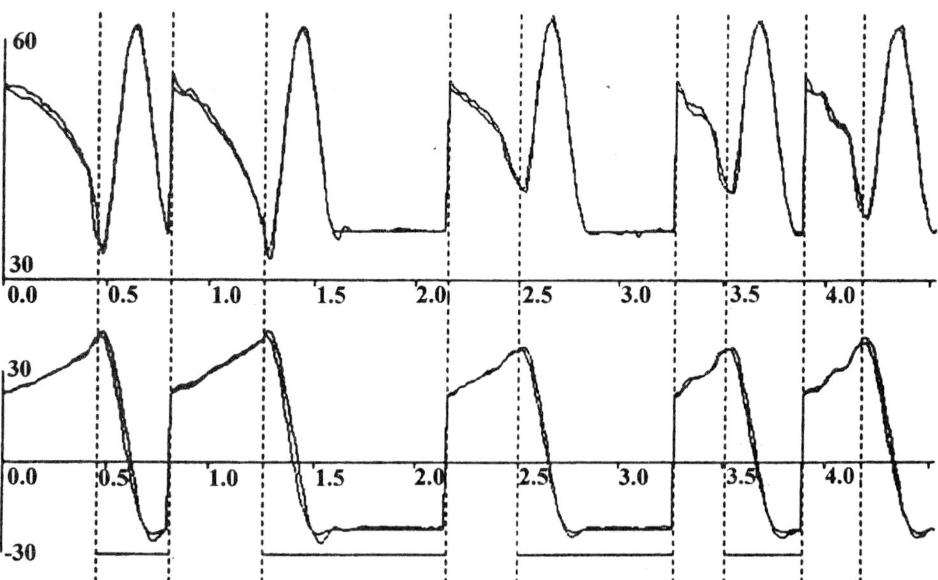

*Fig. 8: Time dependencies of angles (degree vs. second) during an experiment. Measured values and corresponding commanded trajectory are plotted. Horizontal segments mark single-support phases. The upper graph shows the time dependence of knee angle of leg being transferred, and the lower graph - angle between thighs.*

In this figure 8 time dependencies of several joint angles and corresponding commanded trajectories during the walking are plotted. The knee angle of the leg being transferred is plotted in the upper part and the angle between things is plotted in the lower part of the picture. The horizontal segments mark the single-support phases. In this experiment the biped starts from the rest state, makes eight steps (i.e., eight leg transfers) and halts. The first five steps are depicted. The jumps at the beginnings of the double-support phases do not correspond to a real motion , but are merely because of transferring and supporting leg interchange at that time instant. For example, on the upper plot the knee angle of right leg is followed by the knee angle of the left leg and so on, according to the leg role in the step cycle.

As it can be seen, the recorded motion is rather close to the commanded trajectory, meaning that the servo system is quite good. The commanded trajectories are slightly disturbed on the double-support phase (especially on the forth and fifth steps).

The walking of the anthropomorphic mechanism was recorded on film.

## CONCLUDING REMARK TO THE PROBLEM
## OF DESIGN AND CONTROL OF BIPED MECHANISMS

The gait of the biped mechanisms described above is obviously dissimilar to  human locomotion. One of the main differences is that the motion of our biped is planar, whereas human locomotion is spatial. We have shown that a control which would ensure the dynamically stable gait of a biped robot can be designed, and we hope that in the future better mechanisms will be designed whose gait will be more closely resemble human locomotion.

## ACKNOWLEDGEMENTS

The research described in this article was supported by Grant 93-013-16321 from Russian Foundation of Fundamental Research and by Grant No M71000 from International Science Foundation.

# THEORY AND PRACTICE OF MACHINE WALKING


**F. Pfeiffer, Th. Rossmann and J. Steuer**
**Technical University of Munich, Munich, Germany**



Abstract:

In this paper the theory and two examples of machine walking is presented. Part I contents the theory of multi-body dynamics, the kinematics and kinetics of rigid body systems seen at the example of a six-legged roboter and the theory of optimization with constraints. Part II contents two examples of walking robots. First, there is a six-legged walking machine whose kinetics, gait patterns and control system are derived from a stick insect. The second example is a tube-crawling robot with eight legs. It has four legs in the front and four legs in the rear. This construction shall enable it to go through pipes with a diameter between 60 and 70 cm.

# 1   Foreword

In simulating, designing and realizing walking machine, and, as a matter of fact, many other machines, it will make sense, to watch certain rules and sequences of events to assure a successful development. This must not be as perfect as industrial program management, but it helps to establish an efficient research progress and convincing results.

The overall organization follows Figure 1, which contains three main blocks: layout and design, hardware-in-the-loop tests and finally the real machine. All steps for realizing such a walking machine are connected with tests and evaluations with respect to performance according to the basic ideas and requirements, which come so-to-say from first creative intuitions and goals, with respect to confirmations of the goals and the requirements and finally with respect to possible improvements. According to Karl Popper every creative process is an iterative process, where during problem solving new problems and questions come up thus modifying and improving original ideas and goals. Such processes must be controled not to become unstable.

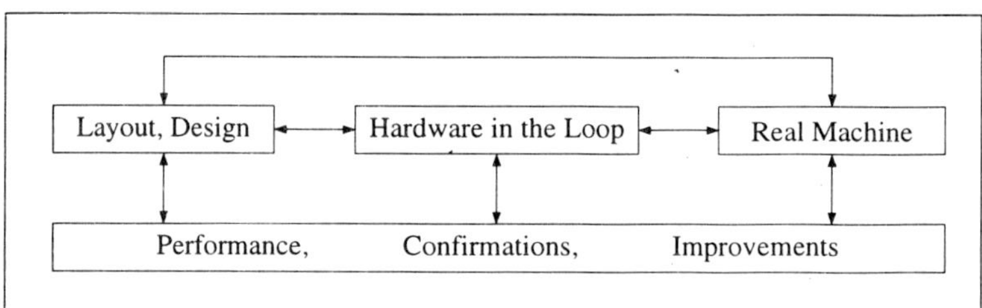


Figure 1.1: Realizing a Walking Machine

With respect to our walking machines the intuitive phase of creating ideas and concepts very much was interconnected with research findings of biologists. They know about mechanics of walking, and they know quite remarkable structures of biological walking control. At the very beginning we were of course aware of the fact that it makes no sense to copy biology. But on the other hand we are convinced that a good combination of biological design ideas and technological possibilities will make a good walking machine.

Therefore, in an early step we started to design a six-legged machine oriented at features of the stick-insect. Layout and design includes on a software basis everything of the future machine: concept and configuration, dynamics and control, gait pattern and stability; simulations again and again to find out the best performance, the best load-to-weight-ratio, the best components from the mechanical side and from electronics. One has to perform trade-offs for sensors and actuators, for design configurations and for shape and materials. The selection of commercial components from external sources follows optimization processes with criteria like load-to-weight, stiffness, stability.

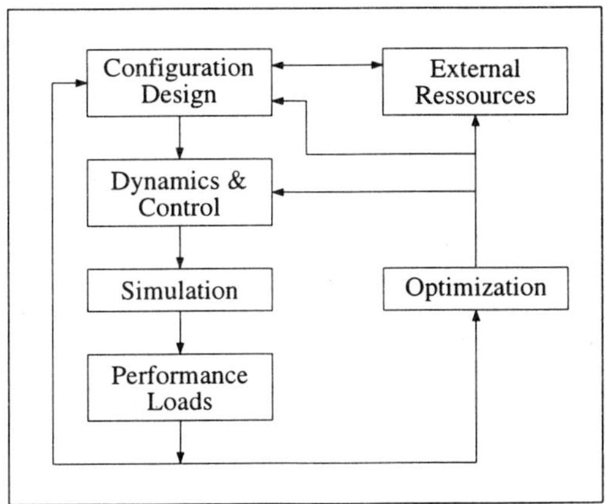


Figure 1.2: Layout and Design

Figure 2 illustrates this research phase. At the end we have a rather complete impression how the machine will operate, what are the difficulties, where do we have to expect the biggest problems.

At this stage it make very much sense to prepare hardware-in-the-loop tests. For a walking machine with the above preparations it is more or less straightforward. In simulations we make the machine walk in the computer with the exception of one leg. This one leg we realize in hardware, establish a test set-up and combine the motion of this one leg in hardware with the simulated motion of the other five legs on the computer.

As a consequence we are able to operate the complete machine, one leg in reality, five legs in simulations. We can test the performance and the control of one real leg

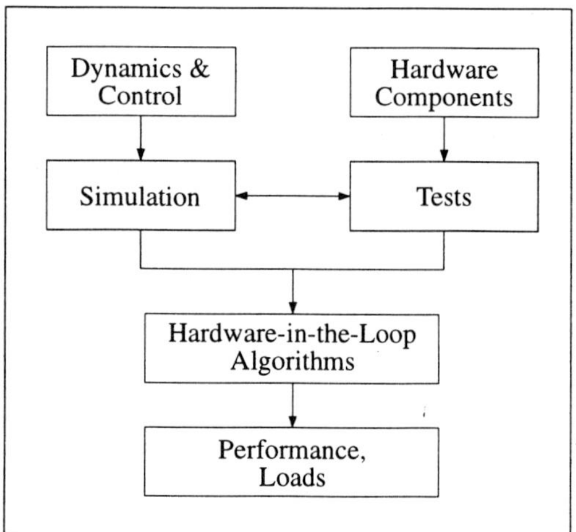


Figure 1.3: Hardware-in-the-Loop Tests

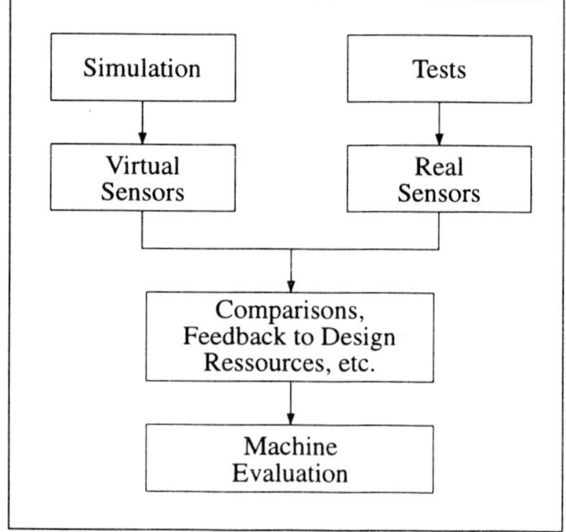


Figure 1.4: Machine Realization

and of the complete machine and find out most of the errors and drawbacks made during layout and design. Especially control performance can be tested, control hardware can be adapted and problems like EMC (electro-magnet compatibility) can be considered. Altogether the two stages layout, design and hardware-in-the-loop tests clear up most of the problems beforehand. The final machine realization looses much of its risks.

On the basis of these beforehand-activities the last step of construction the real walking-machine starts with a set of drawings for both, the mechanical and electronic workshop. Questions of manufacturing, external ressources, integration and assembly have to be answered and handled. From virtual sensors and virtual actuators we proceed to real sensors and actuators. Machine performance will be compared with the design idea, and the whole process of machine testing can be started.

# Part I: Theory of Walking

# 2 Dynamics of Rigid Body Systems

The investigation of general dynamic systems starts with an appropriate formulation of the equations of motion. We consider systems of rigid bodies under the influence of active forces which may be represented by compliance or damping elements, and we restrict their movement by including constraint conditions [6]. In this

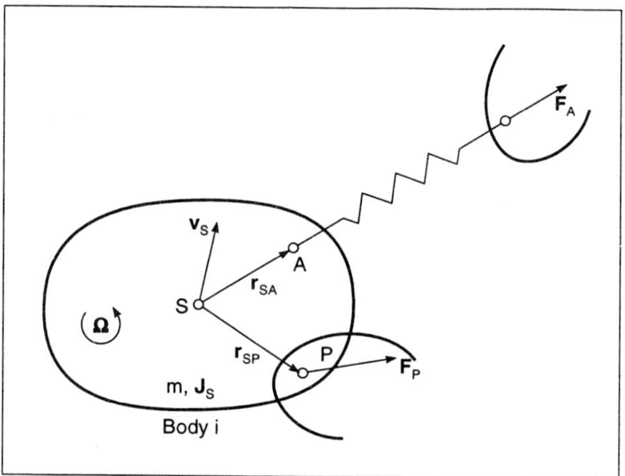


Figure 2.5: Constrained Multibody System

section we derive the equations of motion. A typical body in such a system is shown in Fig. 2.5. If we have $n$ bodies in our system we can write for each body $i$ the equations of the linear and angular momentums, $\dot{p} \in \mathbb{R}^3$ and $\dot{L} \in \mathbb{R}^3$ respectively, as

$$\left\{ \begin{pmatrix} \dot{\boldsymbol{p}} \\ \dot{\boldsymbol{L}} \end{pmatrix} - \begin{pmatrix} \boldsymbol{E} & \boldsymbol{0} \\ \tilde{\boldsymbol{r}}_{SA} & \boldsymbol{E} \end{pmatrix} \begin{pmatrix} \boldsymbol{F}_A \\ \boldsymbol{M}_A \end{pmatrix} - \begin{pmatrix} \boldsymbol{E} & \boldsymbol{0} \\ \tilde{\boldsymbol{r}}_{SP} & \boldsymbol{E} \end{pmatrix} \begin{pmatrix} \boldsymbol{F}_P \\ \boldsymbol{M}_P \end{pmatrix} \right\}_i = \boldsymbol{0} \; ; \tag{1}$$

$$i = 1, \dots, n \; ,$$

with

$$\begin{pmatrix} \dot{\boldsymbol{p}} \\ \dot{\boldsymbol{L}} \end{pmatrix} = \begin{pmatrix} m\boldsymbol{E} & \boldsymbol{0} \\ \boldsymbol{0} & \boldsymbol{J}_S \end{pmatrix}_i \begin{pmatrix} \dot{\boldsymbol{v}}_S \\ \dot{\boldsymbol{\Omega}} \end{pmatrix}_i + \begin{pmatrix} \boldsymbol{0} \\ \tilde{\boldsymbol{\Omega}} \boldsymbol{J}_S \boldsymbol{\Omega} \end{pmatrix}_i \; . \tag{2}$$

In (1), (2) and Fig. 2.5 $S$ denotes the centre of mass of the body under consideration with mass $m$ and inertia matrix $\boldsymbol{J}_S \in \mathbb{R}^{3,3}$ about $S, \boldsymbol{v}_S \in \mathbb{R}^3$ is the absolute velocity of point $S$ and $\boldsymbol{\Omega} \in \mathbb{R}^3$ is the absolute angular velocity of the body. The forces $\boldsymbol{F} \in \mathbb{R}^3$ and moments $\boldsymbol{M} \in \mathbb{R}^3$, which act on the body, are divided into two sets by the indices $A$ for "active" and $P$ for "passive". "Active" forces can be moved along their axis, "passive" can not. For example, $\boldsymbol{F}_A$ means an active force acting on point $A$, and $\boldsymbol{M}_P$ is a passive moment (constraint moment) not related to any point on the body. Finally the terms $\tilde{\boldsymbol{r}}_{SA}$ and $\tilde{\boldsymbol{r}}_{SP}$ are skew symmetric matrices $\in \mathbb{R}^{3,3}$ which express the cross product $\boldsymbol{a} \times \boldsymbol{b}$ by a matrix-vector-multiplication $\tilde{\boldsymbol{a}}\boldsymbol{b}$, and $E$ is the identity matrix in $\mathbb{R}^{3,3}$ (In the following we need one more additional kinematical relation, namely the dependency of the velocities $\boldsymbol{v}_A$ and $\boldsymbol{v}_P$ on $\boldsymbol{v}_S$).

$$\begin{pmatrix} \boldsymbol{v}_A \\ \boldsymbol{\Omega} \end{pmatrix}_i = \begin{pmatrix} m\boldsymbol{E} & -\tilde{\boldsymbol{r}}_{SA} \\ \boldsymbol{0} & \boldsymbol{E} \end{pmatrix}_i \begin{pmatrix} \dot{\boldsymbol{v}}_S \\ \boldsymbol{\Omega} \end{pmatrix}_i \; ; \; \begin{pmatrix} \boldsymbol{v}_P \\ \boldsymbol{\Omega} \end{pmatrix}_i = \begin{pmatrix} m\boldsymbol{E} & -\tilde{\boldsymbol{r}}_{SP} \\ \boldsymbol{0} & \boldsymbol{E} \end{pmatrix}_i \begin{pmatrix} \boldsymbol{v}_S \\ \boldsymbol{\Omega} \end{pmatrix}_i \; . \tag{3}$$

We also assume that the system has only $f$ degrees of freedom due to $(6n - f)$ bilateral holonomic (or nonholonomic) constraints. Thus, we can choose a set of $f$ independent (velocity-)coordinates $\dot{\boldsymbol{q}}$ which describe the system uniquely and fulfills each of the constraints. This set we call the generalized coordinates of our system. It is well known that every velocity, acceleration or variation can be expressed in a linear manner by the corresponding terms of the generalized coordinates, for example we have

$$\begin{pmatrix} \boldsymbol{v}_S \\ \boldsymbol{\Omega} \end{pmatrix}_i = \begin{pmatrix} \boldsymbol{J}_S \\ \boldsymbol{J}_T \end{pmatrix}_i \dot{\boldsymbol{q}} + \begin{pmatrix} \tilde{\boldsymbol{j}}_S \\ \tilde{\boldsymbol{j}}_T \end{pmatrix}_i \; ; \; \begin{pmatrix} \dot{\boldsymbol{v}}_S \\ \dot{\boldsymbol{\Omega}} \end{pmatrix}_i = \begin{pmatrix} \boldsymbol{J}_S \\ \boldsymbol{J}_T \end{pmatrix}_i \ddot{\boldsymbol{q}} + \begin{pmatrix} \bar{\boldsymbol{j}}_S \\ \bar{\boldsymbol{j}}_T \end{pmatrix}_i \; ;$$

$$\begin{pmatrix} \delta\boldsymbol{v}_S \\ \delta\boldsymbol{\Omega} \end{pmatrix}_i = \begin{pmatrix} \boldsymbol{J}_S \\ \boldsymbol{J}_T \end{pmatrix}_i \delta\dot{\boldsymbol{q}} \; . \tag{4}$$

It may be noticed that in the second equation of (4) the arising additional terms when expressing the absolute accelerations $(\dot{v}_S, \dot{\Omega})$ are collected in $(\bar{j}_S, \bar{j}_T)$ and are not further specified. The matrices $(J_B, J_T)$ which are derived from the operation

$$\begin{pmatrix} \partial v_B / \partial \dot{q} \\ \partial \Omega / \partial \dot{q} \end{pmatrix}_i = \begin{pmatrix} J_B \\ J_R \end{pmatrix}_i \quad ; \quad \begin{pmatrix} J_B \in \mathbb{R}^{3,f} \\ J_R \in \mathbb{R}^{3,f} \end{pmatrix}_i \tag{5}$$

are called the "Jacobian of translation of point $B$", where $B$ is any of $(S, A, P)$ and the "Jacobian of rotation" (index $R$), respectively. When we apply the operation (5) to the right hand sides and left hand sides of (3), we get the transformation rule of the Jacobians,

$$\begin{pmatrix} J_A \\ J_T \end{pmatrix} = \begin{pmatrix} E & -\tilde{r}_{SA} \\ 0 & E \end{pmatrix} \begin{pmatrix} J_S \\ J_T \end{pmatrix} \quad ; \quad \begin{pmatrix} J_P \\ J_T \end{pmatrix} = \begin{pmatrix} E & -\tilde{r}_{SP} \\ 0 & E \end{pmatrix} \begin{pmatrix} J_S \\ J_T \end{pmatrix} . \tag{6}$$

Now the virtual power of the system (1) can be formulated as

$$\sum_{i=1}^{n} \left\{ \begin{pmatrix} \delta v_S \\ \delta \Omega \end{pmatrix}^T \left[ \begin{pmatrix} \dot{p} \\ \dot{L} \end{pmatrix} - \begin{pmatrix} E & 0 \\ \tilde{r}_{SA} & E \end{pmatrix} \begin{pmatrix} F_A \\ M_A \end{pmatrix} - \begin{pmatrix} E & 0 \\ \tilde{r}_{SP} & E \end{pmatrix} \begin{pmatrix} F_P \\ M_P \end{pmatrix} \right] \right\}_i = 0 \; ,$$

which with help of the third equation of (4) leads to

$$\delta \dot{q}^T \sum_{i=1}^{n} \left\{ \begin{pmatrix} J_S \\ J_T \end{pmatrix}^T \left[ \begin{pmatrix} \dot{p} \\ \dot{L} \end{pmatrix} - \begin{pmatrix} E & 0 \\ \tilde{r}_{SA} & E \end{pmatrix} \begin{pmatrix} F_A \\ M_A \end{pmatrix} - \begin{pmatrix} E & 0 \\ \tilde{r}_{SP} & E \end{pmatrix} \begin{pmatrix} F_P \\ M_P \end{pmatrix} \right] \right\}_i = 0 \; . \tag{7}$$

At this point we have to remember that the generalized coordinates have been chosen in such a manner that the constraints are fulfilled for any arbitrary $\dot{q}$. Thus equation (7) must hold for every $\delta \dot{q}$ which is only possible if the sum is equal to zero. Using the transformation rule for the Jacobians (6), equation (7) results in

$$\sum_{i=1}^{n} \left\{ \begin{pmatrix} J_S \\ J_T \end{pmatrix}^T \begin{pmatrix} \dot{p} \\ \dot{L} \end{pmatrix} - \begin{pmatrix} J_A \\ J_T \end{pmatrix}^T \begin{pmatrix} F_A \\ M_A \end{pmatrix} - \begin{pmatrix} J_P \\ J_T \end{pmatrix}^T \begin{pmatrix} F_P \\ M_P \end{pmatrix} \right\}_i = 0 \; . \tag{8}$$

The sets of forces and moments with index $A$ and $P$ in (8) should be discussed further. If we have chosen the set with index $P$ in such a manner (principle of d'Alembert and Jourdain) that

$$\sum_{i=1}^{n} \left\{ \begin{pmatrix} J_P \\ J_T \end{pmatrix}^T \begin{pmatrix} F_P \\ M_P \end{pmatrix} \right\}_i \equiv 0 \; , \tag{9}$$

then the dynamics of the system is only influenced by the terms with index $A$,

$$\sum_{i=1}^{n}\left\{\begin{pmatrix} J_S \\ J_T \end{pmatrix}^{T}\begin{pmatrix} \dot{p} \\ \dot{L} \end{pmatrix} - \begin{pmatrix} J_A \\ J_T \end{pmatrix}^{T}\begin{pmatrix} F_A \\ M_A \end{pmatrix}\right\}_{i} = 0 \ . \tag{10}$$

Thus the forces and moments in (9) are not needed to determine the dynamics of our system, and therefore we can use (9) as a definition for what we call passive forces (or constraint forces): Each force or moment $\in \mathbb{R}^3$ (or pairs, triples, ... of forces or moments or combinations of them) which fulfills (9) is called passive and does not influence the dynamics of the system. If we use a set of gerneralized coordinates these terms are not needed in the equations of motion (10).

Finally, a more condensed representation of equation (10) can be written. Substituting (2) into (10) and expressing the resulting accelerations using the second equation of (4) yields

$$\sum_{i=1}^{n}\left\{\begin{pmatrix} J_S \\ J_T \end{pmatrix}^{T}\begin{pmatrix} mE & 0 \\ 0 & J_S \end{pmatrix}\begin{pmatrix} J_S \\ J_T \end{pmatrix}^{T}\ddot{q} + \begin{pmatrix} J_S \\ J_T \end{pmatrix}^{T}\cdot\right.$$

$$\left.\cdot\left[\begin{pmatrix} 0 \\ \tilde{\Omega}J_S\Omega \end{pmatrix} + \begin{pmatrix} mE & 0 \\ 0 & J_S \end{pmatrix}\begin{pmatrix} \bar{j}_S \\ \bar{j}_T \end{pmatrix}\right] - \begin{pmatrix} J_A \\ J_T \end{pmatrix}^{T}\begin{pmatrix} F_A \\ M_A \end{pmatrix}\right\}_{i} = 0 \ .$$

This results in an expression of the form

$$M(q,t)\cdot\ddot{q} - h(q,\dot{q},t) - Q(q,\dot{q},t) = 0 \qquad \in \mathbb{R}^{f} \tag{11}$$

with a symmetric positive definite mass matrix $M \in \mathbb{R}^{f,f}$, a vector $h \in \mathbb{R}^{f}$ which consists of all gyroscopical accelerations and a vector $Q$ which consists of all active moments and forces.

# 3   Kinematics of Walking

In case of the six-legged walking machine different coordinate frames are introduced [19] (see fig. 3.6)

- the inertial coordinate frame I, in which the $_Ix$–axis is parallel to the direction of motion and the $_Iz$–axis is directed vertically upwards

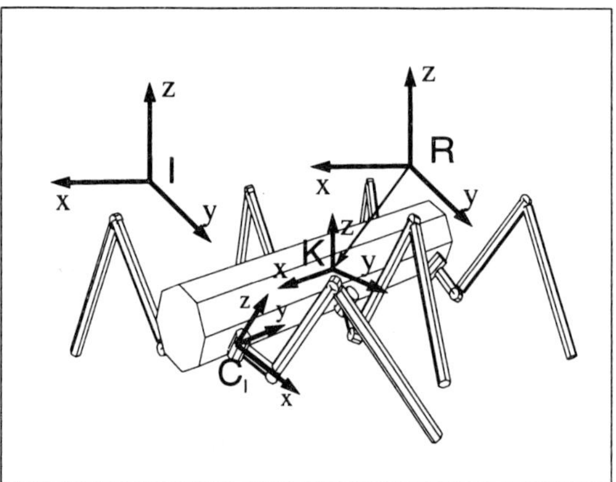


Figure 3.6: Mechanical Model

- a reference frame R which is paraxial to I and shifted with the constant average translational speed $v_0$ relative to I

- the body-fixed frame K, whose $_Kx$–axis marks the longitudinal axis af symmetry of the central body. It is shifted relative to the reference system by the three translational degrees of freedom, $(q_1, q_2, q_3)$, and rotated by the three KARDAN–angles $(q_4, q_5, q_6)$

- the root coordinate frames $(C_l)$ for the first segment (*Coxa*) of each leg, which origins in the connecting joints between the central body and the legs (index $l$ denotes the leg: $l \in \{fl, ml, hl, fr, mr, hr\}$, $f$: front, $m$: middle, $h$: hind, $l$: left, $r$: right).(In biological research, *Coxa* denotes the first leg segment.) The spatial orientations of the of the six $C_l$–frames relative to the body-fixed $K$–frame are obtained by a set of elemantary rotations:

1. Rotation about the $_K z$–axis by the timeinvariant angle $\phi_l$

2. Rotation about the obtained intermediate $y$–axis by the time-invariant angle $\psi_l$

3. Rotation about the $_{C_l} z$-axis, whose orientation relative to the $K$–frame is timeinvariant, by angle $\alpha_l$, denoting the first degree of freedom of each leg.

The three segments of each leg lie in the $_{C_l} x - _{C_l} z$–plane, which will be called *leg plane* in the following. The $_{C_l} x$–axis marks the longitudinal axis of the first leg segment, $\beta_l$ and $\gamma_l$ denote relative angles between the second and first and between the third and second segment, respectively (see fig. 3.7).

To analyse the kinematics of the regarded gait pattern, we investigate the movements of the *tarsi* relative to the body of the insect, measured in horizontal and upright projection for discrete times $t_j, j \in \{1, \ldots, 17\}$ by H. CRUSE [[2]]. *Tarsus* denotes the low end of the last leg segment, the *tarsi* movements relative to the body thus are describec by the vectors $_K \boldsymbol{r}_{G_l T_l}(t_j)$, (see fig.3.6).

Phase charateristics of the leg movement have been investigated by GRAHAM [9]; the following computations are based upon a *tripod gait* on a horizontal plane, the phase lag between the movemants of the *left tripod* and the *right tripod* being exactly hlf the gait period denoted by T.

The motion of the central body can be obtained in following subsequent steps: the vectors $_K \boldsymbol{r}_{ST_l}$, locating the contact points $T_l$ in the body–fixed $K$–frame, are obtained by adding the vector from the center of mass to the connecting joint of the leg $l$, $_K \boldsymbol{r}_{ST_l}$ (which has time-invariant components in the $K$–frame), to the vector of the relative *tarsus* location (see figure 3.8),

$$_K \boldsymbol{r}_{ST_l}(t_j) \;=\; _K \boldsymbol{r}_{SG_l}(t_j) +_K \boldsymbol{r}_{G_l T_l}(t_j). \tag{12}$$

A *left standing triangle* is described by the vectors $_K \boldsymbol{r}_{ST_l}(t_j)$, $l \in \{fl, mr, hl\}$, a *right standing triangle* by the vectors $_K \boldsymbol{r}_{ST_l}(t_j)$, $l \in \{fr, ml, hr\}$ accordingly. During motion on a horizontal plane these triangles are alternately fixed in the inertial $_I x-$ , $_I y$–plane. Thus, the location and orientation of the $K$–frame relative to a given $I$–frame can be derived inversely. Relative to the $R$–frame the motion of the central

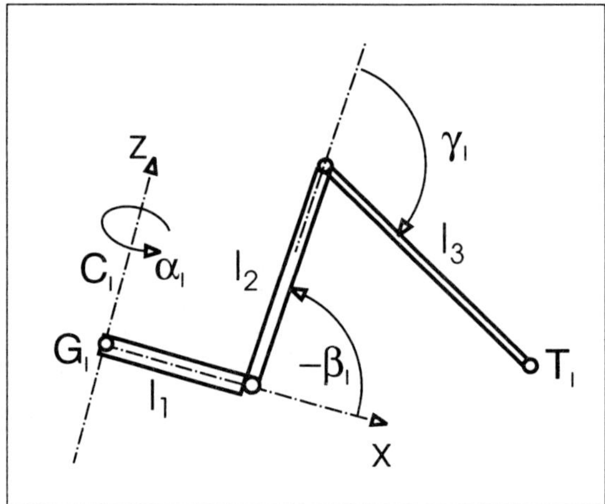


Figure 3.7: Geometry of the legs

body is then described by three generalized coordinates of translation $(q_1, q_2, q_3)$ where

$$_R\boldsymbol{r}_{OS}(t_j)^T := [q_1, q_2, q_3], \tag{13}$$

and three generalized coordinates of rotation $(q_4, q_5, q_6)$, yielding the transformation matrix $\boldsymbol{A}_{KR}$ from the $R$–frame to the $K$–frame:

$$_K\boldsymbol{r} = \boldsymbol{A}_{KR} \cdot_R \boldsymbol{r}, \tag{14}$$

$$\boldsymbol{A}_{KR} = f(q_4, q_5, q_6). \tag{15}$$

The joint angles $\alpha_l, \beta_l, \gamma_l$ are derived by the inverse kinematics from the vectors $_K\boldsymbol{f}_{G_l T_l}(t_j)$ for each leg subsequently.

$$\alpha_l = f(_K\boldsymbol{r}_{G_l}, T_l) \tag{16}$$
$$\beta_l = f(_K\boldsymbol{r}_{G_l}, T_l) \tag{17}$$
$$\gamma_l = f(_K\boldsymbol{r}_{G_l}, T_l) \tag{18}$$

The vector of generalized coordinates $\boldsymbol{q} \in \mathbb{R}^{24}$ is composed of the motion coordinates of the central body $q_1$ to $q_6$ plus the joint angles:

$$\boldsymbol{q}^T = [q_1, \ldots, q_6, \alpha_{fl}, \beta_{fl}, \gamma_{fl}, \ldots, \alpha_{hr}, \beta_{hr}, \gamma_{hr}] \tag{19}$$

It is reasonable to approximate each of the components of $\mathbf{q}$ by a Fourier-series, since the motion of the insect appears smooth and harmonic. Using only the first three

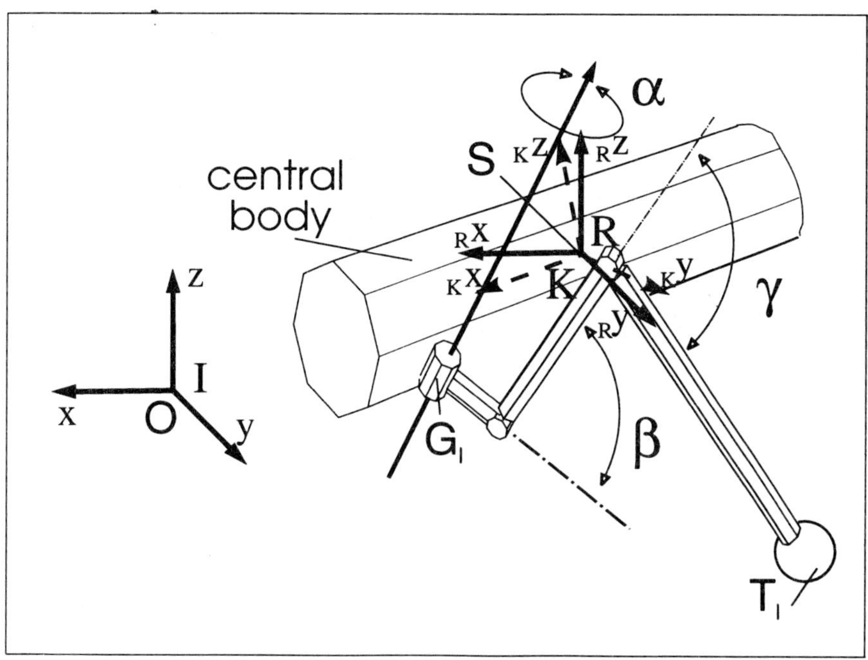


Figure 3.8: Kinematic of the walking machine

frequencies of the Fourier-series, the measured generalized coordinates $q_1$ to $q_6$ and also the joint angles $q_7$ to $q_{24}$ are closely approximated.

$$q_k(t) \approx a_{k_o} + \sum_{m=1}^{3} [a_{k_m} cos(\frac{2\pi mt}{T}) + b_{k_m} sin(\frac{2\pi mt}{T})] k \in \{1, \dots, 24\} \qquad (20)$$

Figure 3.9 shows the movements of the central body over a gait period $T$. The continuous line represents the approximation, the dotted line represents the measurements.

## 4  General Kinetics

To determine active joint torques and contact forces on the ground, the equations of motion are derived from d'Alemberts principle [1]:

$$\int_{(S)} \delta r^T (\ddot{r} dm - d f_e) = 0 \qquad (21)$$

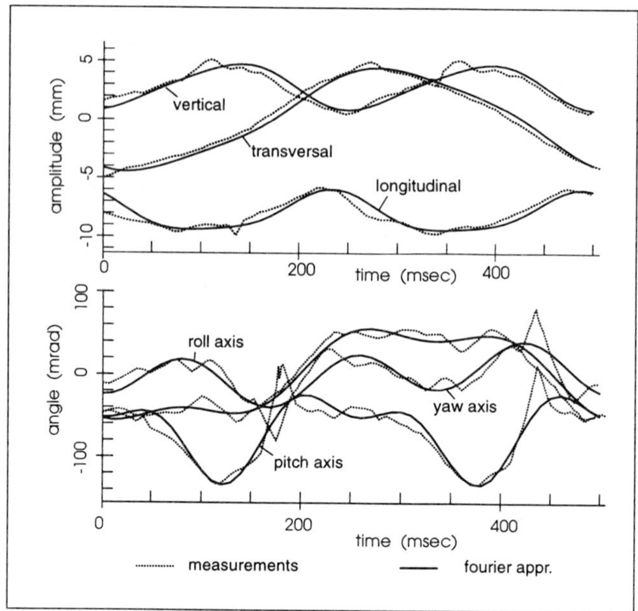


Figure 3.9: Relative Movements of the Central Body

When regarding a rigid multibody system, the evaluation of eq.(21) simplifies to

$$\sum_{p=1}^{p=n} \left[ \boldsymbol{J}_T^T(m\ddot{\boldsymbol{r}} - \boldsymbol{f}_e) + \boldsymbol{J}_R^T(\boldsymbol{I}\dot{\boldsymbol{\omega}} + \tilde{\boldsymbol{\omega}}\boldsymbol{I}\boldsymbol{\omega} - \boldsymbol{t}_e\right] = \boldsymbol{0} \tag{22}$$

where: **r** denotes the vector locating the center of mass of the p-th body, $\boldsymbol{J}_T$ the jacobian matrix of translation, $\boldsymbol{J}_R$ the jacobian matrix of rotation, $\boldsymbol{f}_e$ active external forces, $\boldsymbol{t}_e$ active external torques.

Applying eq.(22) to the walking stick insect yields the equations of motion:

$$\boldsymbol{M}\ddot{\boldsymbol{q}} = \boldsymbol{h} + \boldsymbol{J}_T^T\boldsymbol{f} + \boldsymbol{J}_M^T\boldsymbol{t} \tag{23}$$

where $\boldsymbol{M} \in \mathbb{R}^{24,24}$ denotes the mass matrix, $\boldsymbol{q}$ is given according to eq.(19), and $\boldsymbol{f} \in \mathbb{R}^{18,1}$ is the vector of contact forces,

$$\boldsymbol{f}^T = \left[ f_{lv_x}, f_{lv_y}, f_{lv_z}, \ldots, f_{rh_x}, f_{rh_y}, f_{rh_z} \right], \tag{24}$$

$\boldsymbol{t} \in \mathbb{R}^{18,1}$ is the vector of active joint torques,

$$\boldsymbol{t}^T = \left[ t_{\alpha_{lv}}, t_{\beta_{lv}}, t_{\gamma_{lv}}, \ldots, t_{\alpha_{rh}}, t_{\beta_{rh}}, t_{\gamma_{rh}}, \right], \tag{25}$$

$h \in \mathbb{R}^{24}$ denotes the generalized influence of gravitation, $J_F \in \mathbb{R}^{18,24}$ is composed of the jacobian matrices of translation of the contact points $T_L$ in columns, $J_M \in \mathbb{R}^{18,24}$ accordingly projects the torques $t$ into the space of the generalized coordinates $q$. The vectors $f$ and $t$ are unknown, so that there are 36 unknown quantities with 24 equations.

With $m$ legs in ground contact, $m(m-1)/2$ closed kinematic loops have to be taken into account, yielding an infinite number of solutions for the contact force distribution. For a simulation of the system in the case of unknown accelerations $\ddot{q}$ the active torques $t$ must be given and *Lagrange-multipliers* must be used to include the distance constraints of the contact points on the ground in the equations of motion.

With a complete analysis of the kinematic, however, the desired gait pattern of the walking stick insect is given over time, $q(t)$, and resulting accelerations $\ddot{q}$ are easily acquired by deriving eq.(20) twice with respect to time. In the case of the walking stick insect, the vectors $f$ and $t$ remain unknown. Some supplementary assunptions are therefore necessary to determine torques and forces for the based gait pattern $q(t)$ (see section 6.2).

# 5 Theory of Optimization

## 5.1 Fundamentals of Optimization

- <u>Evaluation of the mimimum of a scalar function:</u>

$$
\begin{aligned}
\text{given:} \quad & f(\boldsymbol{x})\,\text{with} \quad \boldsymbol{x} \in X \subset \mathbb{R} \\
\text{global minimum } \boldsymbol{x}^* : \quad & f(\boldsymbol{x}^*) \le f(\boldsymbol{x}) \quad \forall \quad \boldsymbol{x} \in X \\
\text{local minimum } \boldsymbol{x}^* : \quad & f(\boldsymbol{x}^*) \le f(\boldsymbol{x}) \quad \forall \quad \boldsymbol{x} \in X \cap U_\epsilon(\boldsymbol{x}^*)
\end{aligned}
\tag{26}
$$

$$\text{with } U_\epsilon \text{ an } \epsilon\text{-environment of } \boldsymbol{x}^*.$$

- <u>Necessary condition for a minimum:</u>

$$
0 = df = \left.\frac{\partial f}{\partial \boldsymbol{x}}\right|_{x^*} d\boldsymbol{x} \Leftrightarrow \left.\frac{\partial f}{\partial \boldsymbol{x}}\right|_{x^*} = \boldsymbol{0}
\tag{27}
$$

if the function is convex, this is a necessary and sufficient condition.

- <u>Sufficient condition:</u>
  if the Hessian-matrix:

$$
\boldsymbol{H}(\boldsymbol{x}^*) := \left.\frac{\partial^2 f}{\partial \boldsymbol{x} \partial \boldsymbol{x}^T}\right|_{x^*}
\tag{28}
$$

is positiv definite at the point $\boldsymbol{x}^*$ (see eq.27), then a minimum exists at $\boldsymbol{x}^*$.

## 5.2 Minimization of a function with equality-constraints

*Given:*

$$
f(\boldsymbol{x}) \ \textit{with } \boldsymbol{x} \in X \subset \mathbb{R}^n
\tag{29}
$$

*under the constraints*

$$
\boldsymbol{h}(\boldsymbol{x}) = \boldsymbol{0} \in \mathbb{R}^q; \quad q \le n
\tag{30}
$$

The minimum of $f$ under the constraints $\boldsymbol{h}(\boldsymbol{x}) = \boldsymbol{0}$ is desired. So $(n-q)$ independent variables $\boldsymbol{z}$ with $\boldsymbol{x} = \boldsymbol{x}(\boldsymbol{z})$ remain to describe the problem.

$$f = f(\boldsymbol{x}(\boldsymbol{z})); \quad \boldsymbol{z} \in \mathbb{R}^{n-q} \tag{31}$$

The necessary condition for a minimum is (eq. 27):

$$0 = df = \frac{\partial f}{\partial \boldsymbol{x}} \cdot \frac{\partial \boldsymbol{x}}{\partial \boldsymbol{z}} \cdot d\boldsymbol{z}. \tag{32}$$

Taking the derivative of the constraints (eq. 30) results in:

$$\boldsymbol{0} = d\boldsymbol{h} = \frac{\partial \boldsymbol{h}}{\partial \boldsymbol{x}} \cdot \frac{\partial \boldsymbol{x}}{\partial \boldsymbol{z}} \cdot d\boldsymbol{z}. \tag{33}$$

Because of the independence of the components of $\boldsymbol{z}$

$$\frac{\partial f}{\partial \boldsymbol{x}} \cdot \frac{\partial \boldsymbol{x}}{\partial \boldsymbol{z}} = \boldsymbol{0} \tag{34}$$

$$\frac{\partial \boldsymbol{h}}{\partial \boldsymbol{x}} \cdot \frac{\partial \boldsymbol{x}}{\partial \boldsymbol{z}} = \boldsymbol{0} \tag{35}$$

can be applied.

Thus the *Lagrange-function* can be written:

$$L(\boldsymbol{x}, \boldsymbol{\alpha}) = f(\boldsymbol{x}) + \boldsymbol{\alpha}^T \boldsymbol{h}(\boldsymbol{x}); \boldsymbol{\alpha} \in \mathbb{R}^q \tag{36}$$

Derivation of $L$ with respect to $\boldsymbol{x}$ and $\boldsymbol{\alpha}$ results in:

$$\boldsymbol{0}^T = \frac{\partial L}{\partial \boldsymbol{x}} = \frac{\partial f}{\partial \boldsymbol{x}} + \boldsymbol{\alpha}^T \frac{\partial \boldsymbol{h}}{\partial \boldsymbol{x}} \tag{37}$$

(This is a linear combination of eqs. (34) and (35)) and

$$\boldsymbol{0}^T = \frac{\partial L}{\partial \boldsymbol{\alpha}} = \boldsymbol{h}^T(\boldsymbol{x}). \tag{38}$$

see eq. (30). So $(n+q)$ equations for the determination of the components of $\boldsymbol{x}$ and $\boldsymbol{\alpha}$ are obtained.

## 5.3  Minimization with inequality constraints

*Given:*

$$f(\boldsymbol{x}) \; with \; \boldsymbol{x} \in \boldsymbol{X} \subset \mathbb{R}^n \tag{39}$$

*under the constraints*

$$g(x) \leq 0 \in \mathbb{R}^p; p \leq n \tag{40}$$

The minimum of $f$ under the constraints $g(x) \leq 0$ is desired. At first the *Lagrange-function* is given as:

$$L(x, \beta) = f(x) + \beta^T g(x) \tag{41}$$

Now active and passive constraints have to be separated. Active constraints restrict the function f and passive do not.

Therefore $g(x)$ can be divided in an active part $g_1(x)$ and a passive part $g_2(x)$ .

$$\beta^T g(x) := \beta^T g_1(x) + \beta^T g_2(x) \tag{42}$$

Passive conditions have no effect on the minimum and thus do not have to be considered.

$$g_2(x^*) < 0 \wedge \beta_2 = 0 \tag{43}$$

For active conditions we state:

$$g_1(x^*) = 0 \wedge \beta_1 \leq 0, \tag{44}$$

which yields

$$\frac{\partial L}{\partial x} = 0 = \frac{\partial f}{\partial x} + \beta^T \frac{\partial g}{\partial x} \tag{45}$$

$$\beta_i \cdot g_i(x) = 0 \quad \text{with} \quad \beta_i \geq 0 \quad \forall \quad i = 1, \ldots, p \quad \text{and} \quad g(x) \leq 0. \tag{46}$$

The active constraints now can be treated as equality constraints. (See further actions in chapter 5.2).

## 5.4   Vector-Optimization

*Compute*

$$\min_{x \in X} f(x) \text{ with } x \in \mathbb{R}^n; \quad f \in \mathbb{R}^m \tag{47}$$

*under the constraints*

$$h(x) = 0 \quad h \in \mathbb{R}^q$$

$$g(x) \leq 0 \quad g \in \mathbb{R}^p.$$

Here a vector of functions is to be minimized. In general the solution is not unique, because the individual minimums $x_i^*$ of the component functions $f_i(x)$ are not at the same location. In general

$$x_1^* \neq x_2^* \neq \ldots \neq x_m^* \tag{48}$$

applies. Thus the problem has to be solved using a scalar substitute. No general objective procedure exists to solve this problems uniquely, the solution will always be a compromise between the original minimums of the single components $f_i(\boldsymbol{x})$ of the vector-function $\boldsymbol{f}(\boldsymbol{x})$.

The solution process is called Pareto-optimization.

## 5.5  Pareto-optimization

**Def.:** *A solution $\boldsymbol{x}^* \in \boldsymbol{X}$ is called pareto-optimal, if there is <u>no</u> other vector $\boldsymbol{x}$ with*

$$f_i(\boldsymbol{x}) \leq f_i(\boldsymbol{x}^*) \quad \forall\, i \in \{1,\ldots,m\} \tag{49}$$

*and at least for one $j \in \{1,\ldots,m\}$ applies:*

$$f_j(\boldsymbol{x}) < f_j(\boldsymbol{x}^*). \tag{50}$$

This means that diminishing one $f_i$ results in an increase of at least one of the other $f_j$. The region $\boldsymbol{X}^* := \{\boldsymbol{x}^*\}$ is called pareto-optimal region of the optimization problem (47).

So the substitute for the problem (47) is:

*Compute*

$$\min_{\boldsymbol{x}\in X}\, p(\boldsymbol{f}(\boldsymbol{x}))\ with \quad \boldsymbol{x} \in \mathbb{R}^n; \quad \boldsymbol{f} \in \mathbb{R}^m \tag{51}$$

*under the constraints*

$$\boldsymbol{h}(\boldsymbol{x}) = \boldsymbol{0} \quad \boldsymbol{h} \in \mathbb{R}^q$$

$$\boldsymbol{g}(\boldsymbol{x}) \leq \boldsymbol{0} \quad \boldsymbol{g} \in \mathbb{R}^p.$$

This problem is solvable if a $\tilde{\boldsymbol{x}} \in \boldsymbol{X}^*$ with

$$p(\boldsymbol{f}(\tilde{\boldsymbol{x}})) = \min_{\boldsymbol{x}\in X}\, p(\boldsymbol{f}(\boldsymbol{x})) \tag{52}$$

exists.

Examples for substitute functions $p$ in (51):

i) **Method of objective weighting**

$$p(\boldsymbol{f}(\boldsymbol{x})) := \boldsymbol{w}^T \cdot \boldsymbol{f}(\boldsymbol{x}), \quad \boldsymbol{x} \in \boldsymbol{X} \tag{53}$$

$$\text{with:}\quad 0 \leq w_i \leq 1; \quad \sum_{i=1}^{m} w_i = 1 \tag{54}$$

The problem in this case is to find a normalization for the individual $f_i$'s and to choose suitable weighting factors $w_i$.

## ii) Min-Max-formulation

$$p(\boldsymbol{f}(\boldsymbol{x})) := \max_{i=1,\ldots,m} \left( \frac{f_i(\boldsymbol{x})}{f_{i_o}} \right); \quad f_{i_o} > 0 \quad \forall\, i = 1,\ldots,m \tag{55}$$

Here the individual reference values $f_{i_o}$ have to be chosen. They determine the minimum vector $\boldsymbol{x}^*$.

## iii) Quadratic weighting function

$$p(\boldsymbol{f}(\boldsymbol{x})) := \sqrt{\sum_{i=1}^{m} w_i f_i^2(\boldsymbol{x})}, \quad \boldsymbol{x} \in \boldsymbol{X} \tag{56}$$

$$\text{with:} \quad 0 \leq w_i \leq 1; \quad \sum_{i=1}^{m} w_i = 1. \tag{57}$$

Continue in the same way as in (i).

# Part II: Practice of Walking

# 6   Walking derived from the *stick insect*

## 6.1   Kinetics and Gait Patterns

The basic geometry of a leg is taken from the stick insect Carausius Morosus ([5], [15], [23]). Figure 6.10 gives an indication of the walking machine and of the specific leg design as derived from biology. All leg components move in one plane which

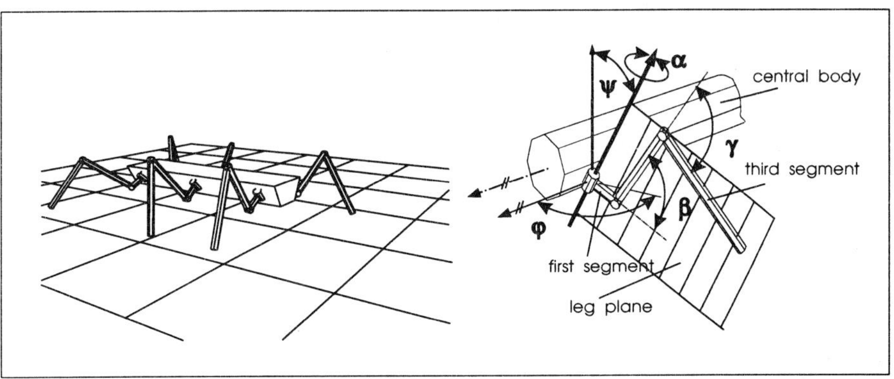


Figure 6.10: Six-Legged Walking Machine and Details of Leg Design

itself rotates around an oblique axis fixed at the central body. The orientation of this axis is given by the two angle $(\psi, \varphi)$, the rotation around it by the angle $\alpha$. The two leg segments (for the stick insect *Femur* and *Tibia*) move in the plane with the two rotation angles $(\beta, \gamma)$.

The coordination of the six legs during walking is mainly laid down in a gait pattern system. Our biological model, the stick insect, applies for walking two patterns, namely the tetrapod gait and the tripod gait. The first one more for low and the second one for higher speeds. Gait patterns are characterized by three parameters *pi, pc, df*. The ipsilateral phase *pi* is the normalized phase lag between two neighbouring legs on the same side of the body. The contralateral phase *pc* marks the normalized phase lag between a leg and its opposite neighbouring leg. The duty factor *df* defines the portion of contact time with the ground related to total walking cycle time of one leg. One gait pattern can conveniently be characterized by one point in the (*pi, pc, df*)-space (Fig. 6.11). In addition this type of presentation is a good basis for stability analysis for different gaits.

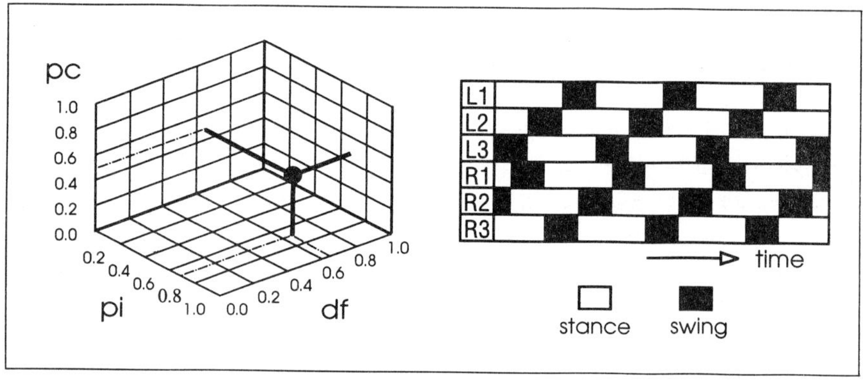


Figure 6.11: The Tetrapod Gait

## 6.2 Kinetics and Criterions for Design-Optimization

The evaluation of design criteria as applied in biological systems greatly profits from the fact that with a prescribed gait pattern the determination of the torques in the leg joints and the forces on the ground leads to an underdetermined system of equations of motion. To make this system solvable one may apply an additional optimization process which gives an opportunity to test several criteria and to adapt these criteria to measured forces from the stick insect [5].

The walking stick insect is modelled as a multibody system with rigid components and altogether 24 degrees of freedom (one central body with 6 DOF, six legs each with 3 DOF). Prescribing the gait pattern we write the equations of motion in an inverse form

$$J_R^T \cdot t + J_T^T \cdot f = M \cdot \ddot{q} + h. \tag{58}$$

$\ddot{q} \in \mathbb{R}^{24}$ is the vector of the accelerations of the generalized coordinates of the MBS, $M$ is the mass matrix, and $J_R$ and $J_T$ are the Jacobian matrices of rotation and translation, respectively. The vector $t \in \mathbb{R}^{18}$ contains the three unknown torques around the angular DOF for each leg, the vector $f \in \mathbb{R}^{18}$ denotes the vector of the ground contact from each leg. The relevant number of unknown forces and torques depends on the gait pattern and thus on the number of legs in a swing phase. With each leg on the ground we have 24 equations (58) and 36 unknowns. This is the worst case. For a synchronization of equations and unknowns we add an optimization process in a Lagrangian form.

We introduce a supplementary criterion $C$ relating forces and torques to each other. This additional criterion $C$ offers the possibility of testing different physical constraints which might be a basis of biological design. The equations of motion must be satisfied with the resulting forces and torques, in the Lagrangian Function $L$ they are coupled to the criterion by a vector of Lagrangian multipliers:

$$L = C(t^2, f^2) + \lambda^T \left[ J_R^T \cdot t + J_T^T \cdot f - (M \cdot \ddot{q} + h) \right] + \lambda^{*T} U f \tag{59}$$

The last expression in eqs. (59) records the fact that some legs may be in a swing phase with no contact forces at the feet. Consequently, the matrix $U$ possesses a 0–1–structure. According to the Lagrangian theorem, the criterion $C$ achieves a minimum for vanishing partial derivates of the Lagrangian function $L$ with respect to all unknown quantities:

$$\frac{\partial L}{\partial t_n} = 0 \quad \wedge \quad \frac{\partial L}{\partial f_n} = 0 \quad 1 \leq n \leq 18$$

$$\frac{\partial L}{\partial \lambda_m} = 0 \quad 1 \leq m \leq 24 \quad \wedge \quad m \in \mathbb{N} \tag{60}$$

$$\frac{\partial L}{\partial \lambda_k^*} = 0 \quad 1 \leq k \leq 3n_a \quad \wedge \quad k \in \mathbb{N}$$

Given the abbreviations

$$\frac{\partial C}{\partial t} = C_1 \cdot t + C_2 \cdot f \; ; \quad \frac{\partial C}{\partial f} = C_3 \cdot t + C_4 \cdot f \tag{61}$$

we finally obtain a linear system,

$$\begin{bmatrix} J_R^T & J_T^T & 0 & 0 \\ 0 & U & 0 & 0 \\ C_1 & C_2 & J_R & 0 \\ C_3 & C_4 & J_T & U^T \end{bmatrix} \begin{bmatrix} t \\ f \\ \lambda \\ \lambda^* \end{bmatrix} = \begin{bmatrix} M\ddot{q} + h \\ 0 \\ 0 \\ 0 \end{bmatrix} \tag{62}$$

which can be solved using numerical methods. Whenever feet lift off the ground, the dimension of this linear system changes accordingly. We investigated five different criteria $C$:

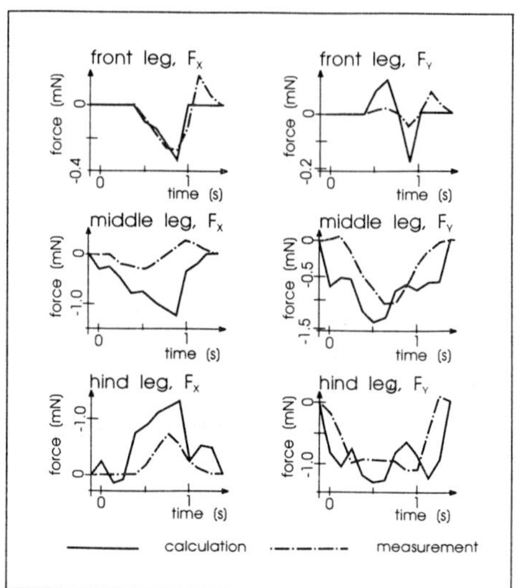


Figure 6.12: Measured and Calculated Contact Forces in the Walking Plane

- Minimization of bending energy loaded upon the legs,

- minimization of interaction forces in the walking plane [22],

- minimal forces in the joints,

- special direction of the main force in each leg,

- minimization of active joint power consumption.

The results of the forces and torques are compared with measurement on the walking stick insect performed by Cruse [2]. The best agreement with respect to these measurements is achieved using the requirement for minimization of bending load in the legs coupled to a minimization of interaction forces in the walking plane with proportion 60:40. Fig. 6.12 shows measured horizontal contact force components for each leg in comparison with their computed simulation values (dash-dotted-lines).

## 6.3   Design of the Walking Machine

The central components of every walking machine are the legs. Therefore, walking machine design means leg design. Moreover, leg design means design of its most important joint, the $\beta$-joint (see Fig. 6.10). Figure 6.13 illustrates the basic design

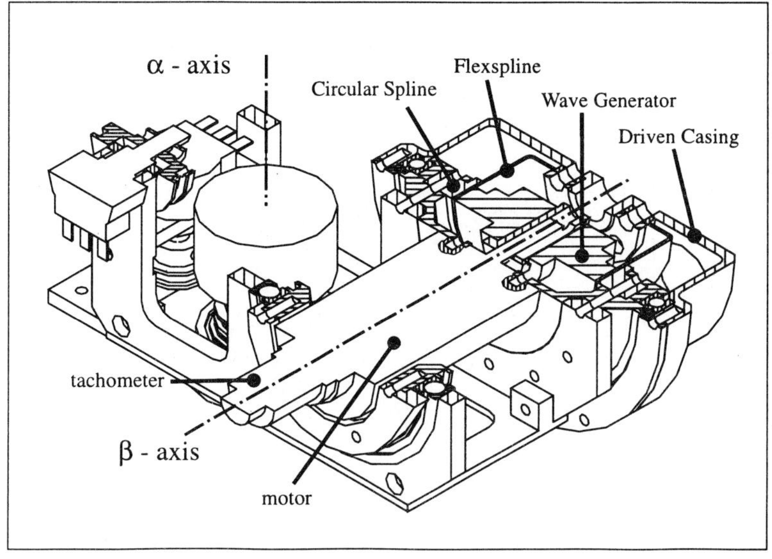


Figure 6.13: Design of the $\beta$-Joint

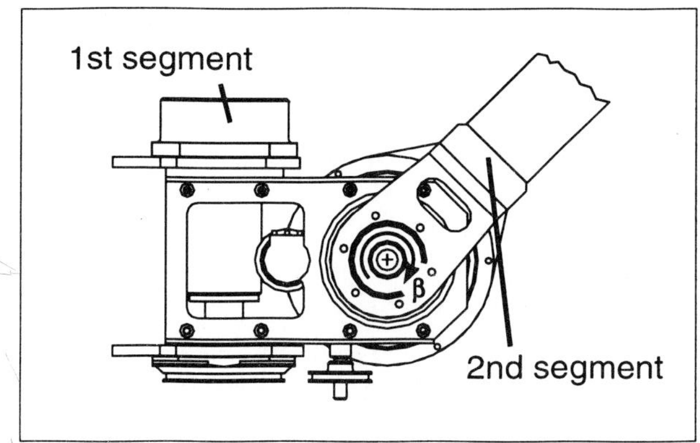


Figure 6.14: Excentric Fastening of the second Leg Segment

features. The main idea of such a direct drive system consists in a direct connection
of the flexspline with the driven casing, which results in a very small weight of the
complete drive system. Another important feature with regard to weight reduction

is the shortest possible distance between the two main axes of the $\alpha$- and $\beta$-joint, which could only be realized by the dense construction of the $\beta$-combination of direct current motor and harmonic drive system. In addition and for realizing a relative

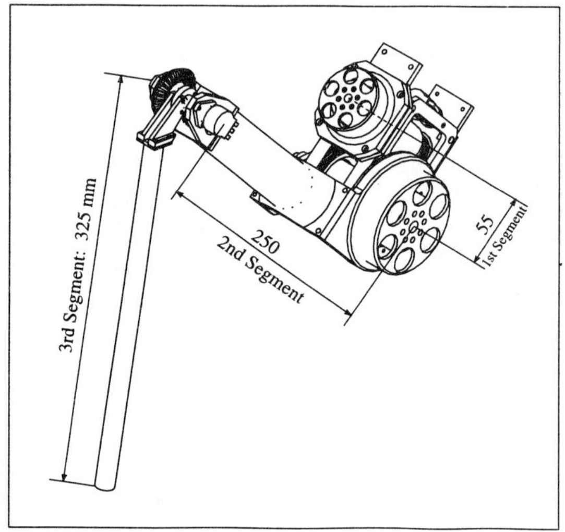


Figure 6.15: Leg with 3 Degrees of Freedom (2.8 kg)

angle of $70^o$ between segment 1 containing the $\alpha$- and $\beta$-joints (Figs. 6.10,6.13) and the second segment an excentric fastening of segment two to the $\beta$-axis was chosen as an optimum solution (Fig. 6.14).

In further reducing any component of the leg construction to its minimum shape taking into consideration the stress limits of stability we could perform a leg with a total weight of together 2.8 kg but a load bearing capacity of nearly 18 kg at the most (Fig. 6.15). The six-legged walking machine has three equal legs on each side where the legs from one side to the other are mirror symmetric. Each leg has the same direct drive systems as described in chapter C. In additon to the tachometer measurement all joints are equipped with potentiometers for angular measurements. For the joints $(\alpha, \beta)$ these potentiometers are driven by pulleys, for the $\gamma$-joint it is driven directly.

The weight of the complete walking machine comes out with 23 kg, about 17.5 kg for the six legs including special fastenings, 1.5 kg for the central body and about 3.5 kg for the electronic and electric equipment. A specially designed fastening component for each leg allows an adaptation of the $\alpha$-axis orientation to different walking requirements in a very wide range, which will be systematically tested experimentally. Figure 6.16 gives an idea of the walking machine design.

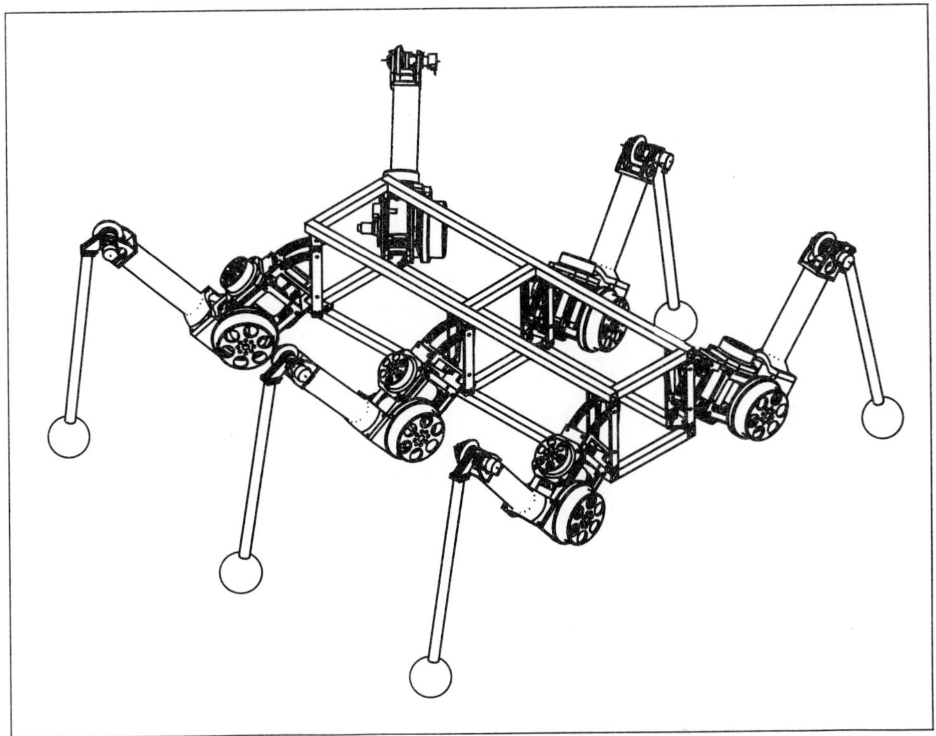

Figure 6.16: The Six-Legged TUM-Walking Machine

# 7   The Control System of the Walking Machine

## 7.1   The Three-Layer Concept

The main ideas taken over from neurobiological research ([2],[3],[4]) are depicted in Fig. 7.17, which follows in its performance very closely to biological behaviour. A global leg coordination module (LCM) is an information level where each leg informs its neighbouring legs about its state as laid down in the decision functions of each single leg controller (SLC) [17].

## 7.2   The Coordination Level

The leg coordination module (LCM) is responsible for setting the landing and lifting points of each leg (In the following AEP = *anterior extreme position* and PEP = *posterior extreme position*). In controlling these points the global behavior of the walking process can be influenced. Although this level is doing a global task, the control mechanism works locally. In figure 7.18 this mechanism is depicted. In this figure it can be seen, that neighbouring legs can shift the AEPs and PEPs by a small amount. Thus e.g. legs can inhibit adjoining legs from lifting of the ground in postponing their PEPs. Each leg gets specific information from the other legs:

- the walking phase (see section 7.3)

- the velocity

- the AEP and PEP-Values

This information is sufficient for each LCM to compute its new AEP and PEP. These values are sent to the middle control level. There is no central supervision.

   The control influences used in this approach have been measured and isolated by neurobiologists ([2],[3],[4]). Up to eight control mechanisms can be implemented in the LCM, the function principle of two of the most important mechanisms numbered I and II are shortly explained in the following: Given that the rostrally neighboured leg is not yet in STANCE phase, the mechanism I inhibits the lifting of the leg in

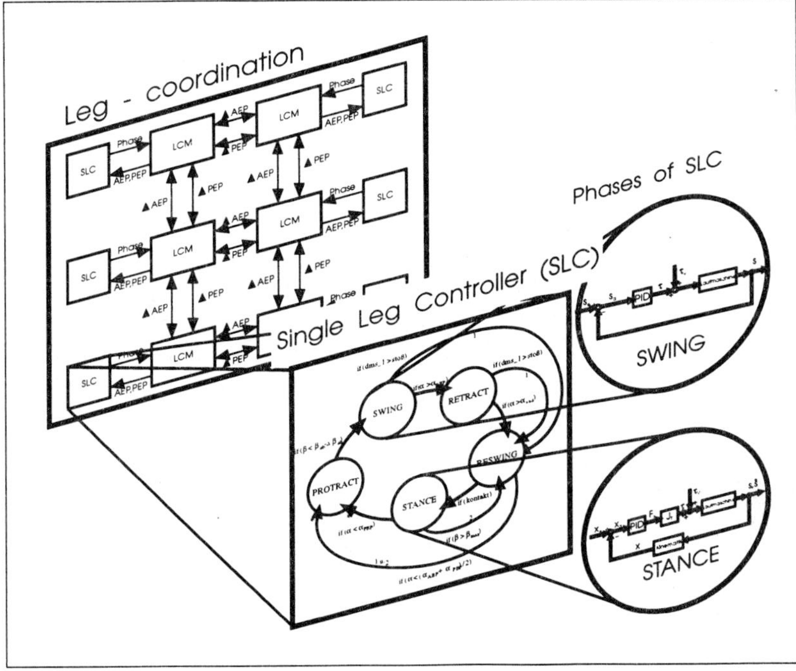


Figure 7.17: Global Control Structure of the Walking Machine

shifhting back the PEP by a certain increment. Similarly, the mechanism II inhibits a start of the lifting phase when the contralateral adjacent leg is not yet back in STANCE phase.

## 7.3  The Single Leg Controller (SLC)

The single leg controller (SLC) is the heart of leg motion performing all decisions necessary to move the leg and to control the various phases. The order of the dirferent phases in a normal step is STANCE, PROTRACT, SWING and RETRACT (see fig. 7.19). The SLC switches between the phases in dependency of the AEP, the PEP and some specific events (e.g. hitting an obstacle). It does some on-line path planning at the beginning of the PROTRACT phase. Moreover the SLC gives to each leg some local intelligence especially needed to manage obstacles, impacts or other unforeseen events.

The single leg controller detects and surpasses obstacles, controls body height and corrects slippage effects. The capability of obstacle avoidance is achieved by

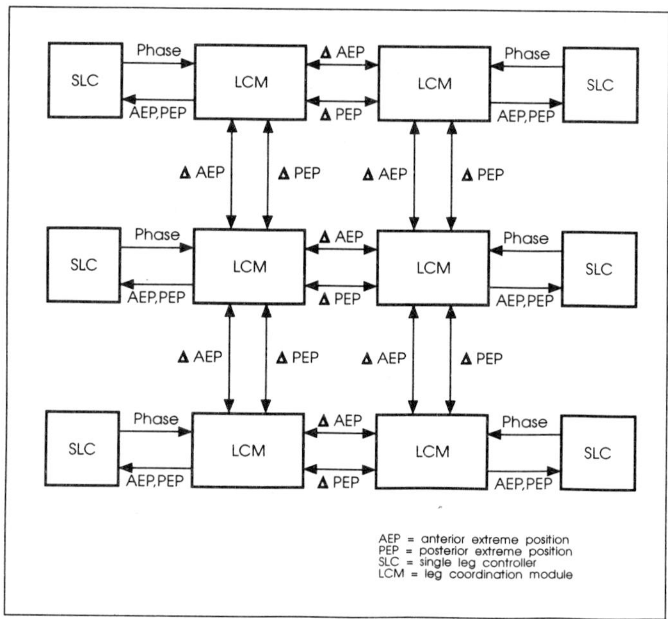


Figure 7.18: The Coordination Mechanism

means of a special detection mechanism and a different approach to general path planning. During SWING phase the SLC monitors the bending load in the leg segments. Whenever the corresponding strain gauge signal exceeds a certain threshold value the obstacle avoidance mechanism is activated. A short RESWING phase is executed followed by a new SWING phase trying to pass the obstacle.

The path planning algorithm for the three leg angles $\alpha, \beta, \gamma$ thereby differs from standard path planning used in robotics. Usually, end effector trajectories are described by time histories of work space or configuration space coordinates. In our approach we describe the dependency of the outer joint coordinates $\beta, \gamma$ in terms of the leg angle coordinate $\alpha$.

$$\gamma = f(\alpha) \quad ; \quad \beta = f(\alpha) \tag{63}$$

Physically, we thereby describe the geometrical shape of the trajectory but not its velocity and acceleration profile. Since the SLC monitors the $\alpha$-movement of the leg plane, $\beta$ and $\gamma$ are cascade-controlled by evaluating their desired values in depend-

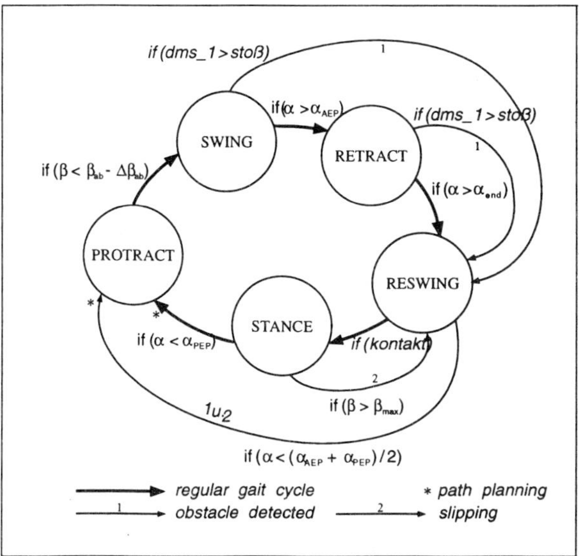


Figure 7.19: The single leg controller

ency of the $\alpha$-value:

$$\beta = f(\alpha) ; \quad \rightarrow \quad \dot{\beta} = \frac{\partial f}{\partial \alpha}\dot{\alpha} + \frac{\partial}{\partial t}f$$

$$\gamma = g(\alpha) ; \quad \rightarrow \quad \dot{\gamma} = \frac{\partial g}{\partial \alpha}\dot{\alpha} + \frac{\partial}{\partial t}g \tag{64}$$

Since these evaluations have to be made on-line and therefore in real time, we demand the foot trajectories to be composed of segments of simple polynomial functions. The so derived trajectories are in good accordance with foot trajectories observed and measured in walking insects.

The path planning algorithm is executed at the beginning of a SWING phase within the 1ms-time slice of an hardware interrupt driven control architecture. Similarly, foot slippage is detected by means of monitoring the $\beta$ angle and its velocity, if necessary a RESWING phase is executed and the foot is moved to a new, legal STANCE position.

The STANCE phase is controlled in cartesian coordinates. The height is controlled in position and the other two directions in velocity. Thus the desired values for the STANCE phase have to be computed from the given kinematic of the central body of the robot. These values are the input for the lowest level controller in the STANCE phase.

## 7.4   Lowest Level Control

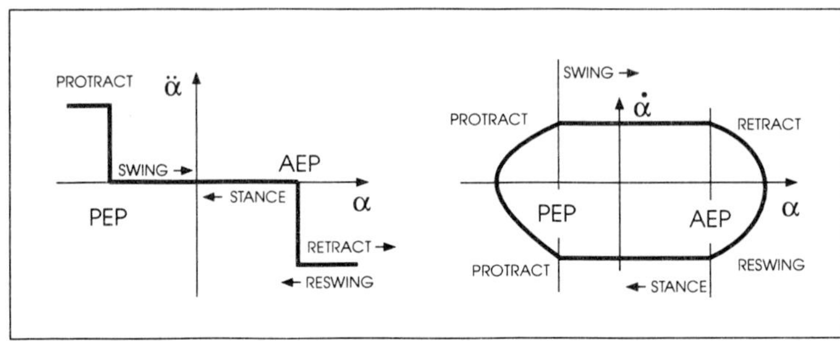


Figure 7.20: Three Step Controller for the $\alpha$-Joint (Leg Plane)

In addition to the two upper levels the leg needs a lowest level control system which typically, and again near to biological performance, consists in a feedforward non-linear decoupling scheme combined with a feedback linear controller. The low level controller for the AIR phase (which includes PROTRACT, SWING, RETRACT and RESWING) resembles a manipulator controller, where on-line path planning is carried through applying eqs. (64). The controllers for the AIR and STANCE phases differ in the controlled coordinates.

During the STANCE phase the leg is in an active support phase and is controlled in cartesian coordinates (see below). In the AIR phase the leg angles are controlled. The accelaration $\ddot{\alpha}$ is given by a three step controller approximating thus the biological behaviour of the controlling neurons (see fig. 7.20). The angles $\beta$ and $\gamma$ are computed at every step from the momentary angle $\alpha$. These two angles are controlled by a linear PD-controller. SWING marks the return movement of the leg to the next ground point and PROTRACT and RETRACT/RESWING denote the high acceleration transition areas from status STANCE to SWING or vice versa, respectively. We furthermore demand piecewise constant angular accelerations which are switched at the anterior extreme position (AEP) and the posterior extreme position (PEP). Fig. 7.20 shows acceleration versus angle and the corresponding phase portrait of the swing movement of the leg plane. The accelaration of the angle $\alpha$ in the STANCE phase is not exactly zero, because it results from the kinematik of the robot central body due to the switching in a cartesian system.

In the STANCE phase the controlled values are in a cartesian system. In this phase the position and velocity of the *tarsus*, this is the end point of the leg, is computed online in the body-fixed coordinate system. The motion in direction of the body axis ($x$-direction) and the motion to the side ($y$-direction) are velocity-PID controlled. The height ($z$-direction) is position controlled. The desired values are given from the single leg controller.

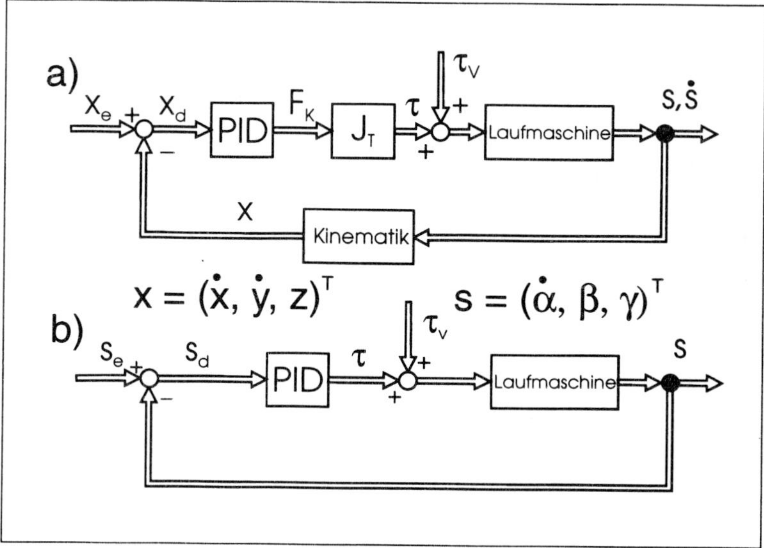


Figure 7.21: Lowest Level Controller for (a) STANCE- and (b) AIR-Phases

# 8   Pipe Crawling Robot

## 8.1   Aim of the Project

Tube systems differ in their pipe diameters, lengthes, the mediums inside, the complexity of the tube arrangement etc.. Different kinds of robots have been developed for inspecting and repairing tubes from inside. They are driven by wheels or chains or they float with the medium. All types of robots have their specific difficulties, for example problems of traction or low flexibility and do not satisfy all requirements expected by the users. The aim of this project is the development of a robot moving forward by feet to study the possibilities and difficulties of legged locomotions in contrast to other systems. The higher flexibility of legs can be used to extend the technical possibilities of moving in tube systems.

## 8.2   Robot Design

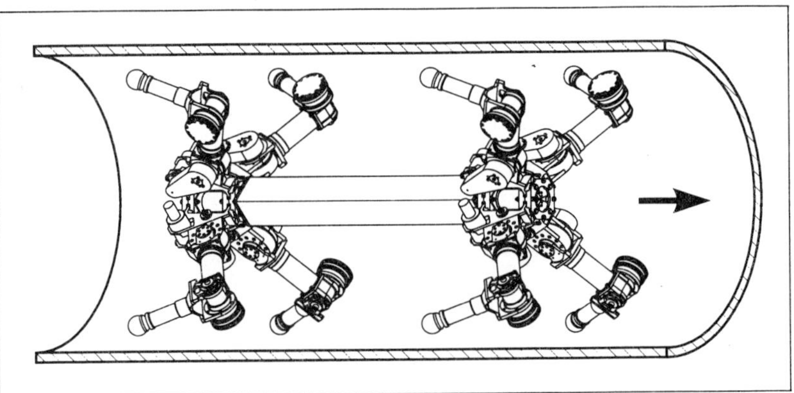

Figure 8.22: Construction of the Pipe Crawling Robot

The robot shown in figure 8.22 has eight legs arranged like two stars. The attachments of the eight legs are located in two planes that intersect at the longitudinal axis of the central body. These planes are called leg planes. Each leg has two active joints, which are driven by DC-motors. Their axes of rotation are orthogonal to the leg planes. This provides each leg with a full planar mobility. The leg is mounted to the central body with an additional passive joint, which allows small compensating movements in the third direction.

The crawler has a length of about $0.75m$ and is able to work in pipes with a diameter of $60 - 70cm$. In each of the eight legs, the distance between the two active joints (hip and knee) is $15cm$ and the length of the last leg segment (from knee to foot) is $17cm$. The highest possible torque of the hip joint is $78Nm$ short term and $40Nm$ permanent. The corresponding values of the knee are $78Nm$ and $20Nm$. In a stretched out position a leg is able to carry 6.5 times its own weight (less than $2kg$) permanently and 12 times for short time operations. Its mechanical design is based on the six legged walking machine [5][17]. The total weight of the crawler is about $20kg$ including the electronic parts. Details of the mechanical design can be found in [11].

The robot is controlled by five Siemens microcontrollers 80C167 CAN, which are installed on the crawler itself. One controller acts as a central unit. Each of the remaining four units controls two opposite legs. The controllers are able to communicate over a CAN bus system.

Each leg has two potentiometers to measure the joint angles and two tachometer generators to measure the angular velocity of the motors. For measuring the contact forces to the pipe a special light weight sensor was developed. With its five axes it does not depend on the exact contact configuration. For future extensions the electronic architecture allows the implementation of further sensors like inclination meters.

## 8.3   Design Optimization

The structural parameters of the robot and the characteristics of the gait influence the capacity and the efficiency of the robot arbitratively. Therefore corresponding optimizations were done by the research team of the Institute for Problems in Mechanics of Russian Academy of Sciences, which takes part in the development of the robot in the scope of the "Koerber-Preis" [18][14]. Two different performance criteria are considered to be maximized: the robot velocity and the thrusting force produced by the legs. Thereby the investigations are restricted to regular motions with given gait patterns. The parameters, which are chosen to be varied are the length of the last segment $l_2$, the begin of the support phase $x$ and the step length $s$. These parameters easily can be changed and therefore are adaptable to different working conditions. The fixed parameters are the dimensions of the central body, the length of the first link, the available joint torques, the mass parameters and the reachable angular velocities of the joints. These parameters are restricted by the available motors and gears or constructional requirements.

## 8.4   Optimization of the Robot Speed

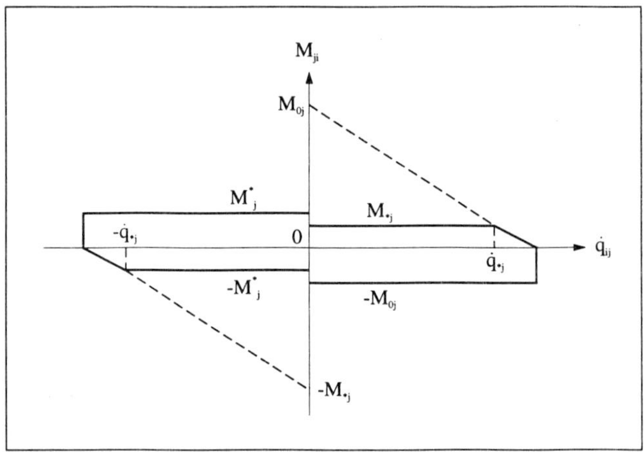


Figure 8.23: Drive Constraints

As performance index for the optimization problem, the robot body velocity $v$ is taken to be maximized. The problem can be formulated by using the following equations:

$$\max_{\boldsymbol{y}}\{v_{max}(\boldsymbol{y}) : \boldsymbol{g}(\boldsymbol{y}) \leq 0\} \tag{65}$$

with:

$$\boldsymbol{y} = (l_2, x, s)^T \tag{66}$$

$$v_{max} = \max\{v : \boldsymbol{h}(v, \boldsymbol{y}) \leq 0\} \tag{67}$$

$$\boldsymbol{g} \leq 0 \quad : \quad \text{constraints of the optimization parameters} \tag{68}$$

$$\boldsymbol{h} \leq 0 \quad : \quad \text{general kinematical or kinetical constraints} \tag{69}$$

Examples for the constraints are a restriction of $l_2$ to be less than the clearance ($\in \boldsymbol{g}$) or the restriction of the needed joint torques $\boldsymbol{T}$ to the permanent available motor torques ($\in \boldsymbol{h}$). The last ones must be determined using the equations of motion. The leg forces $\boldsymbol{F}$ are calculated by minimizing the maximal normal force with respect to the conditions of sticking.

$$M\ddot{\boldsymbol{q}} - \boldsymbol{h} - J_F^T \boldsymbol{F} = J_T^T \boldsymbol{T} \tag{70}$$

In figure 8.23 the constraints for $T_i$ are shown qualitatively. The sloping lines correspond to well-known torque-velocity characteristics for a $DC$ motor, while the horizontal lines reflect the constraints on the maximum admissible current through the motor armature. When crossing the torque axis the minimum and the maximum values of the output torque as well as the slopes of the corresponding lines undergo a discontinuity (jump) due to the Coulomb friction in the gear train.

An algorithm for solving this problem must include two blocks: the block of calculating the function $v_{max}$ and the block of its maximization. Practically, one can calculate $v_{max}$ by computing the robot motion for an increasing sequence of velocities $v = v_k = k\delta v$, where $k = 0, 1, 2, \dots$ and $\delta v$ is a specified (sufficiently small) increment. On each step, the constraints $\boldsymbol{h}$ must be checked. If $v_K$ is the first velocity value violating at least one of the constraints, then $v_{max} = v_{K-1}$ can be approximately assumed or a more exact solution can be determine by bisection. To maximize the function $v_{max}$ with respect to $\boldsymbol{y}$, one can use available algorithms for constrained minimization of multi-variable functions. The choice of the algorithm depends, in particular, on the number of the design variables and on the structure of the problem.

On the basis of the modeling and optimization technique described above the following conclusions can be drawn. The maximum velocity of the regular motion of the robot inside the tube is virtually independent of the angle of the tube inclination and of the orientation of the robot body. The maximum velocity of the robot considerably depends on the parameters $l_2, s$, and $x$ and monotonically increases as the length $l_2$ of the leg second link increases. Optimization of these parameters allows us to obtain a significant gain in the speed of the robot motion inside the tube.

Note for comparison that for $l_2 = 0.15\,m$, $s = 0.30\,m$, and $x = 0.08\,m$ the maximal speed is $v_{max} = 0.079\,m/s$, whereas for the optimal choice of these parameters ($l_2 = 0.25\,m, s = 0.12\,m$, and $x = 0.15\,m$) it is $v_{max} = 0.245\,m/s$, i.e. the speed has increased by a factor of 3.1.

The developed technique for modeling the dynamics of the tube-crawling robot and optimizing its parameters makes it possible to investigate the influence of various parameters on the motion characteristics. However, to make a rational choice of parameters, one should take into account many other factors such as possible wide variation of the friction coefficient, capability of the robot to avoid obstacles, to follow the curved and branching tubes, etc.

### 8.4.1 Maximization of the Propulsion Force

Another important operating characteristic of the robot is the maximum propulsion force, i.e. the maximum total force that can be produced by the supporting feet in the direction of the robot motion. This criterion is especially important for the robot climbing vertically along the tube. In this case it determines the load carrying capacity of the robot. The tube-crawling robot moving along a cylindrical tube is considered, not necessarily at constant speed. The simplifying assumption that the mass of the legs is much less than that of the body and neglect the inertial properties of the leg links is made. This leads to a quasistatic model. For a given configuration and a fixed contact point the maximal propulsion force $F_{max}$ is given by:

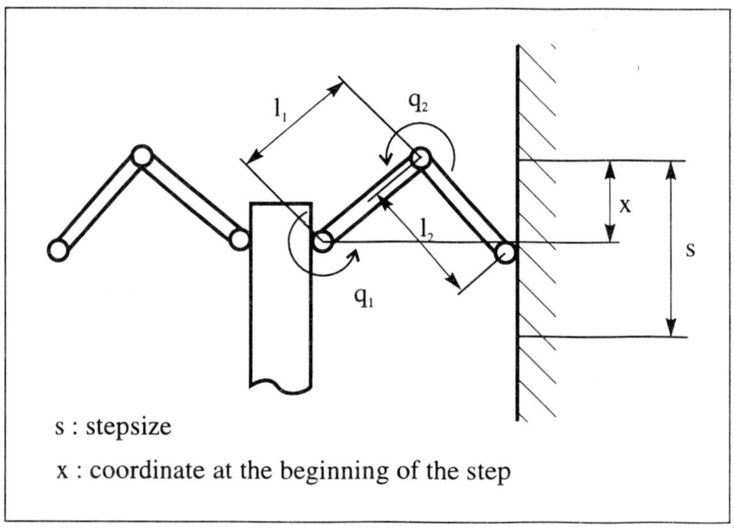


Figure 8.24: Kinematic of the robot

$$F_{max} = \max_{T_1,T_2}\{F_{tan} = f_1 T_1 + f_2 T_2\} \tag{71}$$

with the constraints:

$$|T_1| \leq T_1^0 \tag{72}$$
$$|T_2| \leq T_2^0 \tag{73}$$
$$F_{nor} \geq 0 \tag{74}$$
$$-\mu F_{nor} \leq F_{tan} \leq \mu F_{nor} \tag{75}$$

and:

$$F_{nor} = n_1 T_1 + n_2 T_2 \tag{76}$$

$$f_1 = \frac{\sin(q_1 - q_2)}{l_1 \sin q_2} \tag{77}$$

$$f_2 = \frac{l_1 \sin q_1 + l_2 \sin(q_1 - q_2)}{l_1 l_2 \sin q_2} \tag{78}$$

$$n_1 = \frac{\cos(q_1 - q_2)}{-l_1 \sin q_2} \tag{79}$$

$$n_2 = \frac{l_1 \cos q_1 + l_2 \cos(q_1 - q_2)}{-l_1 l_2 \sin q_2} \tag{80}$$

As performance criterion for a periodic gait it is useful to choose the minimum of $F_{max}$ over the foot positions during the support phase.

This optimization was computed for different sets of parameters e.g. tube diameters or friction coefficients. It is not useful to discuss the different results in more detail. Some aspects about the general behaviour of $F_{max}$ are:

- For each fixed leg position, the maximum friction force $F_{max}$ does not increase with $l_2$.

- As the leg position changes from the fore to the rear extreme position, for a fixed $l_2$, the force $F_{max}$ varies nonmonotonically. Typically, it initially increases, then passes a local maximum and decreases, and then passes a local minimum and increases again. As $\mu$ and the clearance grow, the local maximum tends to move towards the rear extreme position of the foot. For comparatively small $\mu$ the local maximum of $F_{max}$ is its global maximum. As $\mu$ increases, the situation changes, and the global maximum is reached at the rear extreme position.

- For high friction coefficients and large clearances, the rate of the growth of $F_{max}$ during the step considerably exceeds the rate of the decrease of $F_{max}$ with $l_2$. This leads to the following result: if the second link becomes longer, it is possible to shift it backwards and thus to yield a higher $F_{max}$. Hence, the elongation of the leg's second link is advisable if the robot is intended for motion inside tubes of large diameter with high $\mu$. This is true for gas pipe-lines where lubrication of the surface is absent. If the robot is designed for oil pipe-lines, where the tube surface is lubricated, another choice of the length of the second link can turn out to be most rational.

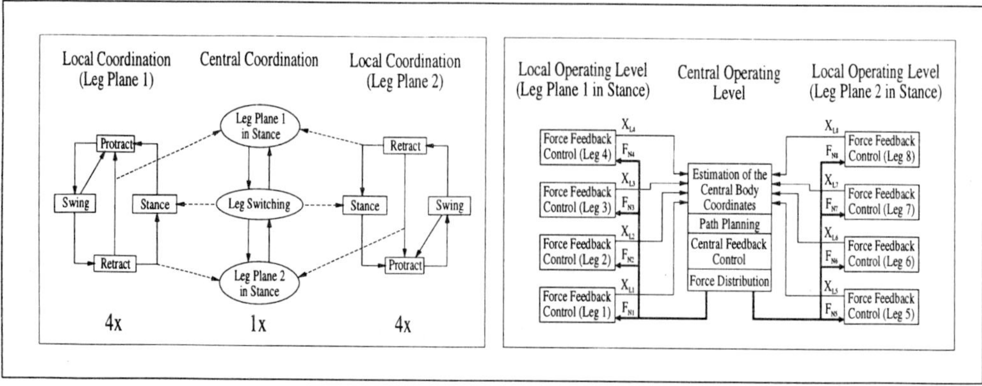


Figure 8.25: Level of Coordination and Operating Level

## 8.5   Control of the Robot

### 8.5.1   Control Structure

The presented control structure enables the robot to move in straight and curved pipes independently of the position inside the tube or the inclination of the tube (from horizontal up to vertical pipes). Considering the experiences with a six legged walking machine [15][23] a structure was chosen that is divided into two hierarchical levels. The upper level encloses the mechanism of coordination. The lower level controls the position and forces (it executes operating functions). Based on this division it is possible to realize a function orientated structure and to leave the solution of problems to the concerned components.

The gait pattern influences the dependencies between the legs and thus affects the coordination and the control structure. Because of the limited leg mobility, a load shift is only feasible from the legs of one leg plane to the legs of the other leg plane. This provides the crawler with full mobility in this plane. Three dimensional movements must be approximated by acting in orthogonal spaces. In other cases the crawler is able to move straight on only (except for special contact positions).

The diagrams of figure 8.25 show the principles of the coordination level and the operating level for the load phase.

- The *central coordination level* coordinates the phase characteristics of the two leg planes. Decisions on switching of the legs under load are made by this component. The legs do not have any autonomy here with the advantage of higher safety from falling. In this aspect the concept differs from other solutions [12][13]. Furthermore, the problems which can only be mastered by a reaction of the whole robot should be solved in this level (e.g. the legs of one plane can not find any contact).

- The *local coordination level* controls the step circle of a single leg, especially the sequence of leg motion phases (stance, protract, swing, retract). It also reacts to disturbances like avoiding small obstacles.

- The *central operating level* controls the position and the velocity of the central body which are estimated from the joint angles of the legs. This is done by changing the leg forces to achieve accelerations for correcting the control errors. For this purpose the local operating level is used. It receives the corresponding setpoint commands. These commands must be created with respect to restrictions like satisfying the condition of sticking or the limitations of the electrical and mechanical components.

- The *local operating level* controls the applied forces during the contact phase and the motions of a single leg during the different air phases. In contrast to the last ones, which are really local problems (legs without contact can be assumed as decoupled), the forces of legs touching the environment are strongly coupled and therefore a strictly local realization can not consider all effects in each configuration. Therefore local means as local as useful.

### 8.5.2 Controller Design

The main problem is the controller design for the load phase of a leg plane. The crawler is a system with geometrical and kinetical nonlinearities. Its several components have many degrees of freedom and are strongly coupled. In accordance with the described structure of the operating level the controller can be presented by the block diagram shown in figure 8.26.

A decentral PID control of the leg forces and the central control of the crawler position was developed by using a multi model design, which is based on linearizations around several leg positions [20]. The qualification of this design was tested by simulations. Nevertheless the system behaviour of this design depends on the actual leg configuration and therefore it can not be optimal in any case. According to this an other design will be presented here, which is based on an input-output-linearization of the inner circuit [21]. The disadvantage of this method is the more complicated and more complex structure. To get system equations which can be handled without loosing the physical context the following simplifications are made, which do not change the characteristic behaviour of the system:

- Motions in the passive joints are not observable and not controllable by the legs of the corresponding leg plane. Therefore these motions are decoupled and

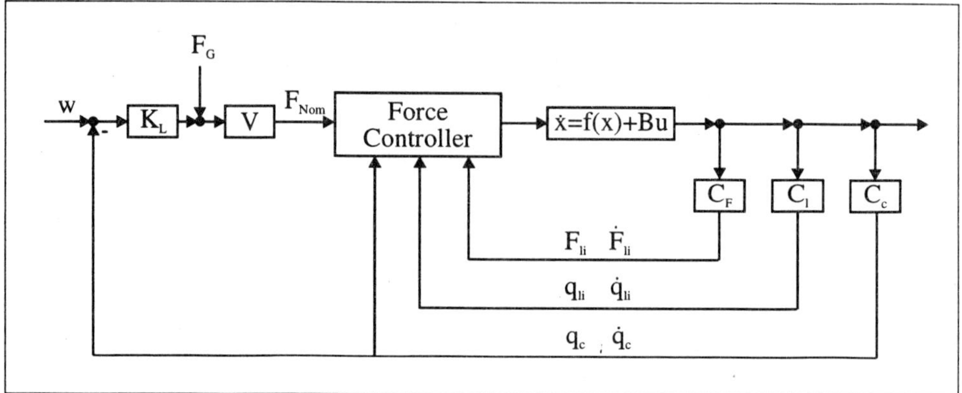


Figure 8.26: Block Diagram of the Operating Level

must not be considered in the controller design. This leads to a planar model with 11 degrees of freedom.

- The damping of the rubber balls (feet) is neglected.

- The masses of the segments are added to the central body and therefore the moments of inertia referred to the leg joints are constant and decoupled from the central body coordinates. Caused of the light weight design the influence of this simplification is less than one per cent.

- The friction in the gears will be compensated by using an observer. The compensation is assumed to be ideal and therefore friction is not considered any further.

Furthermore the central body velocity and the actual direction of gravity are assumed to be known. In reality these variables must also be determined by an observer. This model yields the following equations of motion:

$$M_c\ddot{q}_c = A_c F + mg \tag{81}$$
$$M_{li}\ddot{q}_{li} = J_{li}^T F_{li} - D\dot{q}_{li} + BU_i \forall i = 1, \cdots, 4 \tag{82}$$

Generally the index $c$ denotes the central body and $li$ the $i$-th leg. $M$ are the mass matrices, $q$ the generalized coordinates. The Jacobian $J_{li}$ is the derivative of the leg end point velocity w.r.t. $\dot{q}_{li}$. Analog is $J_{ci}$ the derivative w.r.t. $\dot{q}_c$ (later used). $F$ is the vector of all leg forces and $F_{li}$ that of the $i$-th leg. $U_i$ are the motor inputs with the corresponding input matrix $\boldsymbol{B}$, $m$ the total mass, $\boldsymbol{g}$ the vector of gravity in the plane and $\boldsymbol{D}$ characterizes the dependency of the motor torques on the angular velocities. The matrix $\boldsymbol{A}_c$ depends on $\boldsymbol{q}_{li}$ and $\boldsymbol{q}_c$ and describes the influence of the forces on the central body accelerations.

For the feedback linearization of the inner circuit the leg forces are taken as the system output. They can be calculated using the following equation:

$$\boldsymbol{F}_{li} = \boldsymbol{C}_{li}(\boldsymbol{x}_{li} - \boldsymbol{x}_{lif}) \tag{83}$$

$\boldsymbol{x}_{li}$, $\boldsymbol{x}_{lif}$ are the coordinates of the leg end point and of the touching point at the tube. $\boldsymbol{C}_{li}$ represents the stiffness of the rubber ball.

Recursive differentiation of the outputs leads to the following coherence for the second derivative of the leg forces by using the corresponding equations of motion:

$$\ddot{\boldsymbol{F}}_{li} = \boldsymbol{C}_{li}[\boldsymbol{J}_{li}\boldsymbol{M}_{li}^{-1}(\boldsymbol{J}_{li}^{T}\boldsymbol{F}_{li} - \boldsymbol{D}\dot{\boldsymbol{q}}_{li} + \boldsymbol{B}\boldsymbol{U}_i) + \boldsymbol{J}_{ci}\boldsymbol{M}_c^{-1}(\boldsymbol{A}_c\boldsymbol{F} + m\boldsymbol{g}) + \dot{\boldsymbol{J}}_{li}\dot{\boldsymbol{q}}_{li} + \dot{\boldsymbol{J}}_{ci}\dot{\boldsymbol{q}}_c] \tag{84}$$

It can be seen that all the nonlinearities and interdependences can be compensated by a leg knowing the states of the central body and of the other legs. A single leg only needs its own motors and therefore the system can be viewed as decentral in the sense of the system input.

Based on these results the leg forces can be provided with given linear dynamics, which are determined by the matrices $\boldsymbol{A}_F$ and $\boldsymbol{A}_{\dot{F}}$, by using the following control law $\boldsymbol{U}_i = \boldsymbol{B}^{-1}\sum\boldsymbol{T}_{ij}$, with:

$$\boldsymbol{T}_{i0} = -\boldsymbol{J}_{li}^{T}\boldsymbol{F}_{li} \tag{85}$$

$$\boldsymbol{T}_{i1} = -\boldsymbol{M}_{li}\boldsymbol{J}_{li}^{-1}\boldsymbol{J}_{ci}\boldsymbol{M}_c^{-1}(\boldsymbol{A}_c\boldsymbol{F} + m\boldsymbol{g}) \tag{86}$$

$$\boldsymbol{T}_{i2} = -\boldsymbol{M}_{li}\boldsymbol{J}_{li}^{-1}(\dot{\boldsymbol{J}}_{li} + \boldsymbol{D})\dot{\boldsymbol{q}}_{li} \tag{87}$$

$$\boldsymbol{T}_{i3} = -\boldsymbol{M}_{li}\boldsymbol{J}_{li}^{-1}\dot{\boldsymbol{J}}_{ci}\dot{\boldsymbol{q}}_c \tag{88}$$

$$\boldsymbol{T}_{i4} = -\boldsymbol{M}_{li}\boldsymbol{J}_{li}^{-1}\boldsymbol{C}_{li}^{-1}[\boldsymbol{A}_{\dot{F}}\dot{\boldsymbol{F}}_{li} + \boldsymbol{A}_F(\boldsymbol{F}_{li} - \boldsymbol{F}_{li,nom})] \tag{89}$$

The different inputs can be interpreted as follows: $\boldsymbol{T}_{i0}$ compensates the acting leg forces, $\boldsymbol{T}_{i1}$ the central body accelerations, $\boldsymbol{T}_{i2}$ the leg motion and $\boldsymbol{T}_{i3}$ the motion of the central body. Finally $\boldsymbol{T}_{i4}$ determines the linear behaviour. An interesting property of the system is the fact that the matrix $\boldsymbol{C}_{li}$ is only needed for calculation of $\boldsymbol{T}_{i4}$. This means that only the linear part of the system is affected by errors concerning the ball stiffnesses, which are uncertain values. With some restrictions in choosing $\boldsymbol{A}_F$ and $\boldsymbol{A}_{\dot{F}}$ it can be shown that the linear behaviour is stable for any positive definite matrices $\boldsymbol{C}_{li}$. Closing the inner loop yields the following system equations:

$$\boldsymbol{M}_c\ddot{\boldsymbol{q}}_c = \boldsymbol{A}_c\boldsymbol{F} + m\boldsymbol{g} \tag{90}$$

$$\ddot{\boldsymbol{F}}_{li} = -\boldsymbol{A}_{\dot{F}}\dot{\boldsymbol{F}}_{li} - \boldsymbol{A}_F\boldsymbol{F}_{li} + \boldsymbol{A}_F\boldsymbol{F}_{li,nom} \forall i = 1, \cdots, 4 \tag{91}$$

The remaining internal dynamics of the system correspond to the central body motion. They show a double integrating behaviour and are consequently not asymptotically stable. The task of the outer control circuit is to stabilize it by using the right setpoints for the inner one. For that purpose total forces and torques are determined to compensate gravity and to correct the robot position. These forces must be split into the different legs taking into account the condition of sticking at the tube. This is a highly nonlinear process which can be done by optimization with the target of minimal motor torques. The difficulty in the design of the controller is that the result of the optimization can not be specified analytically. Therefore it is very difficult to take into account the influence of the division on the stability. To overcome this problem a simplification is used which is based on the following considerations. The behaviour of the different leg forces is determined by the eigenvalues of the linear dynamics. It can be assumed that the transient response of the total forces and torques is similar to the several components. Therefore the eight differential equations of the leg forces of the planar system can be substituted by three ones for the resultants ($= \boldsymbol{F}_{res}$) with eigenvalues laying in the same region of the complex plane. Based on these considerations the controller design is done by using the following equations:

$$M_c \ddot{\boldsymbol{q}}_c = \boldsymbol{I} \boldsymbol{F}_{res} + m\boldsymbol{g} \tag{92}$$

$$\ddot{\boldsymbol{F}}_{res} = -\boldsymbol{A}_{\dot{F},res} \dot{\boldsymbol{F}}_{res} - \boldsymbol{A}_{F,res} \boldsymbol{F}_{res} + \boldsymbol{A}_{F,res} \boldsymbol{F}_{res,nom} \tag{93}$$

Couplings are not considered by this method. They can be caused by force distribution. Robustness against these effects can be achieved by choosing the time constants for correcting the robot position not to close to the ones of the force control. In this case the system can be interpreted as one sided decoupled. Investigations in more detail are part of the actual work.. Nevertheless the stability of the closed loop system must be tested with simulations.

## 8.6   Dynamics

A simulation program, which includes all the relevant properties of the robot, was developed. By means of this program it is possible to get informations about the system behaviour and to determine the motor power reserves. Since the elastic eigenfrequencies of the system parts are very high, a modelling as a rigid body system is favourable. The system parts are the central body, the rotors of the motors, the shafts of the gears and the segments of the legs. Different to industrial robots the stiffness of the gears is negligible for the system behaviour. The reasons are the extreme light weight design, the very short lever arms and the small moments of inertia of the segments. The friction of the used Harmonic Drive Gears, which strongly depends on the torque, has great influence on the control and on the loads of the motors (coulomb friction in meshing). For consideration of this effect, "normal torques" are established to calculate tangential friction torques that act against the direction of the rotation. To include sticking without load (effects like No-Load Starting Torque and No-Load Back Driving Torque [10]) an initial tension $\boldsymbol{\lambda}_0$ of the gears is introduced. For sticking under load the transmitted torques are added to the initial tensions. The dynamics are described by the following equations:

$$M\ddot{q} = h + W_N\lambda_N + W_H\lambda_H + H_R(\lambda_{Na} + \lambda_0) \tag{94}$$

$$\ddot{g}_N = W_N^T\ddot{q} + \tilde{w}_N = 0 \tag{95}$$

$$\ddot{g}_H = W_H^T\ddot{q} + \tilde{w}_H = 0 \tag{96}$$

with:

$$H_{Ri} = -\mu_i w_{Ti}\mathrm{sign}(\dot{g}_{Ti}) \tag{97}$$

$$\lambda_{Nai} = |\lambda_{Ni}| \tag{98}$$

$M$ denotes the mass matrix, $h$ is the vector of gyroscopic forces, active moments and active forces. The vector of the generalized coordinates $q$ (its dimension is 62) contains the six degrees of freedom of the central body, the angles of the leg joints and the degrees of freedom of the motors and the gears. $\lambda_N$ is the vector of the normal torques (see above) and $\lambda_H$ the vector of the constraining torques caused by sticking of the gears. Corresponding to this, the constraints are denoted $g_N$, $g_H$ with the Jacobian matrices $W_N$ and $W_H$. Different to usual stick-slip problems, the normal torques can have positive and negative values and therefore are corresponding to normal forces of a bilateral guiding device. The friction torques of the rotating gears are determined by the absolute values of the normal torques, the initial tensions and the friction coefficients $\mu_i$. They are projected into the generalized sliding directions through $w_{Ti}$. As usual, the passing from sticking to slipping is detected by reaching the stick limit $\lambda_{Ti} = \mu(\lambda_{Ni} + \lambda_{0i})$ and from slipping to sticking with the kinematic condition $\dot{g}_{Ti} = 0$. In order to determine the accelerations, the equations are transformed into a linear complementary problem. This can be solved with the Lemke algorithm [7][8].

In addition to the mentioned phenomena, the following ones are part of the simulation model: The contact between legs and ground is realized with a spring-damper element, which represents the rubber balls at the end of the legs. The temperatures of the motors are integrated with a two body model with unlimited caloric conductibility. With these temperatures the torque reserves of the motors can be determined, which are only limited by burning out. Furthermore the motors are changing their behaviour in a not negligible manner caused by the dependence of their coil conductivity on temperature.

The results of a simulation of the whole robot crawling in a vertical tube are presented in figure 8.27. The robot walks about $0.5m$ and makes several steps. In

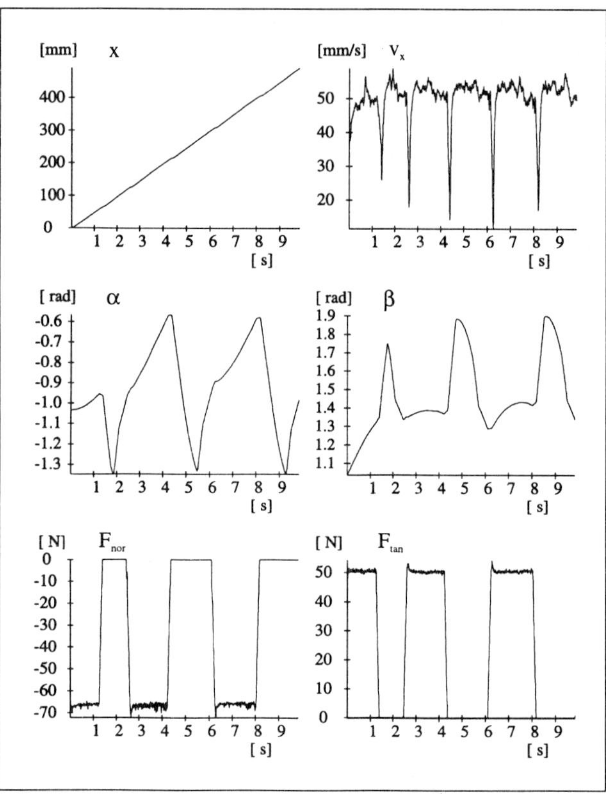

Figure 8.27: Simulation with whole robot

the upper left graph the robot position in direction of the tube axis is shown and in the upper right one you can see the corresponding velocity. In the graphs in the middle row the joint angles of the first leg are displayed. The left graph on the bottom shows the normal force and the right one the tangential forces of the same leg. The steps can easily be detected in the force diagrams. The peaks in the velocity diagram occur during switching of touching legs.

## 8.7  Single Leg Test Setup

For testing the mechanical design and the designed controllers a single leg test setup was built. The leg mounted on a fixed frame can walk on a conveyor-belt, which is motor driven and can be run with different velocities. The mechanical parts and the control hardware is equivalent to that one used in the robot. A picture of this setup is shown in figure 8.29.

For the test setup an extra simulation program is developed. The model is similar to that of the whole robot. In figure 8.28 comparisons of simulation results and measurements are shown. The diagrams on the left side belong to the measurements. The two curves in the graphs correspond to the normal and tangential forces of two steps on the conveyor-belt. In each line a different controller was used. The first one shows steps at a slow speed using a PID controller [20].

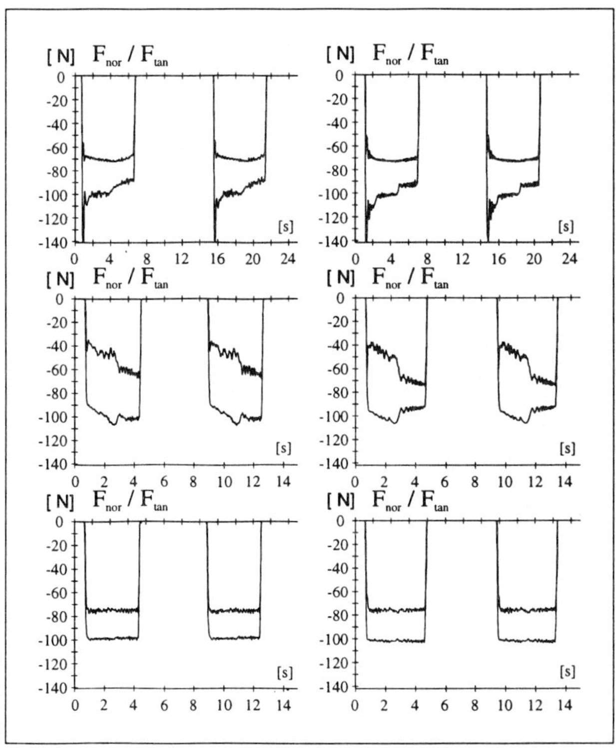

Figure 8.28: Comparison of Measurement and Simulation

Two undesirable properties can be seen. The first one are the high peaks at step beginning and the second the decreasing normal forces in the middle of the steps. This is caused by the gear friction in the knee joint, which changes the direction of rotation. The second and the third line use the controller based on feedback linearization. The difference is that for the third the friction observer is used. The second one is only displayed to illustrate the great influence. It can be seen the compensation works very well. The observer could be used for the PID controller also. In this case it is able to inhibit the decreasing of the force but not the peaks at the beginning. As an excerpt it can be seen that the last controller is qualified for the problem. The curves also show a very good conformity between simulation and measurement.

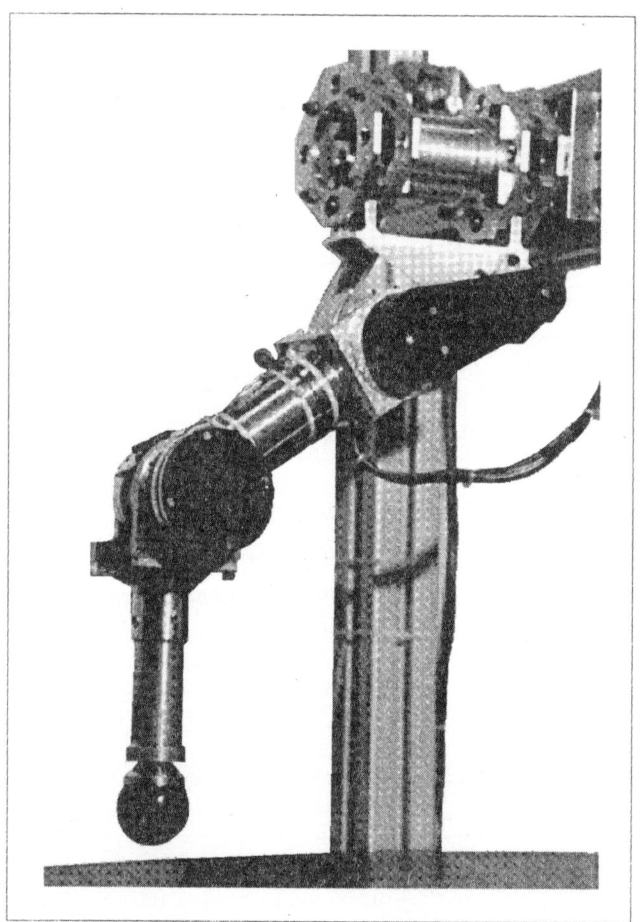

Figure 8.29: Single Leg Test Setup

# 9  Bibliography


## References

[1] Bremer, H.: Dynamik und Regelung mechanischer Systeme, Teubner Verlag, Stuttgart, 1988.

[2] Cruse, H.: The Function of the Legs in the Free Walking Stick Insect, Carausius morosus, Journal of Comparative Physiology, (1976), p. 112.

[3] Cruse, H.: What mechanisms coordinate leg movement in walking arthropods ?, Trends in Neurosciences 13, (1990), pp. 15–21.

[4] Cruse, H.; Dean, J.; Müller, U.; Schmitz, J.: The Stick Insect as a Walking Robot, Proc. Fifth Int. Conf. on Adv. Robotics, Robots in unstructured Environment, Pisa, Italy, June 1991, pp. 936–940.

[5] Eltze, J.: Biologisch orientierte Entwicklung einer sechsbeinigen Laufmaschine, no. 110 in Fortschrittsberichte VDI, Reihe 17, VDI-Verlag, Düsseldorf, 1994.

[6] Glocker, C.: Dynamik von Starrkörpersystemen mit Reibung und Stößen, Reihe 18, Nr. 182, VDI-Verlag, Düsseldorf, 1995.

[7] Glocker, C.; Pfeiffer, F.: Stick-Slip Phenomena and Application, Proc. of Nonlinearity & Chaos in Engineering Dynamics, Symposium, I., ed., 1993.

[8] Glocker, C.; Pfeiffer, F.: Multiple Impacts wich Friction in Rigid Multibody Systems, Nonlinear Dynamics, Kluwer Academic Publishers, (1996).

[9] Graham, D.: A behavioural analysis of the temporal organisation of walking movements in the 1st instar and adult stick insect (carausius morosus), Journal of Comparative Physilolgy, (1972).

[10] Harmonic Drive GmbH: Harmonic Drive Gear Component Sets, HFUC Series, Tech. Rep., Harmonic Drive GmbH, 1993.

[11] Herrndobler, M.: Entwicklung eines Rohrkrabblers mit vollständigen Detailkonstruktionen, Master's thesis, Lehrstuhl B für Mechanik, TU München, 1994.

[12] Neubauer, W.: Locomotion with Articulated Legs in Pipes or Ducts, Proc. of the Int. Conf. on Intelligent Autonomous Systems, Pittsburgh, USA, 1993, pp. 64–71.

[13] Neubauer, W.: A Spider - Like Robot that Climbes Vertically in Ducts, Proc. of the 1994 IEEE/RSJ Int. Conf. on Intelligent Robots and Systems, Munich, 1994, pp. 1178–1185.

[14] Pfeiffer, F.; Chernousko, F.; Bolotnik, N.; Roßmann, T.; Kostin, G.: Tube-Crawling Robot: Modelling and Optimization. To appear in: IEEE Transactions on Robotics and Automation.

[15] Pfeiffer, F.; Cruse, H.: Bionik des Laufens-technische Umsetzung biologischen Wissens, Konstruktion, (1994), pp. 261–266.

[16] Pfeiffer, F.; Eltze, J.; Weidemann, H.-J.: Six-legged technical walking considering biological principles, Robotics and Autonomous Systems, (1995), pp. 223–232.

[17] Pfeiffer, F.; Eltze, J.; Weidemann, H.-J.: The TUM-Walking Machine, Intelligent Automation and Soft Computing, 1 (1995), pp. 307–323.

[18] Pfeiffer, F.; Roßmann, T.; Chernousko, F. L.; Bolotnik, N.: Optimization of Structural Parameters and Gaits of a Pipe-Crawling Robot, IUTAM Symposium on Optimization of Mechanical Systems, Bestle, D.; Schiehlen, W., eds., Kluwer Academic Publisgers, 1996, pp. 231–238.

[19] Pfeiffer, F.; Weidemann, H.-J.; Danowski, P.: Dynamics of the Walking Stick Insect, Proc. of the 1990 IEEE Int. Conf. on Robotics and Automation, Cincinatti, Ohio, May 1990, pp. 1458–1463.

[20] Roßmann, T.; Pfeiffer, F.: Contol and Design of a Pipe Crawling Robot, Proc. of the 13th World Congress, of Automatic Control, I. F., ed., San Francisco, USA, 1996.

[21] Slotine, J.-J. E.; Li, W.: Applied Nonlinear Control, Prentice Hall, Englewood Cliffs, New Jersey, 1991.

[22] Waldron, K.; et al.: Force and Motion Management in Legged Locomotion, IEEE Journal of Robotics an dAutomation, RA-2 (1986).

[23] Weidemann, H.-J.: Dynamik und Regelung von sechsbeinigen Robotern und natürlichen Hexapoden, no. 362 in Fortschrittsberichte VDI, Reihe 8, VDI-Verlag, Düsseldorf, 1993.

[24] Weidemann, H.-J.; Eltze, J.; Pfeiffer, F.: Leg Design based on Biological Principles, Proc. of the 1993 IEEE Int. Conf. on Robotics and Automation, Atlanta, Georgia, May 1993, pp. 352–358.

# DESIGN OF WALKING MACHINES

K.J. Waldron

The Ohio State University, Columbus, OH, USA

## 1. Introduction

The configurations of the electromechanical system, and the information and sensing systems, the geometry of the machine, and the methods used to coordinate its motions all interact intimately. For this reason the design of a legged locomotion system is challenging, quite apart from the technical challenges of understanding the mechanics of legged locomotion. A fundamental question is: What issues should be addressed first? It is reasonable to address the mechanics of the locomotion system first. A fundamental question of approach is whether to use a statically stable or dynamically stable approach to postural control. This is less a hard dichotomy than it might appear since a system with practical scale will require some degree of dynamic stabilization, even if it is designed on statically stable principles.

Once the basic decision of whether to approach the design of the system as fundamentally statically stable, or actively stable has been made, it is natural to next consider the coordination of the leg movements in order to achieve stable operation.

Several comprehensive reviews of the literature on walking and running machines may be found in the literature [1, 2, 3].

## 2. Stability and Gait

*Coordination of Legged Locomotion Systems*

The coordination of a legged system falls into two parts: a phasing problem and a piece wise continuous coordination problem [4].

Because a leg is a discontinuous motion element there is a phase problem in any legged system. That is, it is necessary to decide at what point in the motion cycle a given foot will be placed on the ground, and at what point it will be lifted. The set of placement and lifting phases of all the legs in the system define a *gait pattern*. The number of possible gait patterns increases very rapidly with the number of legs in the system. The issue is almost trivial for a two legged system, is significant for four legs, and exceedingly complex for six, or more legs.

Given a gait pattern and the desired motion of the vehicle body, what motions or forces should the legs be instructed to produce?  One idea is that the desired six axis velocity system is specified, and inverse rate kinematic models of the legs are used to compute the appropriate joint rates for the legs whose feet are on the ground.  This is workable provided not more than three feet are on the ground at any given time, although even in that case it leads to some scuffing and other undesirable effects.  The fundamental reason is inherent in the configuration of any multi-legged system.  In order to achieve full terrain adaptability it is necessary that each leg be capable of at least three degrees of freedom of controlled motion.  This permits the foot to be placed at any point in the three-dimensional working volume of the leg.  The contact between the foot and the ground is best modeled as a three degree of freedom contact in most systems.  There is usually little resistance to rotary motions about axes in the tangent plane at the point of contact.  There may be more resistance to scuffing rotations about the normal at the point of contact, but these motions are still reasonably easy.  Many systems have ankle joints that facilitate some, or all of these rotations.  On the other hand, translatory motion along the common normal is strongly resisted, and there is substantial frictional resistance to translatory motions parallel to the tangent plane.

*Simplified Gait Patterns*

Some practical walking machines use a simplified gait in which the legs are simply divided into two groups, with one group supporting the machine and the other being returned at any time.  This is similar to the tripod gait pattern of a hexapod that is described below.  This has also been described as a "generalized biped" configuration with the individual feet functioning as the "toes" of a super foot.  Machines of this sort are often called frame walkers because they are constructed with two sets of feet mounted on separate frames.  The two frames can translate relative to one another, typically via a roller-rail assembly, to produce the stepping motion.  One frame can also be rotated relative to the other by means of a turntable, to allow the machine to change direction.  Often, the legs have no lateral motion capability and simply slide in the vertical direction.  A six legged frame walker need have only 8 degrees of freedom: vertical sliding of each of the six legs, sliding of one frame relative to the other, and rotation of one frame relative to the other about the turntable axis.  Figure 1 and Figure 2 show a conceptual design of such a machine.  It is the Walking Beam machine that was the subject of a design study by Martin Marietta Corporation [5].

The Dante machine designed by the Field Robotics Center of Carnegie-Mellon University and used to explore the craters of the active volcanoes Mt. Erebus in Antarctica and Mt. Spur in Alaska does have legs capable of independent positioning [6,7].  However, in order to simplify coordination they are used only in two groups.  Thus the mode of operation is similar to a frame walker, although the legs are not mechanically constrained to work together in this case. Rather, they are grouped together in the software.

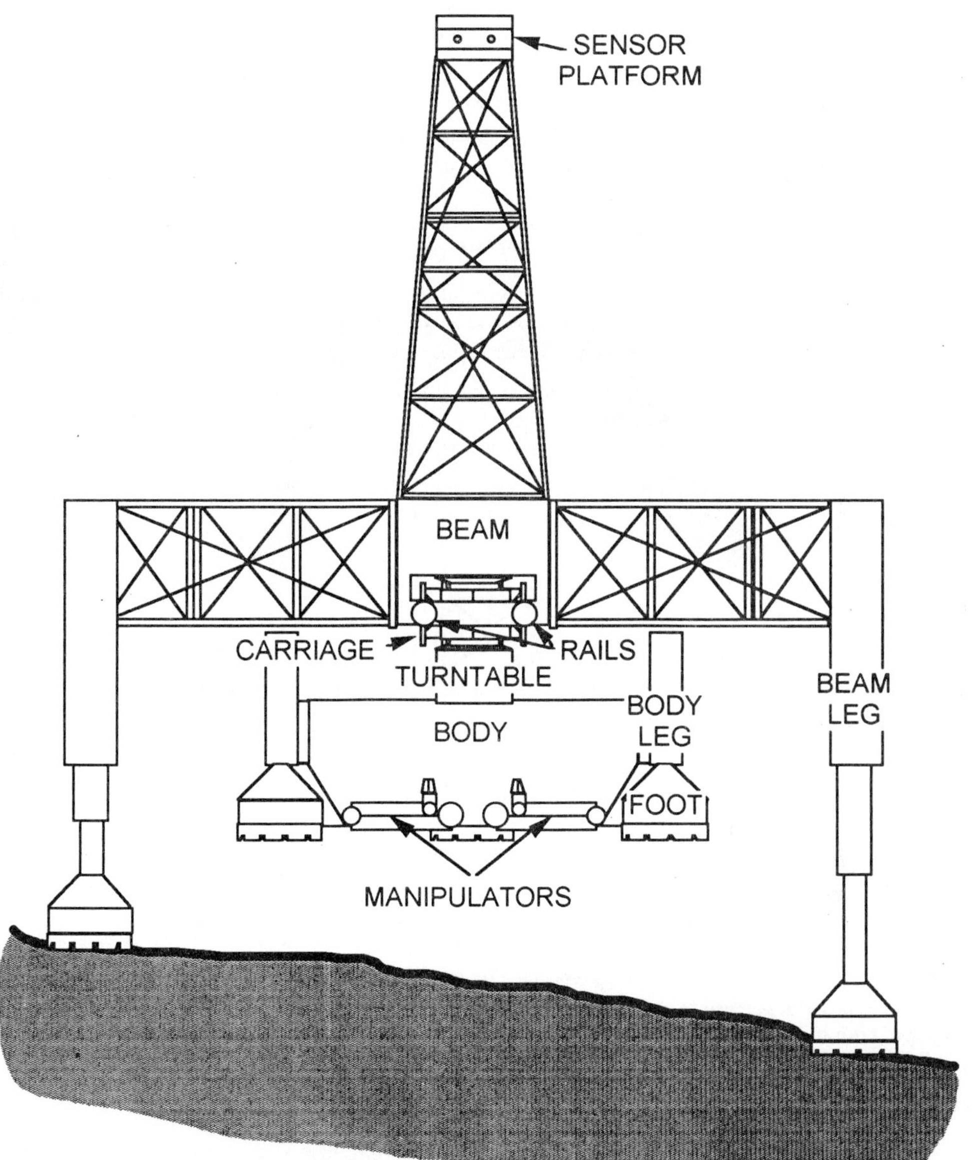



**Figure 1:** The Martin Marietta Walking Beam, also shown in plan view in Figure 2. This is an example of a frame walker in which the machine legs are mechanically segregated into two groups that are alternately used for support and returned. The body translates relative to the beam along longitudinal rails. The body may also be rotated relative to the beam *via* a turntable. The legs simply telescope in the vertical direction

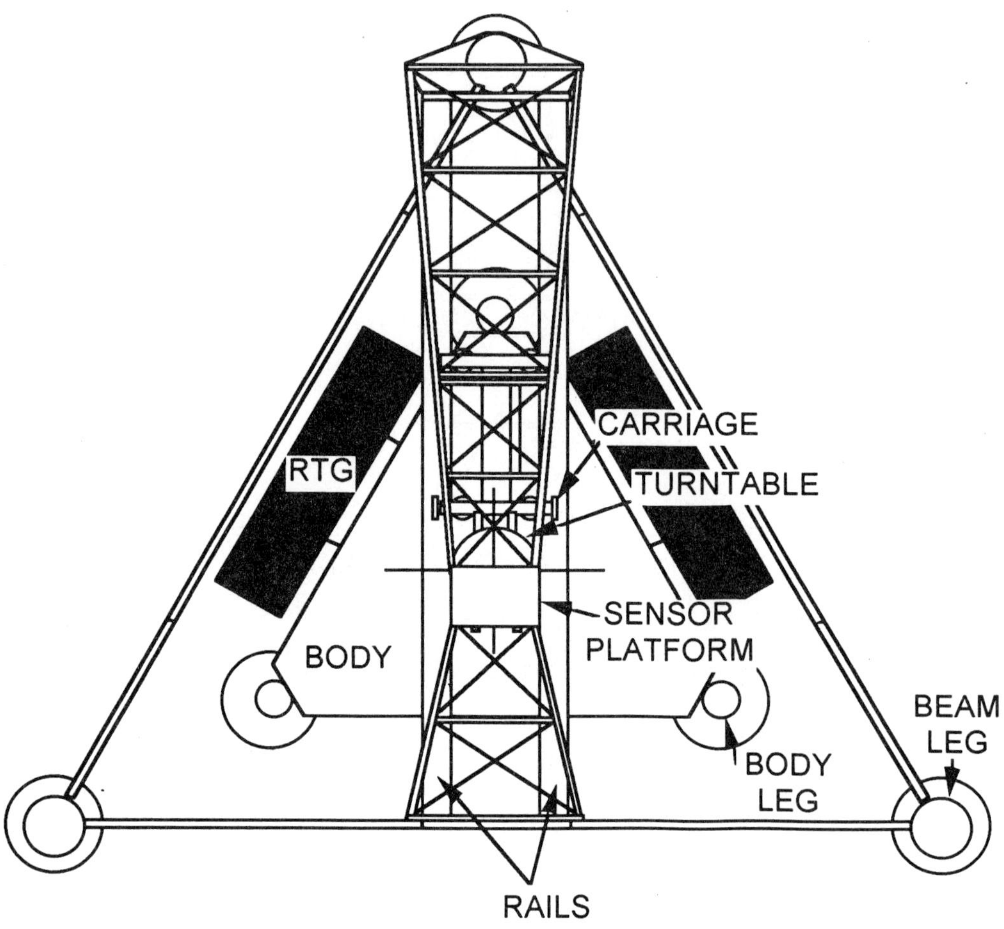


**Figure 2:** A plan view of the Martin Marietta Walking Beam. The direction of motion of the body relative to the beam is vertical in this picture, with the turntable axis at the centroids of the equilateral base triangles of both the body and the beam. The base triangle of the beam had a 6 m side length. The RTG's are radioisotope thermoelectric generators that provide power to the machine.

*Statically Stable Gaits*

A more general approach to coordination of machines that are statically stable is developed below. A machine is statically stable if it would continue to stand stably if all actuators were frozen in position at any time in the motion cycle. There are a great variety of gait patterns that can be used, and quite a few of them are useful in different situations if the machine has fully independently movable legs with at least three degrees of freedom each. Three degrees of freedom is necessary to be able to place the foot at any position within the working volume of the leg.

It is first necessary to define the following terminology [8]:

*Duty factor*, $\beta$,: Time fraction of a walking cycle in which foot is on ground

*Leg phase*, $\phi_i$: Time fraction of walking cycle by which contact of leg I lags that of leg 1

*Stride*, $\lambda$: Distance center of gravity translates during one complete walking cycle

*Stroke*, R: Distance foot is translated relative to body when on ground

*Stroke pitch*, P: Distance between centers of strokes of adjacent legs

An *event* of a gait: Placing or lifting of any foot

*Regular gait*: A gait in which all legs have the same duty factor

*Symmetric gait*: The motions of the legs of any right-left pair are exactly half a cycle different in phase

*Periodic gait*: Similar states of the same leg during successive strokes occur at a constant interval equal to the cycle time.

*Support pattern*: Convex hull of vertical projections of all foot points in support phase

*Longitudinal stability margin*: Is the minimum over the gait cycle of the distances of the center of gravity along its path of motion from the front and rear boundaries of the support pattern

### Wave Gaits

A wave gait for an animal or machine with an even number of legs is a regular, symmetric gait in which the phase difference of successive legs on the same side of the body is equal to the duty factor.

Wave gaits have been shown to be the family of regular, symmetric gaits with optimal longitudinal stability margins, and hence provide the maximum stability at any given speed on easy terrain.

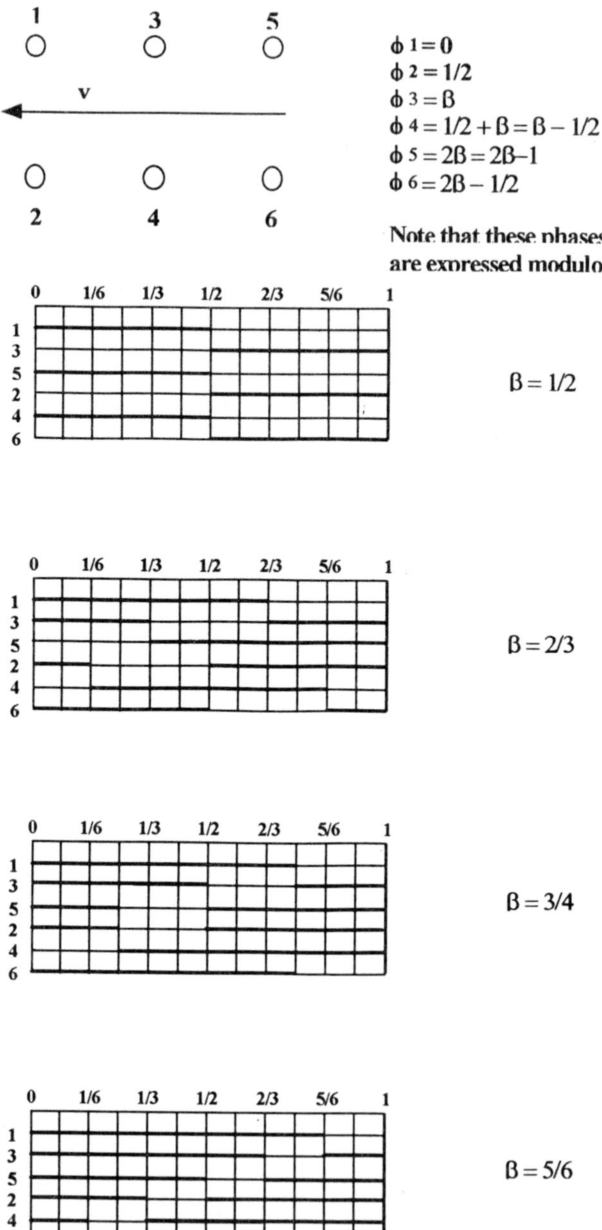



**Figure 3:** Gait diagrams for the wave gaits that have constant numbers of feet on the ground. That is, $2m\beta$ is an even number, 3, 4 and 5 respectively since $2m = 6$.

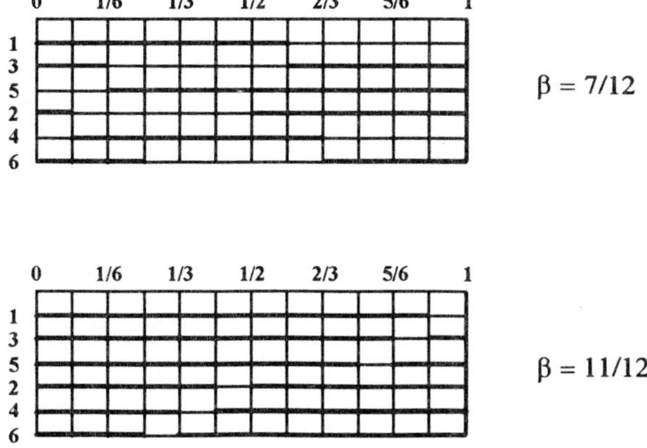

**Figure 4:** Two examples of gait diagrams of wave gaits for which the number of feet on the ground is not constant. That is, $n_{av} = 2m\beta$ is fractional. In fact, $\beta$ may be varied smoothly in the range $1/2 < \beta < 1$ providing continuous control of speed.

*Optimal gait parameters*

The speed that can be achieved with a given walking or running gait is approximately determined by the time taken to *return* the legs to their starting positions. Thus the larger the number of legs in return at any time, the greater the speed.

The average number of feet on the ground is

$$n_{av} = 2m\beta \tag{1}$$

where 2m is the total number of legs and b is the duty factor. For a statically stable gait

$$n_{av} \geq 3$$

so

$$\beta \geq \frac{3}{2m} \tag{2}$$

Also, if T is the cycle time and $\tau$ is the time required to return a leg

$$\frac{\tau}{T} = \frac{1-\beta}{1}$$

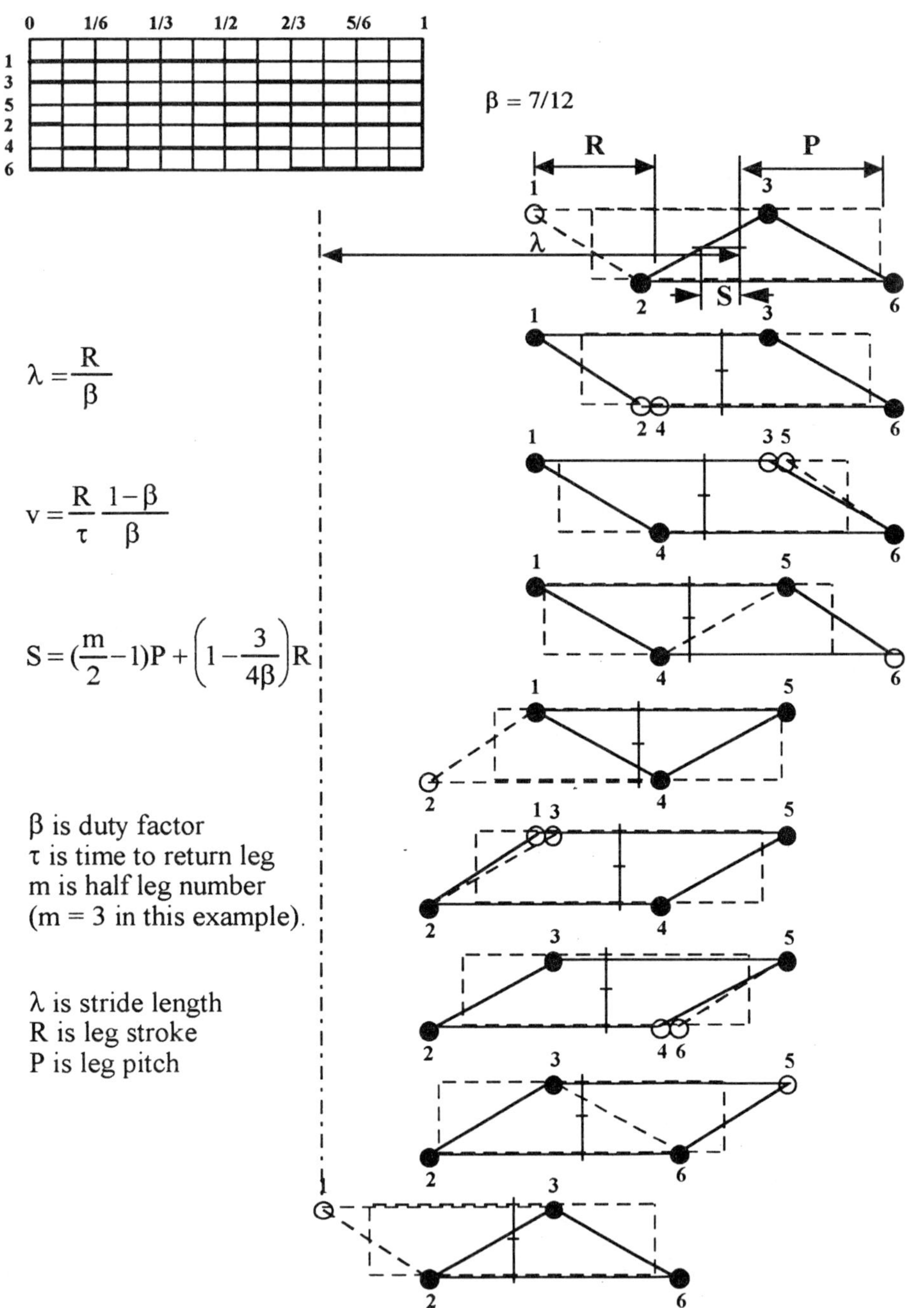



**Figure 5:** Support patterns for one complete gait cycle of a hexapod with β = 7/12.

or

$$T = \frac{\tau}{1-\beta} \qquad (3)$$

The stride, $\lambda$, is related to the leg stroke, R, by

$$\frac{R}{\lambda} = \frac{\beta}{1}$$

or

$$\lambda = \frac{R}{\beta} \qquad (4)$$

The velocity of locomotion, v, is

$$v\frac{\lambda}{T} = \frac{R}{\beta}\frac{1-\beta}{\tau} = \frac{R}{\tau}\frac{1-\beta}{\beta} \qquad (5)$$

*Gait Stability*

For a 2m legged wave gait with $1/2 \leq \beta < 1$, the longitudinal gait stability margin, S, is given by

$$S = \left(\frac{m}{2}-1\right)P + \left(1-\frac{3}{4\beta}\right)R \qquad (6)$$

Where P is leg pitch and R is leg stroke, and

$$R \leq \frac{\beta}{3\beta-2}P \qquad (7)$$

These relationships may be used to design the geometry of a statically stable walking machine to meet speed and stability goals [9].


*Large Obstacle Gaits*

High speed film of insects crossing obstacles that are relatively large compared to their body size reveals that they tend to use the legs on either side of the body in unison, rather than 180° out of phase, as in a wave gait. It is possible to demonstrate theoretically that for near horizontalobstacles, such as voids, the optimum gait in the sense of minimizing the number of discrete leg and body movements is similar to a wave gait in the sense of propagating a wave from the rear to the front of the vehicle, but differs in employing each pair of legs on opposite sides of the body in unison. Further, it is optimal to place the rear feet alongside the middle feet, and the middle feet alongside the front feet since this maximizes the width of the void that can be crossed.

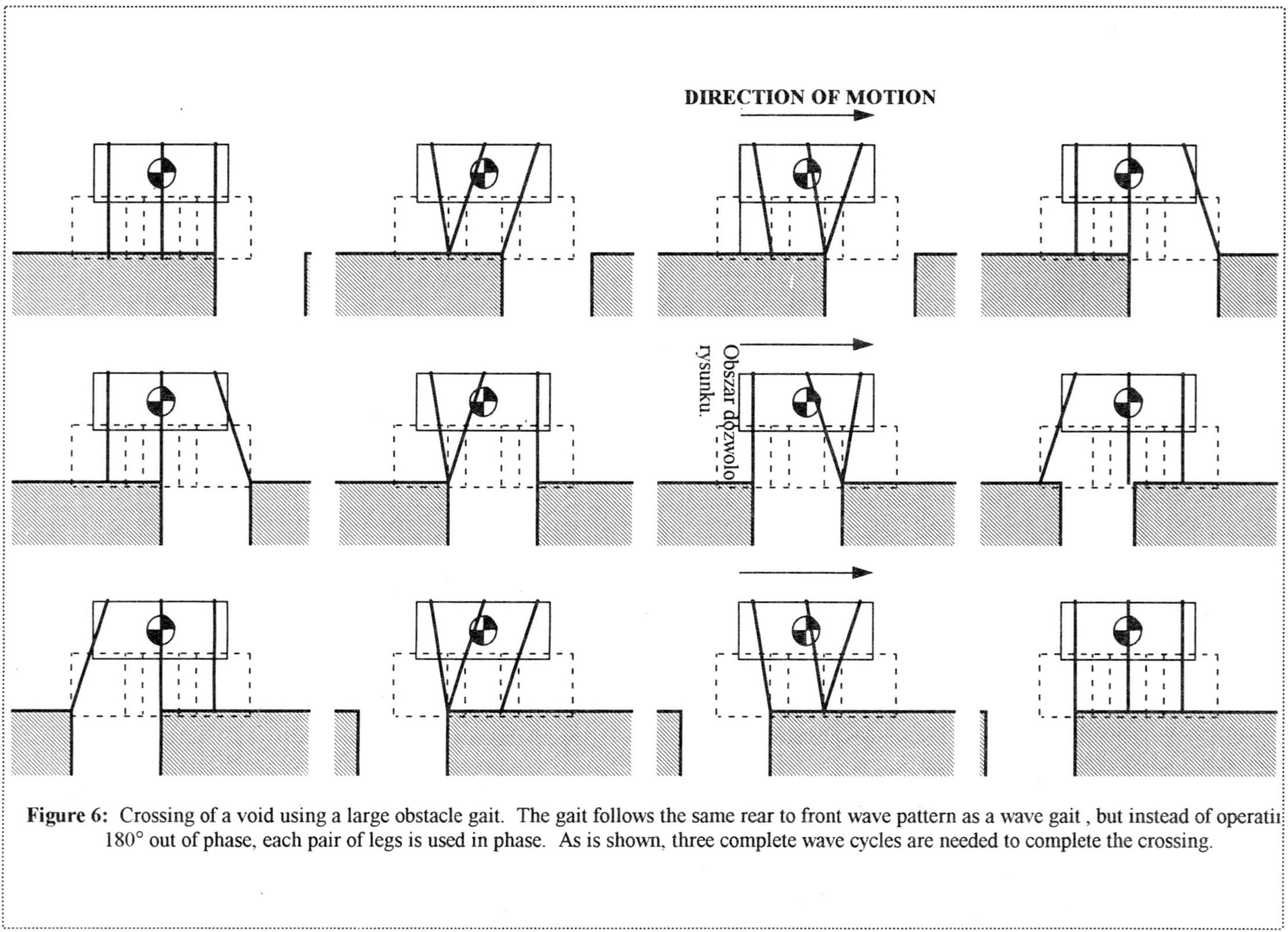


**Figure 6:** Crossing of a void using a large obstacle gait. The gait follows the same rear to front wave pattern as a wave gait, but instead of operati... 180° out of phase, each pair of legs is used in phase. As is shown, three complete wave cycles are needed to complete the crossing.

In the notation used above

$$\phi_2 = \phi_1 = 0$$

$$\phi_3 = \phi_4 = \frac{2}{3}$$

$$\phi_5 = \phi_6 = \frac{1}{3}$$

The motion pattern is shown in Figure 6. It might be noted that three complete wave cycles are needed to complete the crossing. It might also be noted that the gait is discontinuous since some leg movements must be completed without corresponding movements of the vehicle body.

This walking pattern may also be used when crossing an obstacle with vertical relief, such as a vertical step except that in this case it is sometimes necessary to reposition foot pairs while maintaining body position. This can be done by means of shuffling movements, but the economy of movement of the basic gait is then lost. The same basic three motion cycles are needed to cross this type of obstacle, but for maximum geometric performance the body is inclined. It is the inclined position of the body, which shifts the position of the center of mass relative to the working volumes of the legs and thereby creates the need for shuffling in some positions [10].

*Follow-the-leader principle*

It has been observed that animals in difficult terrain never look at their rear feet. Rather, they always place their rear foot immediately alongside the corresponding front foot, or in its footprint. In this manner, the placements of the front feet can be visually selected, and tested by feel and the rear feet can then be placed with assurance. This pattern is also useful for a walking machine in difficult terrain. It minimizes the number of sound footholds that must be identified. This leads to a class of gaits called follow-the-leader gaits characterized by placement of the middle feet alongside the front feet and, in the case of a hexapod, placement of the rear feet in the footprints of the front feet. The large obstacle gait described above belong to this class, and the follow-the-leader property is an important feature from the point of view of vehicle guidance and foothold selection. However, this is only one of a large class of follow-the-leader gaits [4].

In dense fields of moderate sized obstacles it is not possible to use a patterned gait. Various so-called free gaits have been devised. In a free gait the system performs a calculation to optimize stability potential every time it is necessary to choose among actions such as placing feet, and moving the body. It is necessary to have a map of the terrain indicating the areas in which it is, and is not permissible to place the feet.

## Dynamically Stable Gaits

Raibert's method of monopod control provides a simple and effective method of locomotion and postural control of a hopping monopod [11, 12].  This technique lends itself to elaboration for the control of more complex, dynamically stable systems.

The control is broken into two parts: control of velocity by placement of the foot relative to the "center of gravity footprint" at the end of each hop, and control of hopping height by regulating the amount of energy added to the system during each stance phase.

The period, T, of the hopping cycle is related to the maximum height $H_0$ with which the foot clears the ground and the system parameters by the relationship

$$T = \pi \sqrt{\frac{M_2}{K_L}} + \sqrt{\frac{8H_0}{g}} \tag{8}$$

where $K_L$ is the spring stiffness of the leg, $M_2$ is the body mass, and g is the acceleration of gravity.

The total energy associated with motion in the vertical direction is, during the stance phase:

$$E_S = M_1 g y_1 + M_2 g y_2 = \frac{1}{2} M_1 \dot{y}_1^2 + \frac{1}{2} M_2 \dot{y}_2^2 + \frac{1}{2} K_L (k_0 - w + \chi)^2 + \frac{1}{2} K_G y_0^2 \tag{9}$$

where $k_0$ is the rest length of the spring.

During touch-down the leg is suddenly brought to rest  creating an energy loss of

$$E_{TL} = \frac{1}{2} M_1 \dot{y}_1^2 \tag{10}$$

where $\dot{y}_1$ is the velocity of the leg mass center immediately before touch-down. Similarly, at lift-off the system loses vertical energy when the leg is suddenly accelerated to the speed of the body.  A momentum balance before and after lift-off gives this loss as

$$E_{LL} = \frac{M_1 M_2}{2(M_1 + M_2)} \dot{y}_2^2 \tag{11}$$

where $y_2$ is the vertical velocity of the mass center of the body immediately after lift-off.

In order for the system to hop to a desired height H of the body center of mass, the total vertical energy must be:

$$E_H = M_1 g \left[ H - r_2 - (k_0 - r_1) \right] + M_2 g H \tag{12}$$

At any time during stance, Equations 9, 11 and 12 may be used to determine the additional energy, $\Delta E$ required to achieve a desired hopping height

$$\Delta E = E_{H} + E_{LL} - E_{S} \tag{13}$$

The additional energy is provided by extending the leg actuator during stance. The length $\Delta\chi$ by which the leg must extend to add $\Delta E$ is

$$\Delta\chi = \left(w - k_{0} - \chi\right) + \sqrt{\left(w - k_{0} - \chi\right)^{2} + \frac{2\Delta E}{K_{L}}} \tag{14}$$

Note that $w - k_{0} - \chi$ is the current length of the leg spring, and $K_{L}$ is the spring stiffness.

Velocity control is achieved by reference to the *center of gravity print* of the system. This is the vertical projection of the path of the center of gravity during the stance phase. The CG-print for the next stance phase can be computed during the preceding flight phase. Placement of the foot in the center of the CG-print will maintain the current velocity with the gravity moment during stance acting symmetrically. Placement of the foot short of the center of the CG-print will result in an increase in velocity since the gravity moment during stance will act asymmetrically to help rotate the system forward. Placement of the foot beyond the center of the CG-print will result in a decrease in velocity since the gravitational moment will act asymmetrically to tend to rotate the system backward.

The foot is displaced from the center of the CG-print in proportion to the velocity error:

$$x_{0} = x_{2} + \left(vT_{s} / 2\right) + K(v - u) \tag{15}$$

where $x_{0}$ is the position at which the foot is to be placed, $x_{2}$ is the position of the center of gravity at touch-down, $v$ is the horizontal velocity of the body center of mass (during flight), $T_{S}$ is the duration of the stance phase (approximately constant), $u$ is the desired velocity during the next flight phase, and $K$ is a gain. In order to achieve this position, the angle of the leg relative to the vertical at touch-down should be

$$\theta_{1D} = \arcsin\left(\frac{vT_{s} + 2K(v - u)}{2w}\right) \tag{16}$$

A linear servo is used to move the leg to this angle during flight:

$$\tau = K_{P}\left(\theta_{1} - \theta_{1D}\right) + K_{v}\left(\dot{\theta}_{1}\right) \tag{17}$$

where $\tau$ is the torque applied between body and leg, and $K_{P}$ and $K_{V}$ are gains.

It is necessary to apply body attitude corrections during stance phase when ground reaction forces are available. The torque that is applied to correct body attitude is

$$\tau = K_{PS}\left(\theta_{2} - \theta_{2D}\right) + K_{vs}\left(\dot{\theta}_{2}\right)$$

where $\theta_{2D}$ is the desired value of the body angle relative to the vertical, and $\theta_{2}$ is the current value of that angle.

## 3. Coordination of Multi-Legged Walking Machines

*Definition of Coordination*

Coordination is the transformation of the commanded body motion variables into the values to be commanded from the individual actuator servos. In the familiar example of an industrial robot programmed in a point-to-point mode inverse rate control is the basis of the coordination algorithm.

For a multi-legged robotic vehicle force control is most appropriate for those legs in contact with the ground. The reason for this is simple. Think of a four-legged table sitting on an uneven floor. No more than three legs will contact the floor at any time, and there is no way to control the distribution of load among the legs.

The problem then becomes one of translating motions commanded of the vehicle as a whole in a rate controlled mode into force commands to the leg actuators. The system can be thought of as an outer rate control loop and a set of inner force control loops linked via a dynamic model of the system. The dynamic model relates changes in velocity to forces.

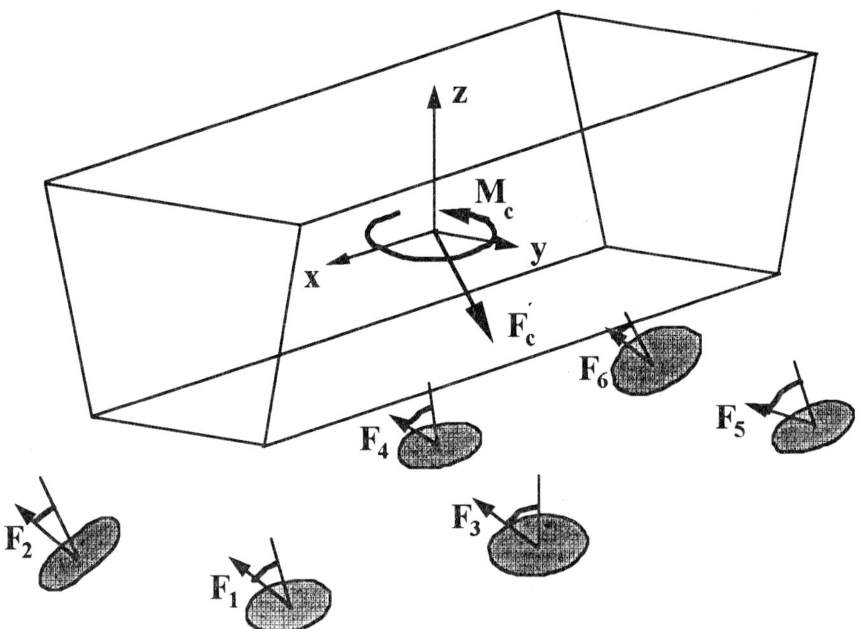


**Figure 7:** The force allocation problem. $\mathbf{F}_c$ and $\mathbf{M}_c$ are the force and moment components of the force system acting on the vehicle body to be equilibrated by the contact forces $\mathbf{F}_i$. The angle between each contact force and the contact normal is a measure of the probability of foot slip.

In the Adaptive Suspension Vehicle system, an inertial sensing package consisting of accelerometers on three orthogonal axes and rate gyroscopes on the same three axes senses body velocity at high bandwidth [13]. This is compared to the operator's commands entered by a six axis joystick, and a six axis rate error system is generated. Division of this system by a characteristic time produces a six axis acceleration system. Multiplication by the effective system inertia matrix and sign reversal produces a six axis inertia force system. When combined with the vehicle weight, this becomes a force system that the legs must be commanded to equilibrate. The coordination problem then becomes one of allocating this force system among the legs that are in contact with the ground, as is indicated in Figure 7.

A reasonable basis for allocation of contact forces among the feet is that the tendency of each foot to slip should be minimized. Since the effective coefficient of friction between foot and ground is never accurately known, the logical strategy is to attempt to minimize the maximum of the angles between the contact forces and the normals to the surfaces at the contact points. This is a non-linear problem, but with a simple linearizing approximation of the friction cone, it can be formulated as a linear programming problem [14]. However, the results of this formulation are somewhat unsatisfactory for the present purpose. Solution *via* the Simplex algorithm, which is the most efficient method for low dimensional problems such as this, yields highly discontinuous functions for the commanded force components. These are not very satisfactory as control inputs. Also, the algorithm is iterative and so the time required for calculation is uncertain, which presents problems in an operation that must be repeated at small, regular time intervals. Thus, the linear programming solution, while useful as a baseline against which to evaluate other techniques, is not attractive for practical implementation.


*Interaction Forces*

Another way of resolving the under constraint of the force field is by constraining the interaction forces between points of contact. The interaction force between two contacts is defined as the difference between the components of the contact forces along the line joining the two contact points [15]. Figure 8 shows two contact points and the components of the contact forces at those two points that are along the line joining the two points, and normal to that line.

Enforcing a requirement that the interaction forces between all pairs of contact points be zero makes physical sense since it removes any tendency for legs to work against each other by pushing together or pulling apart parallel to the ground. It turns out to be feasible to do this and, in fact, this produces a simple and elegant solution. If the interaction force between each pair of contact points must be zero, the geometry of the contact force field becomes homologous with that of the velocities of points in a moving body. Here, the requirement is that the differences between the velocity components along the line joining any two points be zero. This results from the rigidity condition: the distance between any two points in the body must be invariant. We know that the rigidity condition results in the field of velocities of points in a rigid body being helicoidal, with a unique field axis, called the instantaneous screw axis. It follows that the contact force field must also be helicoidal with the geometry shown in Figure 9.

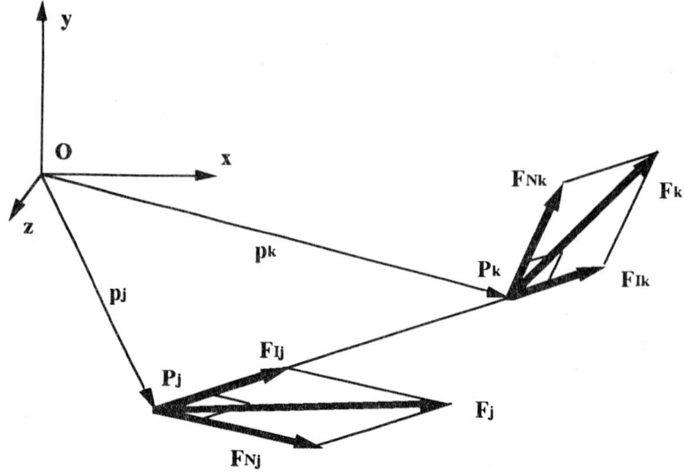



**Figure 8:** The interaction force for the two points $P_j$ and $P_k$ is $F_{Ij}$ - $F_{Ik}$. $F_{Nj}$ and $F_{Nk}$ are the components of the contact forces $F_j$ and $F_k$ that are normal to the line $P_jP_k$. $F_{Ij}$ and $F_{Ik}$ are the components along the line $P_jP_k$.

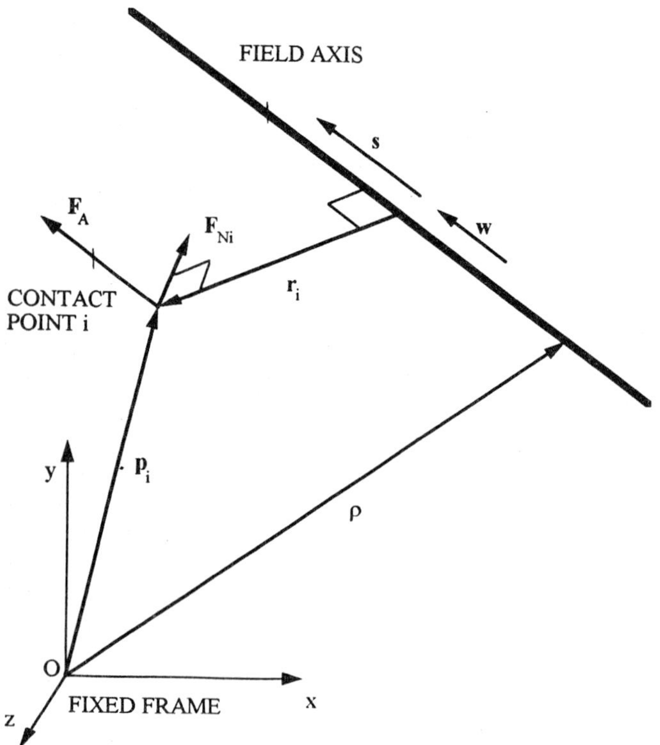



**Figure 9:** The geometry of the helicoidal field of contact forces whose resultant is the commanded wrench $(\mathbf{R}, \mathbf{M})$.

*Determination of Field Parameters*

The geometry of the helicoidal distribution of contact forces is shown in Figure 9 above. The field geometry is characterized by the axis direction, $\mathbf{w}$, the field intensity, s, the field pitch, H, and the location, $\rho$ of any point on the field axis. $\mathbf{w}$ and s may be combined into the field vector, $\mathbf{s} = s\mathbf{w}$.

The contact force at contact point I consists of two components: an axial component $\mathbf{F_A} = H\,\mathbf{s}$ that is the same for all contact points, and a component $\mathbf{F_{Ni}}$ that is normal to the axis and proportional to the distance $r_i$ of the contact point from the axis. $\mathbf{F_{Ni}}$ can be expressed as follows:

$$F_{Ni} = \mathbf{s} \times \mathbf{r}_i = \mathbf{s} \times (\mathbf{p}_i - \rho)$$

where $\mathbf{p}_i$ is the position relative to the fixed reference frame of contact point i. Hence

$$\mathbf{F}_i = H\mathbf{s} + \mathbf{s} \times (\mathbf{p}_i - \rho) \tag{18}$$

where $\mathbf{F}_i$ is the contact force at contact point i.

In order to develop expressions for the field parameters s, H and $\rho$ we note that the resultant of the system of contact forces must be the commanded wrench $(\mathbf{R}, \mathbf{T})$. Consequently

$$\mathbf{R} = \sum_{i=1}^{n} \mathbf{F}_i \tag{19}$$

and

$$\mathbf{T} = \sum_{i=1}^{n} \mathbf{p}_i \times \mathbf{F}_i \tag{20}$$

Substitution for $\mathbf{F}i$ from Equation 18 into Equation 19 gives:

$$\mathbf{R} = \sum_{i=1}^{n} \left\{ H\mathbf{s} + \mathbf{s} \times (\mathbf{p}_i - \rho) \right\} \tag{20}$$

Let $\bar{\mathbf{p}}$ be the position of the centroid of the contact point pattern. Then

$$\bar{\mathbf{p}} = \frac{1}{n} \sum_{i=1}^{n} \mathbf{p}_i \tag{21}$$

Substitution from Equation 21 into Equation 20 gives

$$\mathbf{R} = n\left\{ H\mathbf{s} + \mathbf{s} \times (\bar{\mathbf{p}} - \rho) \right\} \tag{22}$$

Similarly, substitution of Equation 18 into Equation 20 gives

$$\mathbf{T} = \sum_{i=1}^{n} \mathbf{p}_i \times \left( H\mathbf{s} - \mathbf{s} \times \left( \mathbf{p}_i - \rho \right) \right) \tag{23}$$

Using Equation 21 we get

$$\mathbf{T} = n\overline{\mathbf{p}} \times (H\mathbf{s} - \mathbf{s} \times \rho) + \sum_{i=1}^{n} \mathbf{p}_i \times (\mathbf{s} \times \mathbf{p}_i)$$

In order to expand the group

$$\sum_{i=1}^{n} \mathbf{p}_i \times (\mathbf{s} \times \mathbf{p}_i)$$

we apply the identity $\mathbf{a} \times (\mathbf{b} \times \mathbf{c}) = \mathbf{a} \bullet \mathbf{c}\,\mathbf{b} - \mathbf{a} \bullet \mathbf{b}\,\mathbf{c}$ to give

$$\sum_{i=1}^{n} \mathbf{p}_i \times (\mathbf{s} \times \mathbf{p}_i) = \sum_{i=1}^{n} \left( p_i^2 \mathbf{s} - \mathbf{p}_i \bullet \mathbf{s}\mathbf{p}_i \right)$$

$$= \sum_{i=1}^{n} \left\{ \left( x_i^2 + y_i^2 + z_i^2 \right)\mathbf{s} - \left( x_i s_x + y_i s_y + z_i s_z \right)\mathbf{p}_i \right\}$$

$$= \sum_{i=1}^{n} \begin{bmatrix} y_i^2 + z_i^2 & -x_i y_i & -z_i x_i \\ -x_i y_i & x_i^2 + z_i^2 & -y_i z_i \\ -z_i x_i & -y_i z_i & x_i^2 + y_i^2 \end{bmatrix} \begin{bmatrix} s_x \\ s_y \\ s_z \end{bmatrix}$$

Hence

$$\mathbf{T} = n\overline{\mathbf{p}} \times \left( H\mathbf{s} - \mathbf{s} \times \rho \right) + \mathbf{I}_0 \mathbf{s} \tag{24}$$

where $\mathbf{I}_0$ is the inertia matrix, about the origin of the fixed reference frame, of the contact point distribution.

Further simplification is possible using Equation 22 to substitute for the group $H\mathbf{s} - \mathbf{s} \times \rho$

$$H\mathbf{s} - \mathbf{s} \times \rho = \frac{1}{n} \mathbf{R} - \mathbf{s} \times \overline{\mathbf{p}}$$

then

$$\mathbf{T} = \overline{\mathbf{p}} \times \mathbf{R} + \mathbf{I}_0 \mathbf{s} - n\overline{\mathbf{p}} \times (\mathbf{s} \times \overline{\mathbf{p}}) \tag{25}$$

Further, by the parallel axis theorem,

$$\mathbf{I}_0 \mathbf{s} - n\overline{\mathbf{p}} \times (\mathbf{s} \times \overline{\mathbf{p}}) = \mathbf{I}\mathbf{s} \tag{26}$$

where $\mathbf{I}$ is the centroidal inertia matrix of the contact point distribution.

Hence

$$\mathbf{T} = \overline{\mathbf{p}} \times \mathbf{R} + \mathbf{I}\mathbf{s} \qquad (27)$$

which can be inverted to give an expression for **s**

$$\mathbf{s} = \mathbf{I}^{-1}(\mathbf{T} - \overline{\mathbf{p}} \times \mathbf{R}) \qquad (28)$$

Equation 28 may be used to compute **s** from the commanded wrench (**R**, **T**) and the positions of the contact points $\mathbf{p_i}$; $i = 1,..., n$.

Given **s** Equation 22 can be used to obtain an expression for the field pitch H. Taking the scalar product of **s** with both sides of Equation 3.6 gives, after rearrangement

$$H = \frac{\mathbf{s} \bullet \mathbf{R}}{ns^2} \qquad (29)$$

Equation 22 may also be used to develop an expression for the position of the axis $\rho$. Vector multiplication of both sides of the equation gives

$$\mathbf{s} \times \mathbf{R} = ns \times \left(\mathbf{s} \times (\overline{\mathbf{p}} - \rho)\right)$$

$\rho$ can be the position of any point on the axis. Since the axis has direction **s** the product $\mathbf{s} \times \rho$ is not affected by the choice of that point. It is convenient for the present purpose to identify $\rho$ as the position $\rho n$ of the point on the axis at the base of the normal from the origin. That is: $\rho n \bullet \mathbf{s} = 0$. Now

$$\mathbf{s} \times \mathbf{R} = ns \bullet \overline{\mathbf{p}}s - ns^2(\overline{\mathbf{p}} - \rho_n)$$

Rearranging this

$$\rho_n = \overline{\mathbf{p}} - \frac{\mathbf{s} \bullet \overline{\mathbf{p}}s}{s^2} + \frac{\mathbf{s} \times \mathbf{R}}{ns^2}$$

which can be simplified slightly by noting that $\mathbf{s} = s\,\mathbf{w}$:

$$\rho_n = \overline{\mathbf{p}} - \mathbf{w} \bullet \overline{\mathbf{p}}\mathbf{w} + \frac{\mathbf{w} \times \mathbf{R}}{ns} \qquad (30)$$

Equations 28, 29 and 30 allow computation of the field parameters from the commanded wrench (**R**, **T**) and the positions of the contact points $\mathbf{p_i}$; $i = 1,..., n$.

However, for the purpose of computing the contact forces to be commanded from the legs, it is not necessary to explicitly calculate $\rho_n$. All that is needed is the cross product $\mathbf{s} \times \rho$ which can be obtained from Equation 22:

$$\mathbf{s} \times \rho = \mathbf{s} \times \overline{\mathbf{p}} + H\mathbf{s} - \frac{1}{n}\mathbf{R} \, .$$

Substitution of this expression into Equation 3.1 gives

$$\mathbf{F}_i = \mathbf{s} \times (\mathbf{p}_i - \overline{\mathbf{p}}) + \frac{1}{n}\mathbf{R} \qquad\qquad (31)$$

*Relationship to Minimum Norm Solution*

Although the above solution is derived using geometric arguments, it can be shown [15], that the result is identical to that obtained using the Moore-Penrose pseudo-inverse of the system Jacobian to resolve the underconstraint of the contact force system. That implies that the solution is the minimum norm set of contact forces.

## 4. Geometric Design

*Geometric Design of Walking Machines*

There is only one optimal configuration of a serial chain leg in terms of maximizing the working volume for a given length of leg structure. The argument is the same as for an optimal serial manipulator regional structure [16]. Three degrees of freedom are needed to place the foot anywhere in a three-dimensional working volume. Of the three joints, the two most inboard joints must intersect orthogonally. The third joint must be exactly halfway along the leg length, and should be parallel to the second joint (Figure 10). The third, or knee joint needs to be horizontal so that the outboard member is always as close to vertical as possible. This means that the second joint is also horizontal. The choices for the first joint reduce to placing it vertical, relative to the vehicle body, or horizontal and parallel to the longitudinal axis of the vehicle body. These two choices result in the so-called "insect" leg configuration (Figure 10a), and "mammal" leg configuration (Figure 10b).

Although actual walking machine leg hardware is not usually purely serial, but rather has some parallel elements, the configurations shown in Figure 10 nevertheless serve as a good basis for design of leg geometry. Parallel elements are added to provide better strength and stiffness, to allow remote actuation, or to create parallelogram or pantograph action. In all of these cases the basic action of the leg is still usually similar to one of the configurations of Figure 10.

The type of service for which the vehicle is designed is crucial for the layout of the vehicle geometry. Legs work better in some directions than in others. In Figure 10 the preferred direction for both the insect and mammal legs is parallel to the vehicle body longitudinal axis. If the vehicle is to be designed for efficient, relatively long distance locomotion then the preferred operating directions of the legs should all be aligned with the designed direction of locomotion, leading to a bilaterally symmetric vehicle planform. If, on the other hand, the vehicle is to be designed to move in any direction with equal facility, a radially symmetric configuration may be preferable. These two types of planform are illustrated schematically in Figure 11. The insect type legs on the radially

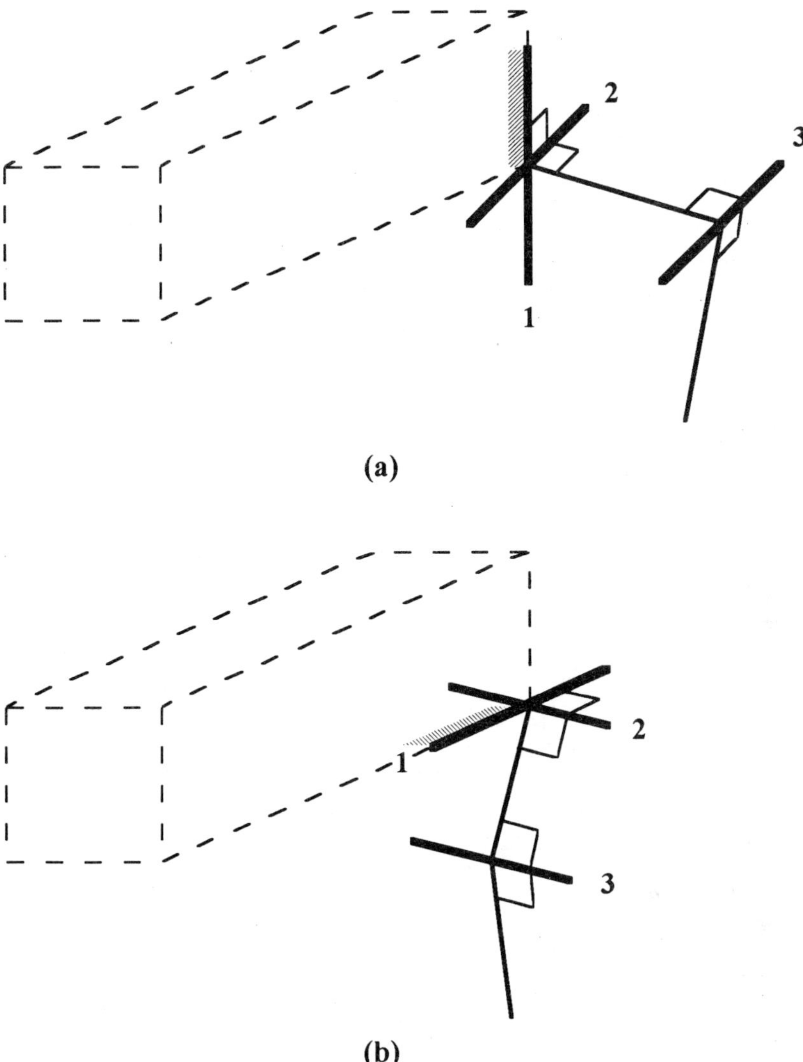

**(a)**

**(b)**

**Figure 10:** The possible configurations of a serial leg that are optimal in the sense of maximizing the working volume of the leg for a given leg length.  Configuration (a) has the first joint axis vertical with respect to the vehicle body reference frame, and is often referred to as the "insect" leg configuration. Configuration (b) has the first joint axis aligned parallel to the longitudinal axis of the vehicle body, and is commonly referred to as the "mammal" leg configuration.

symmetric planform of Figure 11b can swivel about their first axis to perform optimally in any direction of motion.  The mammal type legs of the bilaterally symmetric planform of Figure 11a perform optimally in the preferred direction of motion parallel to the axis of symmetry.

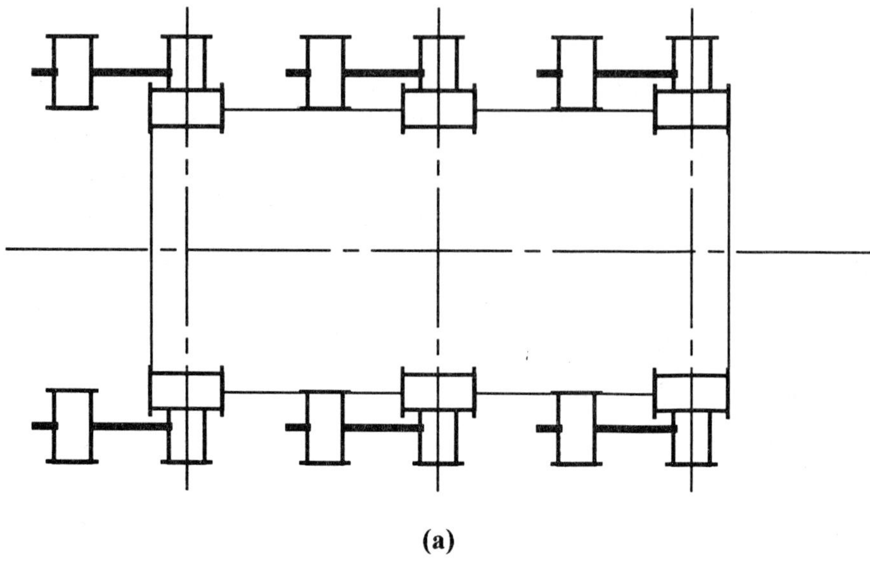

**(a)**

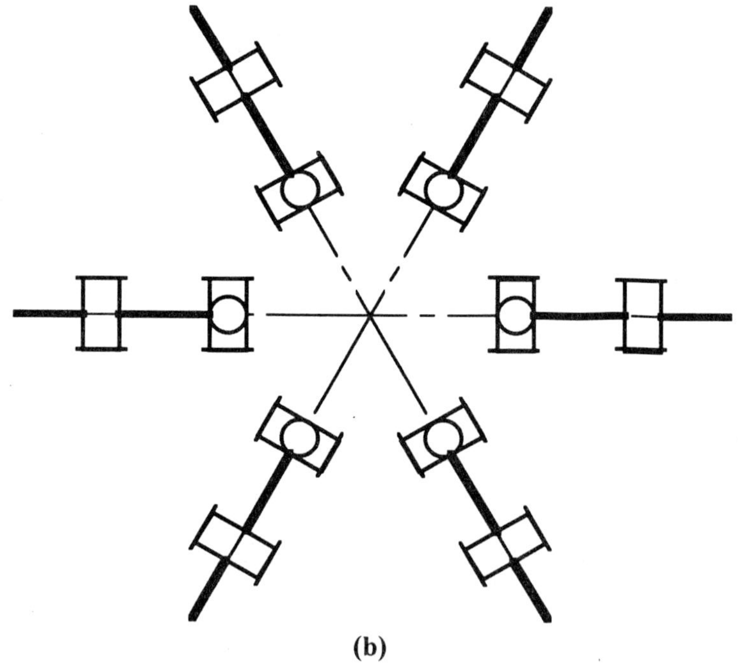

**(b)**

**Figure 11:** Bilaterally symmetric and radially symmetric vehicle planforms.

## 5. Power System and Energy Consumption Issues

There is nothing inherently inefficient in legged locomotion when compared to wheeled locomotion provided they are compared operating on the on the same, unprepared terrain conditions [17]. However, artificial legged locomotion systems have not done well energetically because of inappropriate choices of system configuration. These system configuration issues must be adequately dealt with before self-contained legged vehicles will be possible.

It is very challenging to deliver power efficiently to a large number of independently controllable, interacting actuators.

There are four primary causes of excessive power drain in artificial legged systems:

- Dynamic configuration issues

- Kinematic configuration issues

- Servo control configuration issues

- Accumulated buildup of mechanical and/or electrical system losses

*Dynamic configuration issues*

The primary dynamic system issue is powering alternating motions. If energy is put into driving the forward stroke of a leg, dumped into heat when the leg is decelerated at the end of its stroke, then more energy is put in to drive the return stroke and is, in turn dumped into heat at the end of that stroke the energy used is proportional to

$$\frac{Iv^3}{L^2}$$

where I is moment of inertia referred to the hip joint axis, v is vehicle velocity, and L is leg length. This is the normal system with legs of the "insect" type geometry.

"Mammal" type legs use gravitational oscillation of the leg as a pendulum to minimize the energy used to return the leg. This establishes a preferred return period which must be maintained. Driving at reduced return periods is expensive. Figure 12 shows the power that must be put into a pendulum to oscillate it at frequencies different from its natural frequency. Basically the power cost increases as the cube of the difference between the frequency of oscillation and the natural frequency. This is why animals do not use large variations in leg frequency in any given gait. It is also why a running animal will fold the leg tightly during the return stroke since this reduces the moment of inertia of the leg about the hip and increases the effective natural frequency permitting a faster return stroke. It is also the reason why animals use flight phases when running since the flight phase becomes a way of lengthening the stride while maintaining the same leg period.

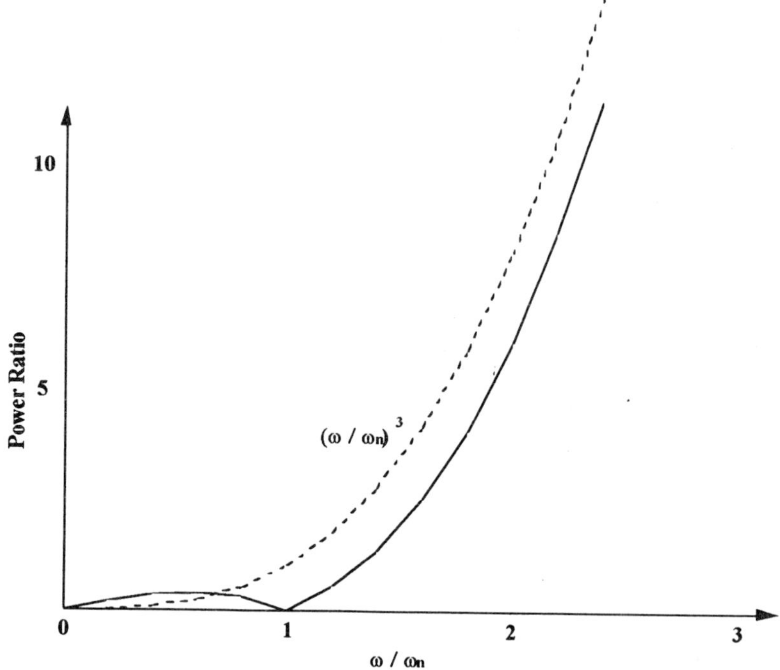


**Figure 12:** Power ratio for an actively driven pendulum as a function of the ratio of the driving frequency to the natural frequency. It is assumed that the system is not regenerative.

*Kinematic configuration issues*

Figure 13 shows the leg action associated with the "geometric work" effect. The "mammal" type leg shown is assumed to be actuated at both the hip and the knee. The body of the vehicle is assumed to be moving horizontally at constant velocity. That is, no energy is being added to the body of the vehicle or extracted from it. As can be seen from the free body diagrams of the leg, and the shank, in the forward position the torque at the hip is in the same direction as the angular velocity of the thigh, so the hip actuator is putting energy into the system. At the knee, the joint torque is opposed to the direction of motion, so the knee joint is acting as a brake and taking energy out of the system. Since no net work is being done, the energy being taken out at the knee is exactly the energy that is being put in at the hip. Unless the power system is configured to allow regeneration, the energy being put in at the hip is being dumped into heat at the knee, creating a very significant energy drain.

In the second position of the leg shown in Figure 13 the situation is reversed. Here the joint torque at the knee is in the same direction as the angular motion about the joint, so energy is being put in at the knee. The torque at the hip is opposed to the direction of motion of the thigh, so the hip actuator is acting as a brake dumping the energy put in at the knee into heat.

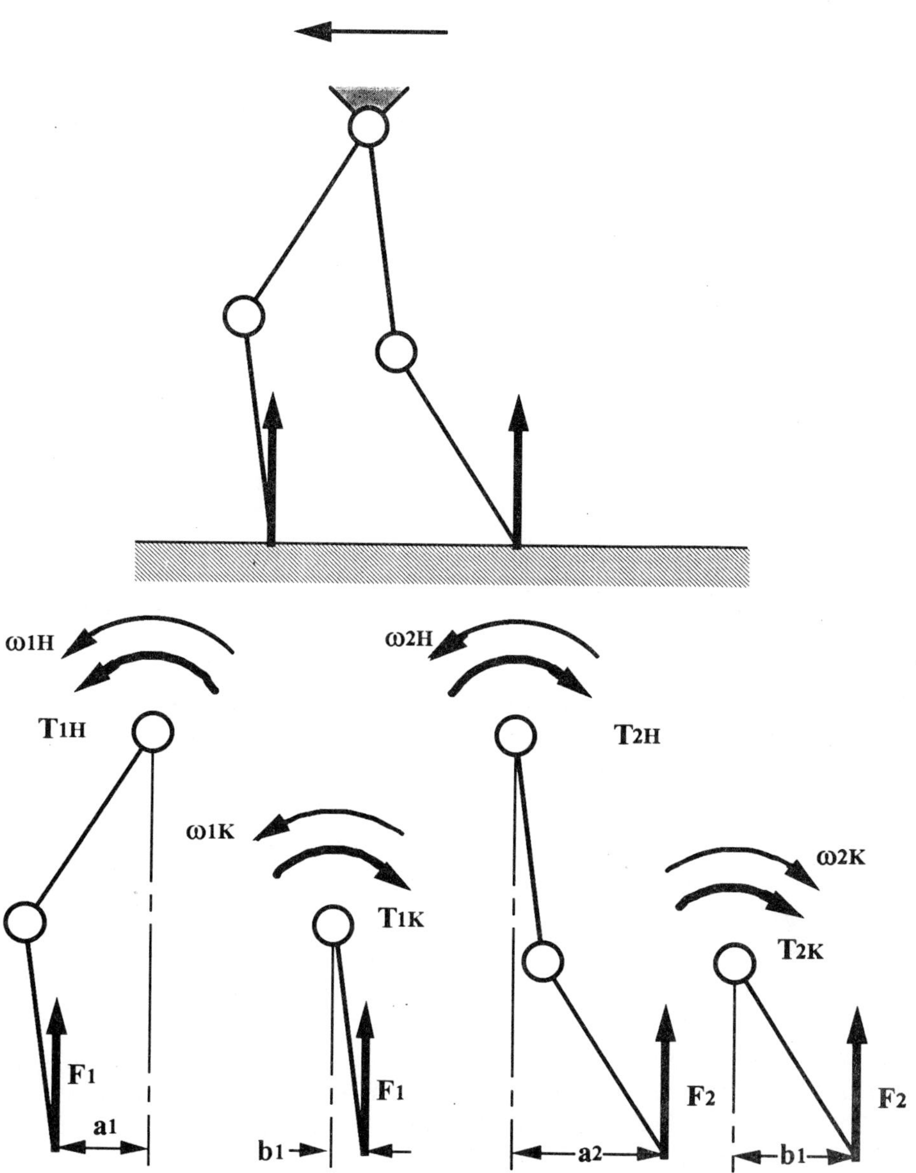


**Figure 13:** Geometric work in a leg in which the hip moves in a horizontal straight line at constant velocity. Since the center of mass of the body does not rise or fall, no net work is done. In both positions the torque at the one joint matches the direction of rotation at that joint. Consequently the actuator at that joint is putting energy into the system. At the same time, the torque at the other joint is opposed to the direction of the joint rotation. Hence the actuator is acting as a brake and removing the same amount of energy from the system as is being put in at the first joint.

In order for geometric work to be avoided, it is necessary to configure the leg so that when the body is moving horizontally at constant velocity, only one actuator needs to be active. This is the motivation for legs with pantograph configuration, and for some other legs that use closed chain geometries.

One can envisage setting up a leg as a four-bar linkage that produces an approximate straight line coupler path. If the ankle joint is placed at that coupler point and the mechanism is mounted to the vehicle body so that the line of coupler point motion is parallel to the longitudinal axis of the vehicle body, this leg can be driven by a single actuator to produce a support stroke without putting energy in or taking it out of the system and the geometric work effect is avoided [4]. However, for operation on uneven terrain it is necessary for the leg to be able to operate at different walking heights. A pantograph leg configuration offers the flexibility of being able to operate without geometric work at a large variety of walking heights.

Figure 14 shows the basic two-dimensional pantograph geometry used in the legs of the Adaptive Suspension Vehicle [4]. The point H is mounted to a slide parallel to the longitudinal body axis (actually a roller-rail assembly) and is actuated by a hydraulic cylinder. When H is moved with point V in fixed position the ankle point, A, moves on a parallel straight line through a distance 5 times the displacement of H. Similarly, V is mounted on a roller-rail assembly in the vertical plane of the leg. Movement of V with H in fixed position produces a vertical motion of A through a distance 4 times the displacement of V.

The third dimension in this case is obtained by swinging the entire leg about an axis parallel to the vehicle longitudinal axis through an angle of plus or minus 20°. For walking in the lateral direction with the body moving horizontally it is necessary to have the vertical actuator active as well as the swing actuator. For this reason there is a geometric work effect when the Adaptive Suspension Vehicle walks laterally. This could be eliminated by the use of a three-dimensional pantograph for the leg mechanism, as in the Titan III [18], but at the cost of a more complex leg mechanism.

Animals avoid the geometric work effect by dispensing with horizontal motion at constant velocity. Rather, when more mechanical energy than is immediately needed is put in by the active muscles, it is stored as an increase in potential or kinetic energy and made use of at another point in the walking cycle. This type of energy management has not yet been attempted in a walking machine, although it can be argued that Raibert's running machines employ a simple form of this principle.

Animals crossing difficult terrain use a follow-the-leader gait in which the rear feet are placed alongside, or in the footprint of the front feet. In this way the animal has only to select sound footholds for the front feet. This strategy is also attractive for walking machines with interactive operators. It is probably a good idea even for autonomous vehicles since it minimizes the number of acceptable footholds that must be identified. It necessitates the use of large obstacle, follow-the-leader gaits which strongly favor a bilaterally symmetric planform. It also necessitates overlapping working volumes between adjacent legs, since otherwise it is not possible to place feet alongside one another.

*Servo Control Configuration Issues*

Many of the strategies used for precise control of mechanical systems are very wasteful of energy. This is not permissible in a walking machine that must carry its own energy source.

For example, traditional electric servo control by means of linear amplifiers results in energy wastage whenever servomotors must operate at relatively low speed and high load. The reason is that the amplifier circuit is fundamentally configured as a potentiometer. The armature current required is determined by the torque that must be produced. The fraction of the supply voltage drop that is not needed to produce speed is dropped across a resistance, converting energy into heat in the form of $I^2R$ loss. The worst case is when the motor must operate at low speed and high load, since the current is high to balance the load torque, and the armature voltage is relatively low. The resistive drop of the amplifier is, therefore high, and the $I^2R$ loss is at its highest.

Phase control, or pulse-width modulation control techniques based on solid state switching are much better, although they do produce high order harmonics in the applied voltage that are, essentially filtered by the motor producing some $I^2R$ losses. These are much more moderate than those of linear amplifiers, and solid state switching control methods should certainly be used if electric actuation is used.

Conventional, pressure regulated, servo-valve controlled hydraulic actuation systems share some of the characteristics of linear amplifier controllers. The load on an actuator determines the pressure drop needed across that actuator. Actuator velocity determines flow through the circuit. Whatever portion of the supply pressure drop is not needed to support the load is accounted for by a throttling pressure drop in the servo-valve. Thus power equal to the product of the volumetric flow and the throttling pressure drop is converted into heat at the valve and carried off in the hydraulic fluid. Here the worst case is when the actuator speed is high and the load is low. Because the speed is high the flow is large, and because the load is low, the actuator pressure drop is low meaning that the throttling pressure drop is a large fraction of the supply pressure drop. This is particularly grievous for a walking machine since these are precisely the conditions that occur during the return of a leg. It is possible for return of the legs to consume several times the energy required to drive and support the vehicle.

A hydrostatic system in which the flow to the actuator is controlled by a variable displacement pump is not subject to this limitation and offers high effective efficiencies. For this reason this type of system is often used in the traction drives of construction machinery. This was the type of actuation system adopted for the Adaptive Suspension Vehicle. The cost is the weight and bulk of a separate variable displacement pump for each actuator.

Both hydrostatic actuation and electric actuation offer the possibility of regeneration: having the actuator act as a generator to return energy to the power system during braking.

This was implemented on the adaptive suspension vehicle. Electric regeneration circuits are complex and the author knows of no occasion when regeneration has actually been used on an electrically actuated walking machine. Although regeneration is attractive if it can be implemented simply, the losses in the system components result in relatively little energy recovery.

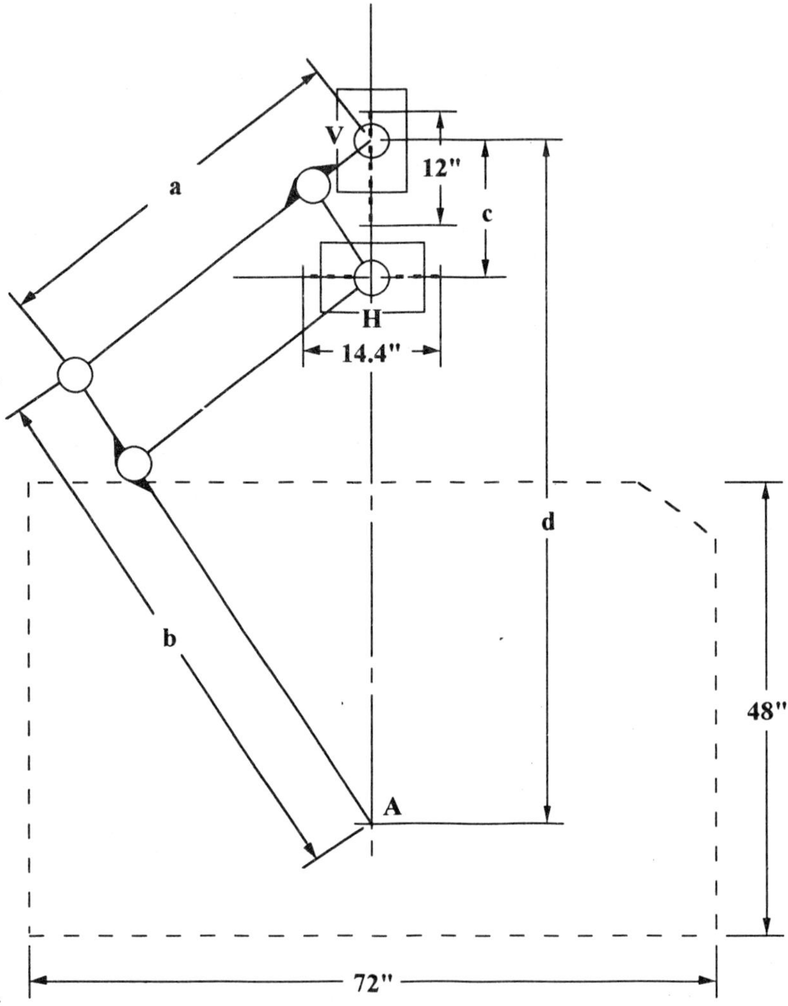



**Figure 14:** The two-dimensional pantograph geometry used in the legs of the Adaptive Suspension Vehicle. The ratio of lengths a/b is 0.7, and that of d/c is 5. The magnification of the stroke in the horizontal direction is 5, and in the vertical direction it is 4.

*Accumulation of System Losses*

Walking machine mechanisms are necessarily complex. Since each component or subsystem in the power train is a source of power loss it is crucial to simplify the system as much as possible. Care must be taken to select components such as bearings and gears, and electric or hydraulic system components to be as efficient as possible. It should be remembered that walking machine systems must function efficiently over a wide range of load and speed conditions. Some electric motors, for example, are very efficient if operated near their optimal operating speed, but are much less efficient when far from their optimal speed. Components that do well under widely varied conditions are to be preferred.

## 6. System Design

Although other philosophies have been vigorously promoted [19] it is productive to envisage the overall control system of a robotic vehicle as a hierarchy of levels. As is indicated in Figure 15, the time and distance scales increase from the lowest level to the highest. The various levels indicated on Figure 15 are defined as follows:

*Navigation:* This level is concerned with obtaining relatively infrequent fixes of absolute position to correct for drift errors in the lower level systems. The function is similar to that of the celestial navigation fixes formerly used for navigation at sea. Since GPS (Global Positioning System) navigation is now available in most terrestrial locations navigation fixes can now be much more frequent and more accurate than formerly. In a planetary rover situation a form of celestial navigation might still be used, possibly in combination with orbiter based instrumentation. The position fixes must be correlated with a map of the terrain to be traversed stored in the vehicles computer. Inertial navigation systems may be used for long distance navigation, but drift corrections are necessary at greater or lesser intervals depending on the quality and cost of the inertial navigation system.

*Path Selection:* This function is selection of the trajectory to be followed by the vehicle over the physical terrain. The sensors used for this purpose are the sensors that the machine uses to model the terrain surrounding it. These are typically video based sensors, although sonar has also been used for this purpose. The processing needed to form a model of the machine's environment can be very complex. Correlation with a stored map is also desirable, and an inertial navigation system may be used for this purpose. The distance scale dealt with here is typically limited by the sensors' field of view.

*Guidance:* This function encompasses local control of interaction with the environment. For a walking machine it would involve analysis of the terrain immediately in front of the machine and selection of acceptable footholds. For a wheeled machine following a road it would include detection of road edges, lane lines, or other markers and steering corrections based on that information. It might also include detection of other vehicles and maintaining station relative to another vehicle. The sensors used include

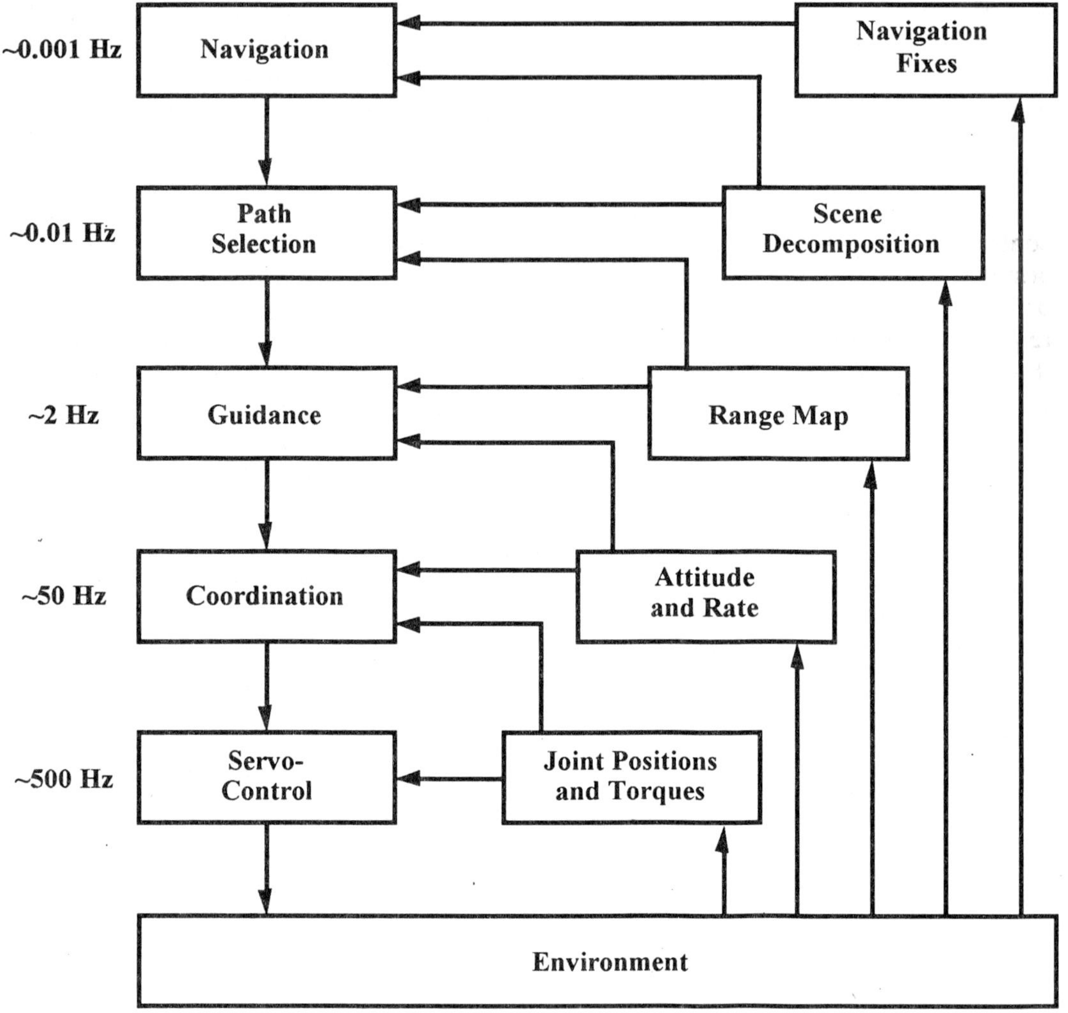



**Figure 15:** Generic hierarchical organization of the control system of a robotic vehicle.

scanning range finders, radar and sonar. The length scale considered here is typically too small for correlation with a stored map, but the system needs to build and store a model of the local terrain.

*Coordination:* For a walking machine, this is the level discussed in Section 2 and Section 3 above. It is the conversion of a motion commanded of the vehicle as a whole to commands to be sent to the actuator servo-controllers. For a walking machine this level is conveniently divided into two sublevels. The first is foot placement based on a gait as described in Section 2, with modifications necessary to ensure that only the acceptable areas for footholds identified at the guidance level are used. The second level is the generation of actuator commands based on a coordination principle such as that described in Section 3 above. Some form of inertial guidance system is useful at this level for direct measurement of vehicle body motions. Information passed up from the sensors used at the servo level may also be used.

*Servo-control:* This is control at the actuator level. As is indicated above, force control is most appropriate when the foot is in contact with the ground, but rate control is best when the leg is being returned. Thus it is necessary to detect when the foot contacts, or leaves the ground and to switch between control modes at those instants. Force control requires sensing actuator force as directly as possible. In a hydraulic machine like the ASV this is straightforward since a differential pressure transducer can be placed across each cylinder. In an electric machine the same result might be achieved by current sensing, possibly combined with load cell information. Position sensing at each actuator is also necessary. Actuator rate sensors will also facilitate faster and more accurate control response during leg return.

It is convenient to divide sensor systems into those that gather information about the environment in which the machine is operating, and those that monitor its internal condition. It is convenient to borrow the biological terms for *exteroceptive sensors:* those that observe the environment, and *proprioceptive sensors:* those that sense the machine's internal parameters. It may be observed that exteroceptive sensor information is predominantly used in the higher levels of the hierarchy, while proprioceptive sensors are dominant at the lower levels. This is not universally true, since an inertial navigation system, which is a proprioceptive system, may also be used at the highest levels.

Depending on the degree of autonomy desired, the functions of the higher levels of the hierarchy might be fulfilled by human operators. For example, the Adaptive Suspension Vehicle system lacks the navigation and path selection levels of the hierarchy because these functions are fulfilled by the human operator.

## Summary

In this chapter some of the configuration design considerations of walking vehicles have been addressed. More detailed treatments of specific topics can be found in many of the references cited below.

Those of us who have had the experience of designing artificial walking machines have found it beneficial to study biological systems and try to understand the principles upon which they operate. In view of the success of machines like Raibert's hopping machines [11, 12], the Adaptive Suspension Vehicle [13, 4], Dante [6, 7] and others, there may be principles that have been learned in the design of artificial systems that can throw light on the fundamentals of biological locomotion.

## References

[1]     McGhee, R.B., "Vehicular Legged Locomotion," Advances in Automation and Robotics, (Ed. G.N. Saridis), Jai Press, Greenwich, Conn. 1985.

[2]     Kumar, V. and Waldron, K.J., "A Review of Research on Walking Vehicles," Robotics Review, (Ed. O. Khatib, J. Craig, and T. Lozano-Perez), The MIT Press, Cambridge, Massachusetts, (1989), pp. 243-266.

[3]     Waldron, K.J., "Terrain Adaptive Vehicles," Special Combined Edition Trans. ASME Journal of Mechanical Design / Journal of Vibration and Acoustics, Vol. 117(B), (1995), pp. 107-112.

[4]     Song, S.M. and Waldron, K.J., Machines That Walk:  The Adaptive Suspension Vehicle, MIT Press 1988.

[5]     Bare, J. E., Chun, W. H., Garrett, F. L., Gothard, B. M., Morgenthaler, D. G., Price, R. S., Spiessbach, A. J., Stout, B., and Waldron, K. J., "Mars Rover/Sample Return (MRSR) Rover Mobility and Surface Rendezvous Studies - Task 2 (FY89)" Final Report to Jet Propulsion Laboratory, California Institute of Technology on Contract 958073, Martin Marietta Space Systems Co., 1989.

[6]     Monastersky, R., "The Inferno Revisited," Science News, Vol. 141, (1992), pp. 376-378.

[7]     Bares, J. E. and Whittaker, W. L., "Configuration of Autonomous Walkers for Extreme Terrain," International Journal of Robotics Research, Vol. 12, No. 6, (1993), pp. 535-559.

[8]     Song, S.M. and Waldron, K.J., "An analytical Approach for Gait Study and Its Application on Wave Gaits," International Journal of Robotics Research, Vol. 6, No. 2, (1987), pp. 60-71.

[9]     Song, S.M. and Waldron, K.J., "Geometric Design of a Walking Machine for Optimal Mobility," Trans. ASME J. Mechanisms, Transmissions and Automation in Design, Vol. 109, No. 1, (1987), pp. 21-28.

[10]    Wang, S.L., The Study of a Hexapod Walking Vehicle's Maneuverability Over Level Ground and Obstacles and its Computer Simulation, MS thesis, Department of Mechanical Engineering, Ohio State University 1983.

[11]    Raibert, M.H., Legged Robots that Balance, MIT Press 1986.

[12]    Raibert, M.H., Brown, H.B. and Murthy, S.S., "3-D Balance Using 2-D Algorithms," First International Symposium of Robotics Research, (Eds. Brady, M., Paul, R.P.), MIT Press, (1984), pp. 279-301.

[13]    Pugh, D.R., Ribble E.A., Vohnout V.J., Bihari, T.E., Walliser, T.M., Patterson, M.R., Waldron, K.J., "Technical Description of the Adaptive Suspension Vehicle," International Journal of Robotics Research, Vol. 9, No. 2, (1990), pp. 24-42.

[14]   Klein, C. A. and Chung, T. S., "Force Interaction and Allocation for the Legs of a Walking Vehicle, IEEE Transactions on Robotics and Automation, Vol. RA-3, No. 6, (1987), pp. 546-555.

[15]   Kumar, V. and Waldron, K.J., "Force Distribution in Closed Kinematic Chains" IEEE Transactions on Robotics and Automation, Vol. 4, No. 6, (1988), pp. 657-664.

[16]   Vijaykumar, R., Waldron, K.J., and Tsai, M.J., "Geometric Optimization of Manipulator Structures for Working Volume and Dexterity," International Journal of Robotics Research, Vol. 5, No. 2, (1986), pp. 91-103.

[17]   Bekker, M. G., Introduction to Terrain-Vehicle Systems, University of Michigan Press, Ann Arbor 1969.

[18]   Hirose, S., "A Study of Design and Control of a Quadruped Walking Vehicle," International Journal of Robotics Research, Vol. 3, No. 2, (1984), pp. 361-368.

[19]   Brooks, R.A., "A Robust Layered Control System for a Mobile Robot," IEEE Journal of Robotics and Automation, RA-2, (1986), pp. 14-23.